The
DASH Diet for
WEIGHT LOSS

Thomas J. Moore, MD

with Megan C. Murphy, MPH, and Mark Jenkins

||||||||||||||||||||||||||||||||||||||||||||||||||||||||||||||||||||||||||||||||||||||||||||||||||||||||||||||||||||||||

GALLERY

New York London Toronto Sydney New Delhi

The
DASH Diet for
WEIGHT LOSS

Lose Weight and Keep It Off—
the Healthy Way—
with America's Most Respected Diet

This publication contains the opinions and ideas of its author. It is intended to provide helpful and informative material on the subjects addressed in the publication. It is sold with the understanding that the author and publisher are not engaged in rendering medical, health, or any other kind of personal professional services in the book. The reader should consult his or her medical, health or other competent professional before adopting any of the suggestions in this book or drawing inferences from it.

The author and publisher specifically disclaim all responsibility for any liability, loss or risk, personal or otherwise, which is incurred as a consequence, directly or indirectly, of the use and application of any of the contents of this book.

Gallery Books
A Division of Simon & Schuster, Inc.
1230 Avenue of the Americas
New York, NY 10020

Copyright © 2012 by Thomas J. Moore, M.D.

All rights reserved, including the right to reproduce this book or portions
thereof in any form whatsoever. For information address Gallery Books Subsidiary
Rights Department, 1230 Avenue of the Americas, New York, NY 10020.

First Gallery Books trade paperback edition December 2012

GALLERY BOOKS and colophon are registered trademarks of Simon & Schuster, Inc.

For information about special discounts for bulk purchases,
please contact Simon & Schuster Special Sales at
1-866-506-1949 or business@simonandschuster.com.

The Simon & Schuster Speakers Bureau can bring authors to your live event.
For more information or to book an event contact the Simon & Schuster Speakers
Bureau at 1-866-248-3049 or visit our website at www.simonspeakers.com.

Designed by Katy Riegel

Manufactured in the United States of America

20 19 18 17 16 15 14 13

The Library of Congress has cataloged the hardcover edition as follows:

Moore, Thomas J.
    The DASH diet for weight loss : lose weight and keep it off—the healthy way—
with America's most respected diet / Thomas J. Moore, Megan C. Murphy, Mark Jenkins.
    p. cm.
    Includes index.
    1. Weight loss.   2. Nutrition.   3. Exercise.   4. Self-care, Health—Popular works.
I. Murphy, Megan C.   II. Jenkins, Mark, 1962–   III. Title.
RM222.2.M5677   2012
613.2′5—dc23   2011045086

ISBN 978-1-4516-6936-7
ISBN 978-1-4767-1471-4 (pbk)
ISBN 978-1-4516-6937-4 (ebook)

I dedicate this book to my family,

for their support, encouragement, and love

Acknowledgments

I would like to thank Mitali Shah, MS, RD, LDN, Lin Pao-Hwa, PhD, and especially Diana Cullum-Dugan, RD, LDN, for their expert help in designing the meal plans and recipes; Caroline Apovian, MD, for providing advice based on her many years overseeing weight-management programs; and Diana Lehman and Diana Cullum-Dugan for their editorial assistance.

I would also like to acknowledge my fellow researchers in the original DASH research studies. Without their collaboration, there would be no DASH Diet to write about. Laura Svetkey, MD, and her team at Duke University Medical Center; Larry Appel, MD, and his colleagues at Johns Hopkins University; George Bray, MD, and his team at Pennington Biomedical Research Center/Louisiana State University; William Vollmer, PhD, and colleagues at Kaiser Permanente Center for Health Research; Eva Obarzanek, PhD, and her colleagues at National Heart, Lung, and Blood Institute; and the friends and colleagues who made up my team at the Brigham and Women's Hospital/Harvard Medical School.

Finally I would like to acknowledge the nearly 1,000 volunteers who participated in the DASH studies, in which we learned that the

DASH eating plan provides so many important health benefits. And to thank the 18,000 people who have enrolled in the DASH for Health program, who taught me what works—and what doesn't—when it comes to weight loss, and who allowed me to share those findings with you, the readers of this book.

Contents

Preface   xi

PART 1. A Diet Whose Time Has Come

1. Why This Book Is Different   3
2. The Science of Weight Loss   11
3. The DASH Diet for Weight Loss:
   A Diet Whose Time Has Come   15

PART 2. Into Action

SECTION I. WHAT YOU EAT

4. Your First Three Steps   33
5. The Food Groups: Going Hi-Lo-Slo   42
6. Challenging Foods: Snacks, Drinks, and Mixed Dishes   82
7. What About Salt?   95
8. The Importance of Food Tracking   100
9. Is Meal Planning the Answer for You?   104
10. Vegetarians, This Diet Is for You, Too   109

SECTION II. HOW MUCH YOU MOVE

11. Walking Your Way to Weight Loss   122
12. Ramping Up Your Fitness Program   127
13. Increasing Lifestyle Exercise   131

SECTION III. BUILDING YOUR SKILLPOWER

14. Create Realistic Goals You Can Reach   138
15. Use Your Tools   143
16. Employ Visualization Techniques   145
17. Practice Conscious Eating   149
18. Ask for Support   153
19. Conquer Emotional Eating   156
20. Stave Off Cravings   159
21. Learn How to Go Grocery Shopping   162
22. Make Your Kitchen Weight-Loss Friendly   164
23. Learn How to Dine Out and Still Maintain
     Weight-Loss Goals   167

SECTION IV. DOING IT FOR LIFE   175

SECTION V. FREQUENTLY ASKED QUESTIONS   181

PART 3. Meal Plans
SECTION I. MEAT-EATER MEAL PLANS   215

SECTION II. VEGETARIAN MEAL PLANS   271

PART 4. Recipes   333

Appendix A. Calculating Your Daily Calorie Target   363
Appendix B. The DASH for Health® Program   367
Appendix C. Scientific Papers About the DASH Diet   369
Index   375

Preface

IN AUGUST 1993, fifty researchers gathered together in an overheated hotel conference room in Bethesda, Maryland, to design what would come to be known as the DASH study.

The initials "DASH" stand for Dietary Approaches to Stop Hypertension. The fifty researchers represented five research teams. There was Laura Svetkey, MD, and her team from Duke; George Bray, MD, and his team from the Pennington Center in Louisiana; Larry Appel, MD, and his team from Johns Hopkins; Bill Vollmer, PhD, and his team from Oregon Health Sciences Center; and my team from Harvard. The National Heart, Lung, and Blood Institute had selected these five teams from among forty applicants. Our task was to design an eating pattern that would lower blood pressure.

The teams had never worked together before. In fact, most of us did not even know one another. But it became clear from the very beginning that we were willing and eager to work together to design the "perfect" diet. By the end of that first meeting, we had agreed on a rough outline of the diets we would test and how we would test them. And I was honored that the group had selected me as the chairman of the overall study.

But it took another twelve months before we were ready to start testing the first research volunteer. That's how long it took to design a study as complex and tightly controlled as the DASH study. DASH was a "feeding study"—that means we gave the research volunteers all of their food for the entire eleven weeks of the study. Volunteers were going to be studied simultaneously in North Carolina, Maryland, Louisiana, and Massachusetts. To be sure that the study was being conducted in the same way at all four sites and that the subjects at all sites were eating the same foods, we prepared careful menus and recipes that would be served in each location. We even worked with food companies that agreed to ship food items (such as bread, crackers, soup, and fruit) from the same production batch to all of our four sites so that the study volunteers were in fact eating identical foods. Samples of each recipe and meal were prepared, ground up, and chemically analyzed so that we were sure exactly what was in the foods. In addition, researchers at each site received identical training on how to measure blood pressure, how to weigh subjects, and how to measure body fat. We wanted to be absolutely sure that all four sites were feeding subjects the same food and measuring the effects of the diet in an identical way.

Once the study was designed, the four sites enrolled 459 volunteers in two and a half years. We tested three different diets. One third of the subjects ate a typical American diet. One third of the subjects ate a typical American diet enriched in fruits and vegetables. And the rest of the subjects received what is now called the DASH Diet. When the results were analyzed, the DASH Diet lowered systolic blood pressure by nearly 11 points—about as much as a typical antihypertensive medication and, in fact, far more than we researchers expected.

Since we first published these results in 1997 in the *New England Journal of Medicine,* many other studies have shown additional benefits of the DASH Diet. We know that it lowers blood pressure in people with high blood pressure, but we also now know that the DASH Diet reduces the development of hypertension, heart failure, heart attacks, and kidney stones, and even reduces the risk of developing colon cancer. Studies have shown that people who eat the DASH Diet "feel better." One study even showed that the DASH Diet improves the ability to think clearly! And—most important for this book— the DASH Diet has also proven to be a *very effective tool for those who want to lose weight.*

So although DASH started off as a diet to lower blood pressure, with all this additional scientific evidence, the US Department of Agriculture now recommends the DASH Diet as the ideal eating pattern for all Americans. And a recent *U.S. News & World Report* ranking rated the DASH Diet as the "#1 Best Overall Diet" when compared to twenty other popular diets such as Weight Watchers, Jenny Craig, and South Beach.

But I often hear the comment, "It's fine that the DASH Diet shows all those benefits when it's tested in a study where volunteers are being given all of their food by the study staff. But how does the DASH Diet work in real life, when people need to select and prepare their own food?"

We're happy to say that it works just fine. Dietitians and nutritionists routinely recommend the DASH Diet to people who are interested in improving their eating habits, who have specific medical conditions that would benefit from DASH, and who want to lose weight. People like the DASH Diet because it is easy to understand. It is about real foods, not special supplements or meals that you have to buy from a specific manufacturer. You can shop for the DASH Diet at the same stores where you've always shopped, and it allows you to follow either a meat-eater or vegetarian diet.

The DASH Diet started out as a tightly controlled scientific study but has turned into something much larger. Doctors, nutritionists, government agencies, and organizations such as the American Heart Association are recommending the DASH Diet. Now we want to get the 150 million Americans who would benefit from the DASH Diet to try it and stick with it.

We hope this book will be part of that solution.

Part 1

A Diet Whose Time Has Come

1

Why This Book Is Different

YOU BOUGHT this book because you want to lose weight on the DASH Diet for Weight Loss, and you are probably anxious to get started. If you just can't wait another minute, you will find detailed instructions on how to get started in Part 2 of this book. But please do read these first three chapters, whether now or later. In these initial pages you will find plenty of reasons to believe in this weight-loss program.

The DASH Diet for Weight Loss is different from any other weight-loss program out there. Our eating recommendations are based on the DASH Diet, which is backed by extensive scientific evidence and is endorsed by leading health care organizations.

I've incorporated our scientific discoveries into the diet as well as lessons from ten years of using DASH to help thousands of people lose weight and get healthier. Our nutrition advice is highly customized for every calorie level—including yours. Finally, this is a weight-loss diet of satisfying, real foods that you can stick to for the long term.

Let's answer some key questions you probably have:

MEDICAL ADVICE

The diet and exercise advice we give in this book is based on established and proven medical evidence. But it may not be appropriate for everyone. We encourage you to ask your doctor about any planned changes in your eating or exercise habits. Your doctor knows your medical condition better than anyone and can give you the best advice about whether the DASH Diet and moderate exercise are right for you.

And if you have any known food allergies or reactions, you should avoid those foods even if they are listed among the DASH recommended items.

- WHAT'S SO SPECIAL ABOUT THE DASH DIET?
- HOW DOES THE DASH DIET WORK?
- WHERE IS THE EVIDENCE THAT THE DASH DIET CAN HELP YOU LOSE WEIGHT?
- HOW IS THE DASH DIET FOR WEIGHT LOSS DIFFERENT FROM OTHER WEIGHT-LOSS PROGRAMS?

WHAT'S SO SPECIAL ABOUT THE DASH DIET?

The DASH Diet is rich in fruits, vegetables, low-fat dairy foods, and whole-grain products. It is reduced in red meat, animal fats, and sugar. "What's so special about that?" you ask. "My parents were telling me to eat that way years ago." True. But what's different about DASH is that we have determined through research the combination of servings from each of eight key food groups you should eat each day. And the number of servings differs depending on your size and calorie needs. We will give you the specific number of food servings that are right for you.

Another thing that's special about the DASH Diet is that it is recommended as an ideal eating pattern for all American adults by the US Department of Agriculture (USDA). The American Heart Association recommends the DASH Diet, too. And in 2011, a team of nutrition experts rated twenty popular diets for *U.S. News & World Report* and selected the DASH Diet as the number one best overall diet.

But it isn't high rankings that make the DASH Diet so special. It is special because it is backed by a mass of scientific proof that shows that eating the DASH Diet can provide real and important health benefits.

The DASH Diet was designed by a team of medical and nutrition scientists and funded by the National Institutes of Health. Our goal was to design an eating pattern that would lower blood pressure. (The name "DASH" stands for Dietary Approaches to Stop Hypertension.) We spent a full year designing the diet and then tested it in a study involving 459 people. We found that the DASH Diet lowered blood pressure as well as a typical high blood pressure medication did. We published those results in the *New England Journal of Medicine,* and the DASH Diet is now part of most standard guidelines for preventing and treating high blood pressure here in the United States and around the world.

As we looked more closely at the data, we found that the DASH Diet did more than just lower blood pressure. It also lowered blood cholesterol levels. And it showed evidence of protecting bone strength. People eating the DASH Diet even reported that they felt better!

Since that original study, our team and others have found additional benefits of the DASH Diet. In fact, there are now more than 100 scientific articles that attest to the benefits of eating the DASH Diet. To mention just a few:

- The DASH Diet combined with a reduced salt intake lowers blood pressure even more than either maneuver alone.
- The DASH Diet prevents the onset of high blood pressure.
- The DASH Diet reduces the occurrence of heart attacks (by 18 percent) and strokes (by 24 percent).
- It reduces the risk of developing heart failure by 37 percent.
- It reduces the development of kidney stones by 45 percent.

- It reduces the risk of developing colon cancer by 20 percent.
- It reduces the risk of developing diabetes (a very important benefit at this time, when the frequency of diabetes in America is skyrocketing).
- It even helps people *think* more clearly!

There is more scientific evidence to support the DASH Diet than any other eating pattern. And that's why it is recommended by the USDA, the American Heart Association, *U.S. News & World Report*, and others. But I always tell my patients, don't be impressed that the DASH Diet is so highly rated—be impressed with the evidence that inspired those ratings. The DASH Diet truly is the eating pattern that will protect your health for life.

HOW DOES THE DASH DIET WORK?

In brief: We don't know.

The cholesterol-lowering effect may be due to the reduced amount of animal fat in the DASH Diet (from less meat, whole milk, full-fat cheeses, and so on). But the cause of the other benefits is really unknown. If we could identify the "magic bullet" in the DASH Diet, we could synthesize it, put in a pill, and just give that to people. Certainly that would be easier than convincing people to change their eating habits! Unfortunately, that "magic bullet" has not been found.

Take blood pressure as an example. We originally designed the DASH Diet to lower blood pressure. So in our design, we tried to incorporate all of the nutrients that earlier studies had suggested might lower blood pressure—elements such as a high potassium content, calcium content, and magnesium content. But then we did a separate study where we gave those minerals as individual supplements and in combination to a group of 300 women. We found that even combining all three of these "magic bullets" lowered blood pressure by only about 2 points. That's much less than the effect of the DASH Diet.

Foods are very complex combinations of minerals, vitamins, antioxidants, fiber, protein, and some other substances we don't even know about yet. It is likely that this *combination* of nutrients leads to the benefits of the DASH Diet. Or maybe, once we adopt the DASH Diet, we are no longer eating a lot of *unhealthy* stuff. We really don't know.

As a scientist, I would of course very much like to know how the DASH Diet achieves its benefits. But as a physician, I can be satisfied just knowing that it *does* provide these benefits and keeps people healthy.

WHERE IS THE EVIDENCE THAT THE DASH DIET CAN HELP YOU LOSE WEIGHT?

Every day, dietitians all over the country are teaching people the DASH Diet to help them lose weight. In part they do this because the DASH Diet is such a healthy eating pattern, as I've just described. But there's also proof that the DASH Diet is an effective diet for weight loss.

A group of my DASH colleagues conducted a study to see if people could lose weight on the DASH Diet. They recruited subjects and divided them into two groups. One group of research subjects was given advice about weight loss but no further instruction. The other group was taught the DASH Diet and was encouraged to exercise regularly. Over a period of eighteen months, the DASH Diet group had regular meetings with dietitians to reinforce the weight-loss advice. Both groups were shooting for a goal of fifteen pounds of weight loss. At the end of eighteen months, the DASH group had lost an average of nine and a half pounds, significantly more weight loss than the "advice only" group. And 25 percent of the DASH group hit their target goal of losing fifteen pounds or more. These results, published in the *Annals of Internal Medicine,* clearly demonstrate that the DASH Diet can be an effective part of a weight-loss plan.

I took a different approach to studying whether people can lose weight on the DASH Diet. Rather than test this in a traditional controlled scientific study (which typically involves only a small number of subjects), I wanted to test it on a much larger number of subjects in a real-life setting. So I developed an online program to teach the DASH Diet and began offering it in 2002. (We will discuss this pro-

|||||||||||||||||||||||||||||

DASH Frequently Asked Question

Almost every week in the newspaper I read about a new study about how to lose weight. Often these studies contradict one another. What should I believe?

Please see the answer to FAQ 1 in Section V,
Frequently Asked Questions.

gram, called DASH for Health, in Appendix B at the end of this book.) Since it began, over 18,000 people have enrolled in the program. Many of these people have successfully lost weight and have kept it off. And what we have learned from these 18,000 people—what does and what does not work for weight loss—forms the basis of much of the advice in this book.

HOW IS THE DASH DIET FOR WEIGHT LOSS APPROACH DIFFERENT FROM OTHER WEIGHT-LOSS PROGRAMS?

The most important difference between this program and others—the DASH Diet is backed by scientific evidence. You can be confident you are getting healthier. Your blood pressure will be lower and your cholesterol levels will be healthier. You will be eating foods that have been linked to a lower incidence of heart disease, cancer, osteoporosis, and diabetes. If you follow the DASH eating plan, you will get healthier if you lose a lot of weight, a little bit of weight, and even if you lose no weight at all.

And second, the DASH Diet for Weight Loss uses proven techniques to help you change your eating habits and follow the DASH Diet. These are tricks and tools that we have learned from the more than 18,000 people who enrolled in the DASH for Health program—people just like you. The tips, tricks, and techniques they have shared with me over the years provide the "skillpower" you need to start on and stick to the DASH Diet for Weight Loss. I'm very pleased that some of the participants in the program volunteered to share their specific advice and experiences in this book. Most diet books offer generic advice about eating fewer calories and exercising more. Our advice is very specifically tailored to helping *you* follow the DASH Diet.

The DASH Diet for Weight Loss offers in-depth meal plans carefully tailored to the number of calories you should be eating to lose weight. These meal plans have been created by a team of qualified health professionals under my direction. There is a meal plan for you if you are a 140-pound-woman who works a desk job or if you are an ex–football player who works on a construction site all day—and there's a program for you, too.

Then there is the food itself. The DASH Diet for Weight Loss focuses on "high volume–low calorie" foods, which nutritionists understand are essential to any weight-loss program. These foods have fewer calories relative to their size. As an example, a wedge of watermelon has far fewer calories than an equivalent-sized piece of chocolate. The greater sense of fullness you get from large volumes of low-calorie foods is the reason nutritionists recommend focusing on these foods if you are trying to lose weight.

We have taken this established concept and developed it by focusing also on how hard you have to work to eat a particular food. Foods that need more chewing and take longer to eat are beneficial if you are trying to lose weight. That's because if the foods take longer to eat (and if you also focus on eating more slowly), then it is more likely your "fullness signal" will be triggered and you won't eat as much as you would if you were eating small amounts of very-high-calorie foods that can be eaten very quickly.

We've combined these food characteristics into an easy-to-remember slogan, Hi-Lo-Slo: HIgh volume, LOw calorie, SLOw to eat. We will refer to this slogan throughout this book.

INTRODUCING HI-LO-SLO FOODS

High Volume: Take up a lot of space on your plate and in your stomach so you feel satisfied

Low Calorie: Low in calories relative to how bulky they are

Slow Ingestion: Require a relatively long time to eat, therefore allowing your fullness signal to be activated

I will recommend that you avoid eating large amounts of high-density foods such as most red meat, full-fat cheese, and sweets like chocolate and pastries. However, in the DASH Diet for Weight Loss, no foods are out of bounds and you can include small amounts of high-density foods in Hi-Lo-Slo food combinations and recipes.

One of the distinguishing characteristics of Hi-Lo-Slo foods is that most of them are high in fiber. Fiber stays in your digestive system longer and provides a feeling of fullness on fewer calories.

Finally, our emphasis is on the long term—losing excess weight and keeping it off. A person can lose weight for a few weeks on almost any diet. All you have to do is eat fewer calories than you burn each day and you'll lose weight. That's the easy part. The hard part is keeping that weight off. That's where most diet programs fail. To have a meaningful effect on health, a diet has to be healthy and allow you to lose the excess weight and keep it off. And that long-term emphasis—*keeping it off*—is an important part of what this book is about.

To better understand how this diet will help you achieve your goals, the next chapter will take a closer look at the metabolic process we call "weight loss."

2

The Science of Weight Loss

THE FUNDAMENTAL REASONS why we lose or gain weight are based on a principle in physics: the law of conservation of energy. If the rest of this chapter were all about mathematical equations, no one (including me) would ever read it. But the fundamentals of weight loss are important to understand, so let me put it in the form of a story.

Bob loved cars. He was especially proud of his Chevrolet Bel Air. He bought it new in 1954. In the early years, he did a lot of long-distance traveling, so he installed an extra-large 100-gallon gas tank. Now, however, he only drives it to and from work, which he does every day, seven days a week.

This is Bob's daily habit: Every morning he stops at the gas station at the end of his street, buys coffee and a newspaper, and puts one gallon of gas into the Bel Air. He drives to work and back, and the next day he repeats the same habit. Bob drives ten miles to work and ten miles home every day (twenty miles total). The Bel Air goes twenty miles on a gallon of gas, so every day he adds a gallon of gas and burns a gallon of gas. Everything comes out even.

This worked perfectly for many years until a coworker told Bob that a new road had just opened that provided a shorter route for his commute. The new road was five miles to work and five miles home, reducing Bob's total commute from twenty miles to ten. Always interested in saving time, Bob immediately started using the new road, but he kept his other habits: every day a cup of coffee, a newspaper, and one gallon into the Bel Air. After using the new road for three months, he noticed that the Bel Air was struggling. It didn't have its usual pep, and its rear end was dragging. Why was this happening? Bob's commuting distance had decreased from twenty to ten miles per day, but he was still adding a full gallon of gas every day. So basically, the Bel Air was burning only half of the gas Bob was adding each day. The other half gallon was being stored in that oversize gas tank. After three months of the new commute, the Bel Air was lugging an extra forty-five gallons of gas in its tank. (Bob eventually figured this out.)

Now let's connect the Bel Air story to the notion of weight gain and weight loss in a person. Let's say the person is Bob himself. The Bel Air is Bob's body. Both the Bel Air and Bob need fuel: the fuel for the Bel Air is gasoline; the fuel for Bob is the food he eats. The fuel for the Bel Air is measured in gallons; the fuel for Bob is measured in calories. How much fuel we need each day depends upon how much physical work we do. For the Bel Air, that was typically twenty miles per day. It's not so easy to measure human work in miles because we perform work of many types. Often, we measure the amount of work we do in a day as the number of calories we use to accomplish it. The part of the story when Bob reduces his commute from twenty miles to ten miles is like what happened to Bob when he moved from adolescence into adulthood. His activity level dropped and he became more sedentary. If he continued to eat the same amount of food even as his activity dropped, the same thing would happen to Bob that happened to the Bel Air. He began to fill his tank with excess fuel (fat). He lost his pep and his rear end was dragging.

So what could Bob do to fix this situation? He could start by reducing how much fuel he adds each day to the level that he needs. If Bob would cut back to the number of calories that he uses up each day,

Cars	How Do They Compare?	People
Bel Air	The machine	Bob's body
Gas	Fuel	Food
Gallons	Fuel measurement	Calories
Miles driven	Measure of "work" performed	Calories burned
Gas tank	Excess fuel storage	Body fat
No pep, rear end dragging	Result of excess fuel stored	No pep, rear end dragging *plus* obesity, diabetes, heart disease, arthritis, sleep apnea, and many more problems

he wouldn't gain more weight, but he wouldn't lose weight, either. To lose weight—to use the fuel we already have stored away as fat—we need to burn more fuel than we consume. There are two ways to do this. We can reduce the amount of fuel that we eat each day or we can increase the amount of fuel that we burn each day. And of course, the best answer is to do both.

Here's a little math. If Bob both eats and burns 2,500 calories per day, his weight would stay the same. He could lose weight by reducing his calorie intake by 500 calories a day to 2,000 calories. His body will get the extra calories it needs by "borrowing" them from his stored body fat. If Bob eats 2,000 calories a day for a week (while burning 2,500), he will lose one pound in that week (–500 calories/day × 7 days = 3,500 calories, and there are 3,500 calories in one pound of fat).

And he could lose more weight by increasing his activity (the calories he burns) by another 500 calories per day. Again, he will have to go to his fat stores for this fuel. He will have to borrow another 500 calories of fuel from those fat stores each day. Doing the math, we see that burning an extra 500 calories each day for a week will result in another pound of weight loss (–500 calories/day × 7 days = 3,500 calories, or one pound).

If Bob could consistently reduce food calories by 500 per day *and* burn 500 calories more per day through exercise, he could burn 7,000 fat calories per week, which would be a weight loss of two pounds of fat.

So all through the rest of this book we will be talking about cutting back on calories and increasing how many calories we burn through exercise. On the basis of this story, you can see that you can actually lose weight by doing either calorie-cutting or exercise. But the most reliable and fastest way to lose weight safely is to do both.

3

The DASH Diet for Weight Loss: A Diet Whose Time Has Come

WHEN I SAT DOWN to start researching and writing this book, I was reminded that I have been studying the effects of food on health for over twenty years. In that time, the national concern about overweight and obesity has become a full-blown emergency. Americans are spending $60 billion per year on diet products, pills, and programs. And as a society we spend $75 billion per year on obesity-related health care. What particularly struck me as I started gathering the latest data on overweight and obesity was how fast things are going down hill. In the 1970s, fewer than half of Americans were overweight or obese (47 percent); now two-thirds of us are (66 percent). The number of "obese" people has doubled, from 15 percent of Americans to 30 percent. Whatever we are doing now to halt obesity, it isn't working.

WHERE DO YOU FIT IN?

What do these terms mean: "overweight" and "obese"? How do we define an unhealthy weight? And where do you fit in? We can't use simple body weight to determine whether someone "weighs too much." A 5-foot-tall man may be very overweight at 160 pounds while someone 6 feet 6 inches could be considered lean at 210 pounds. We needed a way to assess weight according to how tall a person is. And that's where body mass index (BMI) comes in. BMI takes both your weight and height into account. Using the table on page 17, you can learn your BMI.

Or if you like doing a little math and want your precise BMI, use this formula:

$$\text{BMI} = \text{weight (in pounds)} \times 703/ \text{ height (inches)} \times \text{height (inches)}$$

Here is how we classify BMIs:

Underweight: BMI between 16.5 and 18.4
Normal: BMI between 18.5 and 24.9
Overweight: BMI between 25 and 29.9
Obese: BMI 30 or more

So when I say that 66 percent of Americans are now overweight or obese, I mean that 66 percent have BMIs greater than 25. Because the health risks of being obese increase as a person gets heavier and heavier, we put obese people in subcategories:

Class I obesity: BMIs between 30 and 34.9
Class II obesity: BMIs between 35 and 39.9
Class III obesity: BMIs 40 and above

Unfortunately, those highest BMI subcategories are growing faster than ever. The Centers for Disease Control and Prevention informs us that 4.7 percent of Americans now have a BMI greater than 40, up

TABLE 3.1 What's Your BMI?

Find your weight in pounds in the left column (if you are between two weights, pick the lower one). Find your height in inches in the top row. Your BMI is in the box where your weight row and your height column intersect.

Weight (pounds)	Height (inches)																		
	58	59	60	61	62	63	64	65	66	67	68	69	70	71	72	73	74	75	76
100	21	20	20	19	18	18	17	17	16	16	15	15	14	14	14	13	13	13	12
105	22	21	21	20	19	19	18	18	17	16	16	16	15	15	14	14	14	13	13
110	23	22	22	21	20	20	19	18	18	17	17	16	16	15	15	15	14	14	13
115	24	23	23	22	21	20	20	19	19	18	18	17	17	16	16	15	15	14	14
120	25	24	23	23	22	21	21	20	19	19	18	18	17	17	16	16	15	15	15
125	26	25	24	24	23	22	22	21	20	20	19	18	18	17	17	17	16	16	15
130	27	26	25	25	24	23	22	22	21	20	20	19	19	18	18	17	17	16	16
135	28	27	26	26	25	24	23	23	22	21	21	20	19	19	18	18	17	17	16
140	29	28	27	27	26	25	24	23	23	22	21	21	20	20	19	19	18	18	17
145	30	29	28	27	27	26	25	24	23	23	22	21	21	20	20	19	19	18	18
150	31	30	29	28	27	27	26	25	24	24	23	22	22	21	20	20	19	19	18
155	32	31	30	29	28	28	27	26	25	24	24	23	22	22	21	20	20	19	19
160	34	32	31	30	29	28	28	27	26	25	24	24	23	22	22	21	21	20	20
165	35	33	32	31	30	29	28	28	27	26	25	24	24	23	22	22	21	21	20
170	36	34	33	32	31	30	29	28	27	27	26	25	24	24	23	22	22	21	21
175	37	35	34	33	32	31	30	29	28	27	27	26	25	24	24	23	23	22	21
180	38	36	35	34	33	32	31	30	29	28	27	27	26	25	24	24	23	23	22
185	39	37	36	35	34	33	32	31	30	29	28	27	27	26	25	24	24	23	23
190	40	38	37	36	35	34	33	32	31	30	29	28	27	27	26	25	24	24	23
195	41	39	38	37	36	35	34	33	32	31	30	29	28	27	27	26	25	24	24
200	42	40	39	38	37	36	34	33	32	31	30	30	29	28	27	26	26	25	24
205	43	41	40	39	38	36	35	34	33	32	31	30	29	29	28	27	26	26	25
210	44	43	41	40	38	37	36	35	34	33	32	31	30	29	29	28	27	26	26
215	45	44	42	41	39	38	37	36	35	34	33	32	31	30	29	28	28	27	26
220	46	45	43	42	40	39	38	37	36	35	34	33	32	31	30	29	28	28	27
225	47	46	44	43	41	40	39	38	36	35	34	33	32	31	31	30	29	28	27
230	48	47	45	44	42	41	40	38	37	36	35	34	33	32	31	30	30	29	28
235	49	48	46	44	43	42	40	39	38	37	36	35	34	33	32	31	30	29	29
240	50	49	47	45	44	43	41	40	39	38	37	36	35	34	33	32	31	30	29
245	51	50	48	46	45	43	42	41	40	38	37	36	35	34	33	32	32	31	30
250	52	51	49	47	46	44	43	42	40	39	38	37	36	35	34	33	32	31	30
255	53	52	50	48	47	45	44	43	41	40	39	38	37	36	35	34	33	32	31
260	54	53	51	49	48	46	45	43	42	41	40	38	37	36	35	34	33	33	32
265	56	54	52	50	49	47	46	44	43	42	40	39	38	37	36	35	34	33	32
270	57	55	53	51	49	48	46	45	44	42	41	40	39	38	37	36	35	34	33

Table 3.2			
Body Weights of People of Various Heights in the Three Classes of Obesity			
	Obesity Class I (BMI* 30–35)	Obesity Class II (BMI 35–40)	Obesity Class III (BMI above 40)
Height (inches)	Weight (pounds)		
62	164–191	191–218	More than 218
66	186–216	216–247	More than 247
70	207–243	243–278	More than 278
72	233–272	272–311	More than 311

*BMI (body mass index) compares weight to height and is used as a measure of "fatness." See Table 3.1 for a full range of BMIs.

from 2.9 percent a decade earlier. That's 9 million Americans! Table 3.2 shows you what BMI "looks like."

WHY WE WORRY ABOUT OBESITY

Obesity can lead to problems in physical health, mental health, and even in our work lives.

Let's look first at how obesity affects life expectancy. We have known for some time that obese people die earlier of heart disease and stroke than nonobese people. To take a broader look at obesity and the risk of dying, a 2010 study in the *New England Journal of Medicine* examined *all causes* of death, not just heart disease and stroke. Researchers at the National Cancer Institute and several leading centers around the world analyzed the relationship between BMI and *overall* mortality in 1.46 million adults. They found the lowest mortality rate among people with BMI between 22.5 and 25. Compared to people with a BMI of 25, there was a 30 percent increase in mortality for every 5-point increase in BMI, all the way up to a BMI of 50.

Beyond an increase in the risk of dying, obesity causes multiple health problems. Some health problems are related specifically to the excess body fat. Arthritis is one example, in which excess weight accelerates damage inside hips and knees and contributes to osteoarthritis. Sleep apnea is another, in which excess fat around the neck compresses the airway.

Just as troubling is the fact that excess body fat changes our metabolism, which can trigger a host of other serious health problems. Obesity leads to what is called "metabolic syndrome." Metabolic syndrome is a combination of three or more obesity-related health conditions, and is known to increase an individual's risk of heart attacks and strokes. If you have three or more of the following health conditions, you also have metabolic syndrome:

Large waist circumference (more than 40 inches in men, more
     than 35 inches in women)
High blood sugar
High blood pressure
Elevated blood triglyceride levels
Low HDL cholesterol levels (that's the "good" cholesterol)

MEDICAL PROBLEMS ASSOCIATED WITH
OVERWEIGHT AND OBESITY INCLUDE:

Diabetes
Hypertension
Heart disease
Stroke
Certain cancers, including breast and colon
Depression
Osteoarthritis
Sleep apnea (periodic cessation of breathing while asleep)

Let's look more closely at diabetes, one of the most serious obesity complications. It is no coincidence that as the rate of obesity is rising, so is the frequency of diabetes. In 1995, 3.3 percent of American adults had diabetes. In 2009, that figure doubled to 6.6 percent. And diabetes is a devastating disease with devastating consequences. Diabetes causes heart attacks and strokes. It is also the leading cause of kidney failure and blindness.

What about how body weight affects mental health? This is more complex. There is scientific evidence that obese people have a greater risk of psychological problems, especially depression. And the reverse applies too: people with depression may overeat and become obese. Whether obesity is the cause of depression or its result, it is clear there is a very important connection between body weight and mental health. In people with underlying psychological problems, it is important to treat those problems at the same time that we work on weight loss.

Finally, what about obesity and work life? There is abundant evidence that obese people suffer several types of discrimination in the workplace. Obese job applicants are less likely to get hired, even though they may have the same skills and qualifications for the job. Employers rate the job performance of obese employees more critically, and pass out stricter disciplinary action to obese workers. And obese women are paid less than their healthy weight counterparts—up to 12 percent less in some studies. Obese men do not seem to suffer from this type of wage discrimination.

So with all of this evidence that being overweight or obese creates problems in our physical and mental health as well as at work, how is it that we continue to get fatter and fatter?

CAUSES OF OBESITY

How human beings put on weight, lose weight, and regulate our weight is a highly complex process, but the most important principle is encapsulated in the acronym *CICO—calories in, calories out*. Put another way: if you ingest more calories than you burn through physical activity, you will put on weight; if you burn more calories than you ingest, you will lose weight. I explained this in the previous chapter using Bob-and-the-Bel-Air analogy.

The reason our citizens are putting on weight and becoming

Figure 3.1

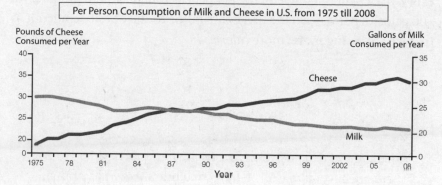

Per Person Consumption of Milk and Cheese in U.S. from 1975 till 2008

Source: adapted from USDA, Economic Research Service

Compared with 1975, Americans in 2008 drank 10 less gallons of milk per year and ate 15 more pounds of cheese. Both are healthy dairy foods, and eaten in appropriate amounts are important in the DASH Diet. But here's a clue that this trend isn't so healthy. Ever since 2002, mozzarella cheese has been the most consumed cheese in the United States. What does that tell you? It says that the cheese Americans are eating is mostly on pizza, and pizza is not an overall healthy food product.

overweight and obese is because they are eating more and being less active.

It doesn't take much to disrupt the balance between the calories we eat and the calories we burn, an imbalance that can lead to progressive weight loss or weight gain. Given the environment in which we live, weight *gain* is a much more likely scenario.

Daily calorie intake increased between 1970 and 2000 by 168 calories for men and 335 calories for women, according to the government's National Health and Nutrition Examination Survey (NHANES). That increase seems quite small—the equivalent of a 16-ounce soda or two, or one or two small candy bars. But it is enough to explain the exploding rates of obesity.

Let's run the numbers to see what would happen if you ate only 100 more calories per day than what's necessary to maintain your current weight:

100 extra calories per day = weight gain of a little less than one pound per month

This would add up to a little more than a ten-pound weight gain every year. And of course many people eat much more than an extra 100 calories per day. So the first contributor to the obesity epidemic is that we are eating more: more *calories in*.

ECONOMICS CLASS

Americans didn't just decide one day to start eating more. There are several reasons why our calorie intake has dramatically increased, some of which has to do with plain old economics:

- The cost of producing food has declined.
- The greatest decline in food costs has been for foods that are high in calories and fast to eat (so-called calorie-dense foods like burgers, chocolate, and ice cream).
- The price of fresh fruits and vegetables, fish, and dairy products has increased much faster than the price of sugar and sweets, fats and oils, and carbonated beverages.
- Preparation of food at home is happening less often due to technology such as the microwave and frozen dinners, not to mention home delivery of high-calorie foods.
- There has been a rapid increase in the number of fast-food restaurants and other "inexpensive" options for eating out.

PHYSICAL ACTIVITY HAS DECLINED

The news gets worse because it's also true that we are exercising less. That's fewer *calories out*. Experts don't know exactly how much less physical activity we are doing on average, but the fact that we are exercising less is not in doubt.

There are several reasons why Americans are doing less physical activity:

- At work, technology allows us to accomplish the same goals with less effort.
- We drive more, walk less.
- There are many more sedentary activities available (Internet, video games, TV).
- There's less physical education taught in the schools than there used to be.
- More of us have desk jobs than farming and factory jobs.

A 2011 study by the Trust for America's Health and the Robert Wood Johnson Foundation showed that in fourteen U.S. states, people were less physically active than they were just a year ago. Despite the focus on fitness and health in our culture, only two U.S. states (Texas and California) saw an increase in physical activity. In those places where physical activity rates have remained at the same low levels, the news is dismal. According to the Labor Department, on average less than 16 percent of Americans exercise every day, about one-fifth of the number who sit and watch TV.

A TOXIC FOOD ENVIRONMENT

Another major cause of the obesity epidemic is that we live in a "toxic food environment."

We are almost always surrounded by large amounts of inexpensive foods that are quick to eat—and which appeal to our primitive desires for fatty, sugary, salty sustenance.

There is almost never a time in the day when such foods aren't easily available to us. We can pull over on the highway for fast food, wander down the hall at work to a vending machine for a candy bar or bag of potato chips, or hoist ourselves off the couch between TV commercials to head to the freezer for a tub of ice cream.

Figure 3.2

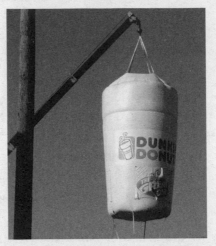

This new size coming to a store near you!

Everywhere, advertisements urge us to eat more, drink more, and participate in ways to be less active.

Our ancestors would be amazed at the huge amounts of food available to us at every turn—giant bottles of soda from convenience stores, towering hamburgers from fast-food joints, tubs of pasta at family restaurants.

Perhaps it's not surprising that portions are getting bigger—we have to fill the larger glasses, bowls, and plates being manufactured. In the 1990s, the standard size of a dinner plate went from ten inches to twelve inches. Cups and bowls also got larger. This is significant. Larger plates, bowls, and silverware influence how much we eat. A study in the *American Journal of Preventive Medicine* described how, when people were given larger bowls and spoons, they served themselves larger portions of ice cream and were also more likely to eat the whole portion.

It is in fact this increase in portion sizes of common foods that is the defining symptom of the toxic food environment. The government's National Heart, Lung, and Blood Institute (NHLBI) did a study of how much portion sizes have increased in the last twenty years, and the results were astonishing.

Food	Twenty Years Ago	Today
Table 3.3		
Portion Inflation: Twenty Years Ago and Today		
Pizza	2 slices = 500 calories	1 slice = 850 calories
Coffee	8-ounce cup = 45 calories with cream and sugar	12 to 32 ounces = up to 700 calories if it's a latte or a loaded mocha!
Movie popcorn	5 cups = 270 calories	1 tub = 630 calories
Bagel	3-inch diameter = 140 calories	5- to 6-inch diameter = 350 calories and higher!
Fast-food cheeseburger	333 calories	590 calories
Soda	8-ounce bottle (original size) = 97 calories	20-ounce bottle = 242 calories

Source: National Heart, Lung, and Blood Institute

Nowhere have portion sizes increased more dramatically than at fast-food restaurants. Portion sizes at fast-food chains are two to five times larger than when items were first introduced. For example, when McDonald's first opened its doors in 1955, it offered one choice of hamburger, and that weighed just 1.6 ounces. Now the chain's largest burger weighs in at a whopping 8 ounces—*500 percent larger*. The Big Mac, once the behemoth of burgers, now seems quite puny compared to menu items at other establishments with names like Triple Whopper, Colossal Burger, and the Western Bacon Six Dollar Burger.

Our perspective has become so distorted by the enormous portions we see when we eat out that we've started to make bigger meals for ourselves in our own kitchens. A study found that people pour themselves about 20 percent more cornflakes and 30 percent more milk than twenty years ago.

How to explain this behavior?

Some experts believe we are a product of evolution—our ancestors were so hungry for so much of the time that when they had the opportunity to eat, they gorged themselves. Translate this to modern times when food has become so plentiful, and if it's there, people will eat it. Many of our citizens have become powerless in the face of the food they are surrounded by.

A PERFECT STORM

This combination of factors—increased calorie consumption, decline in physical activity, and a toxic food environment—has created a perfect storm so powerful it has become incredibly difficult for many people to maintain an appropriate weight. No matter that the goal is so desirable; no matter that society places such a premium on thinness; and no matter that we are constantly being told by the government, our doctors, and our loved ones to lose weight—*it feels like an impossible task.*

||||||||||||||||||||||||||||||

DASH FAQ

Could a weight-loss pill be right for me?

**Please see the answer to FAQ 2 in Section V,
Frequently Asked Questions.**

A DIET WHOSE TIME HAS COME

If it's hard to lose weight, keeping it off is even harder. Many weight-loss diets succeed in helping people lose weight—but only for the short term. No matter what promises are made, these extreme diets (sometimes known as "fad diets") are difficult to follow for very long. Either the foods are so restrictive or the preparations so unfamiliar that they are too difficult to stick to. When you return to a more real-life eating pattern—as you inevitably will—the weight almost always comes right back. Even worse, many people end up heavier than they were before they started. The problem is that those who lose weight on these extreme weight-loss programs don't learn healthy eating habits and when they fall off the wagon, they end up right back where they started, or in a worse position.

I don't consider any weight-loss program successful unless it helps you keep the weight off in the long term. To do this, the program has to stress eating habits that can be maintained long after the initial weight loss takes place. That's why the DASH Diet for Weight Loss teaches you a way of eating that can last you through life.

As I outlined in Chapter 1, it is this and several other reasons why this weight-loss program is right for anyone who wants to lose weight, keep it off, and get a lot healthier in the process. As you prepare to embark on the action portion of the DASH Diet for Weight Loss, let's review this diet's credentials:

It is endorsed by reputable health organizations such as the American Heart Association and the US government's Food and Drug Administration, and is taught at medical schools as the healthiest eating plan available.

It is based on real science, including the results of the original DASH Diet study and over 100 follow-up published papers.

The emphasis is on Hi-Lo-Slo foods, which makes the food content ideal for a weight-loss program.

You get healthier as you lose weight on the eating plan that is at the heart of the diet, and you will be eating foods that have been linked to a lower incidence of heart disease, cancer, osteoporosis, and diabetes.

It's easy to follow, thanks to how the diet is explained—you figure out what your target calorie number is, then find the meal plans that match that number or follow the simple guidelines to create your own eating program.

The foods are familiar and easy to find, and almost nothing is out of bounds.

It has been used successfully by hundreds of thousands of people, including over 18,000 who enrolled in an interactive online weight-loss and health program I have run since 2002. Some of the success tips from those people are included in this book.

ONWARD!

We've spent some time introducing the DASH Diet for Weight Loss in the preceding three chapters that make up Part 1 of this book. This has been the prelude to putting the principles of the program into practice. Armed with the knowledge about how this weight-loss program is so different and why you need it, you are now prepared to take the steps necessary to get started on losing weight and getting healthier. Onward!

Part 2

Into Action

YOU ARE BEGINNING the most important part of the book. This is the "how-to" section, where you learn to put principles into practice. So that it doesn't seem overwhelming, I am going to break it down into manageable sections—small bites, if you will.

The first section is about the foods in the DASH Diet: What You Eat. I have divided this section into the following chapters:

- Your First Three Steps
- The Food Groups: Going Hi-Lo-Slo
- Challenging Foods: Snacks, Drinks, and Mixed Dishes
- What About Salt?
- The Importance of Food Tracking
- Is Meal Planning the Answer for You?
- Vegetarians, This Diet Is for You, Too

Then I discuss the importance of exercise: How Much You Move. I will show you how to increase your weight loss by making physical activity part of your life. The chapters are:

- Walking Your Way to Weight Loss
- Ramping Up Your Fitness Program
- Increasing Lifestyle Exercise

Third, I show you how to put all this into action. This section contains important behavior change strategies I call skillpower. I break this down into:

- Create Realistic Goals You Can Reach
- Use Your Tools
- Employ Visualization Techniques
- Practice Conscious Eating
- Ask for Support
- Conquer Emotional Eating
- Stave Off Cravings
- Learn How to Go Grocery Shopping
- Make Your Kitchen Weight-Loss Friendly
- Learn How to Dine Out and Still Maintain Weight-Loss Goals

I then provide you with the inspiration to keep all those new, healthy habits over the long term in a section called Doing It for Life. And last, but definitely not least, I answer people's Frequently Asked Questions about the DASH Diet.

4

Your First Three Steps

THE BASIC ELEMENTS of learning how to structure your own eating system is as easy as one, two, three:

1. Determine your "calorie target"—how many calories you need to consume per day.
2. Learn the number of servings from each food group you should eat every day for your calorie target.
3. Learn what counts as a serving, and understand the concept of Hi-Lo-Slo foods.

Here's more on these three steps.

STEP 1: DETERMINE YOUR CALORIE TARGET

Refer to the Table 4.1 (Women: Calorie Intake Target per Day for Weight Loss) or Table 4.2 (Men: Calorie Intake Target per Day for Weight Loss) to find how many calories you should be eating each day to lose weight. Read down the left column to find your current weight. If your weight is midway between two weights, use the lower

Table 4.1 Women: Calorie Intake Target per Day for Weight Loss				
Weight (pounds)	Sedentary*	Light activity*	Moderate activity*	Heavy activity*
100	1,200	1,200	1,200	1,326
110	1,200	1,200	1,210	1,404
120	1,200	1,200	1,280	1,481
130	1,200	1,200	1,350	1,559
140	1,200	1,203	1,419	1,636
150	1,200	1,265	1,489	1,714
160	1,200	1,326	1,559	1,791
170	1,200	1,388	1,629	1,869
180	1,202	1,450	1,698	1,946
190	1,256	1,512	1,768	2,024
200	1,310	1,574	1,838	2,101
210	1,364	1,635	1,907	2,179
220	1,418	1,697	1,977	2,257
230	1,472	1,759	2,047	2,334
240	1,526	1,821	2,116	2,412
250	1,579	1,883	2,186	2,489

* Activity Level Definitions:
  Sedentary: little or no exercise
  Light activity: light exercise/sports one to three days a week
  Moderate activity: moderate exercise/sports three to five days a week
  Heavy activity: hard exercise/sports six to seven days a week

weight. Then read across the table to the column that matches your *typical activity level*. There you will find your weight-loss calorie target.

The calorie levels in these tables are a good approximation for overweight and obese people of average height (64 inches for women and 69½ inches for men) and who are about age 50. If you are taller and/or younger than that, the table will give you a lower calorie level than you actually need, so you might lose weight faster, but your DASH servings will be more limited and so harder to stick with. If you

		Table 4.2		
		Men:		
		Calorie Intake Target per Day for Weight Loss		
Weight (pounds)	**Sedentary***	**Light activity***	**Moderate activity***	**Heavy activity***
100	1,200	1,304	1,533	1,763
110	1,200	1,366	1,603	1,841
120	1,200	1,427	1,673	1,918
130	1,236	1,489	1,742	1,996
140	1,290	1,551	1,812	2,073
150	1,344	1,613	1,882	2,151
160	1,398	1,675	1,951	2,228
170	1,452	1,737	2,021	2,306
180	1,506	1,798	2,091	2,383
190	1,560	1,860	2,161	2,461
200	1,614	1,922	2,230	2,538
210	1,668	1,984	2,300	2,600
220	1,722	2,046	2,370	2,600
230	1,776	2,107	2,439	2,600
240	1,829	2,169	2,509	2,600
250	1,883	2,231	2,579	2,600

* Activity Level Definitions:
  Sedentary: little or no exercise
  Light activity: light exercise/sports one to three days a week
  Moderate activity: moderate exercise/sports three to five days a week
  Heavy activity: hard exercise/sports six to seven days a week

are shorter or older, the table will give you a higher calorie estimate than you need, so you won't lose weight as fast.

Calculate your daily calories using the equation in Appendix A if you are in one or more of these categories, or if you would just like to calculate the precise calorie needs for your own height, weight, age, and activity level:

You are younger than 40.
You are older than 60.

You are a woman shorter than 60 inches or taller than 68 inches.
You are a man shorter than 66 inches or taller than 74 inches.

The calorie levels in these tables are calculated to provide 500 calories per day less than you need to maintain your current weight. This
degree of calorie reduction will result in a weight loss of one pound
per week. Reducing calories more than this creates a diet that is too
restrictive. People just get too hungry and are unable to stick with the
diet long enough to hit their desired weight goal. To lose weight faster,
we recommend increasing your activity level. This is covered in detail
in Section II, How Much You Move.

You will notice that we don't recommend calorie levels below
1,200 or above 2,600. It is very difficult to eat a balanced diet with
sufficient nutrition at less than 1,200 calories per day. Diets lower in
calories than 1,200 per day should be supervised by a physician or di-
etician. And to follow our DASH eating plan at 1,200 calories per day,
you need to pay very special attention to choosing Hi-Lo-Slo foods.
These foods are highlighted in Chapter 5. Following our meal plans is
another great way to learn Hi-Lo-Slo foods.

Our highest calorie level, 2,600, is actually more than a 500-calorie-
per-day deficit for some people. But we don't recommend more than
2,600 calories for anyone who wants to lose weight; 2,600 calories provides all of the nutrients and foods you will need to feel satisfied.

STEP 2: LEARN THE NUMBER OF SERVINGS FROM EACH FOOD GROUP YOU SHOULD EAT EVERY DAY FOR YOUR CALORIE TARGET

Now that you know your weight-loss calorie target (from Table 4.1 or
4.2 or because you calculated it in Appendix A), refer to the calorie
target levels in Table 4.3. Find your calorie target in the left column.
Read across that row to see how many DASH servings per day you
should be eating from each of the food groups.

If your calorie target is between two levels, choose the lower calorie level. So if you need 1,768 calories per day, follow the servings goals
in the 1,600 calorie row.

					Meat/ Fish/ Poultry/ Eggs	Nuts/ Seeds/ Legumes	Added Fats	Sweets
Table 4.3								
How Many Servings Should You Eat Each Day from the DASH Food Groups?								
Calorie Target	**Vegetables**	**Fruits**	**Grains**	**Dairy**	**Meat/ Fish/ Poultry/ Eggs**	**Nuts/ Seeds/ Legumes**	**Added Fats**	**Sweets**
1,200	4	3	5	2	1½	¼	½	½
1,400	4	4	5	2	1½	¼	½	½
1,600	4	4	6	2	1½	¼	1	½
1,800	4	4	6½	2½	1½	½	1½	½
2,000	4	4	7	2½	1½	½	2	½
2,200	4	5	8	3	2	½	2½	1
2,400	5	5	9	3	2	½	3	1
2,600	5	5	10	3	2½	1	3	1½

What if you are a vegetarian? Good news—with some modifications, this diet can be eaten by vegetarians, too, while retaining all the weight-loss and health benefits. See Chapter 10 for a full description of how to adapt the DASH Diet to a vegetarian pattern. But very briefly: replace your servings of meat with eggs and foods from the nuts/seeds/legumes group. These foods include beans and tofu (legumes), as well as seitan and tempeh (meat substitutes).

STEP 3: LEARN WHAT COUNTS AS A SERVING IN EACH FOOD GROUP

Examples of DASH Diet for Weight Loss serving sizes are given in Table 4.4, Serving Sizes in the Eight DASH Food Groups. If you eat more than the quantity in a single serving, always count it as more than one serving when you track your food intake for the day. If you eat less, count it as less than one serving. Serving sizes don't have to be exact, though try to stay as close as possible to what counts as a serving size. More details on serving sizes are given in Chapter 5, The Food Groups: Going Hi-Lo-Slo.

You won't need to weigh and measure your food forever. With a

Table 4.4

Serving Sizes in the Eight DASH Food Groups

DASH Food Group	1 Serving Equals
Vegetable	1 cup* raw leafy vegetables ½ cup raw nonleafy vegetables ½ cup cooked vegetables (cut up or mashed) ¾ cup vegetable juice (preferably low-sodium)
Fruit	1 medium whole fruit ¼ cup dried fruit ½ cup fresh, frozen, or canned fruit ¾ cup 100% fruit juice
Grain (and grain products; preferably whole-grain)	One 1-ounce slice bread 1 ounce dry cereal ½ cup cooked rice 1 ounce cooked pasta (about ½ cup)
Dairy (low-fat or nonfat)	1 cup milk 1 cup yogurt 1½ ounces cheese ½ cup cottage cheese
Meat (also fish, poultry, and eggs)	3 ounces cooked meat, fish, or poultry 3 eggs 6 egg whites ¾ cup egg substitute
Meat alternatives (count as 1 DASH serving of meat/fish/poultry)	3 ounces seitan 9 ounces tofu 4 ounces tempeh ½ cup dehydrated TVP (textured vegetable protein)
Nuts/seeds/legumes	⅓ cup nuts 2 tablespoons seeds ½ cup cooked legumes 2 tablespoons peanut butter
Added fat (and oil)	1 teaspoon regular soft margarine, butter, or oil 1 tablespoon regular mayonnaise, salad dressing, or sour cream 2 tablespoons "lite" or reduced-fat mayonnaise, salad dressing, or sour cream
Sweets	1 tablespoon maple syrup 1 tablespoon granulated sugar 1 tablespoon jelly or jam ½ cup gelatin dessert 1 ounce candy (jelly beans, chocolate chips, etc.) ¾ cup sugared lemonade, punch, or soda 3 pieces hard candy ½ cup sherbet 1 Popsicle

* A note about cup measures: Some foods, such as yogurt, gelatin desserts, ice creams, sherbets, and canned fruit, are bought in "cups" of varying sizes. When we refer to cups, we mean the standard American 8-fluid-ounce measure.

little practice, you will get very good at recognizing how much a serving is, especially when you are at home and using your usual plates and bowls. To teach yourself how to recognize a serving, it's a good idea to start off by actually measuring foods for a few days. For this, you'll need:

- A set of dry measuring cups
- A liquid measuring cup
- A set of measuring spoons
- A food scale (available at most grocery stores and some pharmacies)

Here are some useful tips for eyeballing servings:

- ½ cup of food is about the size of a bar of hand soap when piled on a plate. In a small bowl, it is the amount that would fill a cupcake wrapper.
- ⅓ cup is about the amount that would fit in the palm of your hand (see Figure 5.5 to see what one serving of nuts looks like in the palm of a hand).
- 1 cup is about the size of a tennis ball or baseball.
- 1 teaspoon (when you are measuring butter, mayonnaise, or peanut butter) is about the size of your fingertip.
- 1 tablespoon is about the size of an egg yolk.
- 2 tablespoons is about the size of a Ping-Pong ball.
- 3 ounces of meat, fish, or boneless poultry is about the size of a deck of cards.
- 1½ ounces of cheese is about the size of a 9-volt battery (the rectangular kind that you put in your smoke detector).

THE IMPORTANT DIFFERENCE BETWEEN
A "SERVING" AND YOUR "PORTION"

These two terms have very different meanings in this book and in the DASH Diet. And it is an important difference.

When we say a "serving," we mean a *specific amount of food*. So for example, a serving of cooked vegetables is ½ cup. And a serving of milk is 1 cup. As you can see in Table 4.3, a person who needs 2,600 calories eats more servings each day than one who needs 1,200 calories. But *the size of the serving is the same for everyone*. Learning what a serving of food is in each DASH food group is the first step in learning to follow the DASH Diet.

When we say your "portion," we mean the *amount you choose to eat at a meal* or snack.

So a serving is the same for everyone. Your portion is what you decide.

Think of it this way: Let's say two women have the same calorie targets and are following the same DASH goals, and let's say their goal for vegetables is to eat 4 servings per day. Let's also say they only eat their vegetables cooked. One serving of cooked vegetables is ½ cup. Their 4 servings would be 2 cups total (4 × ½ cup).

The first woman decides to have vegetables for lunch and for dinner, so she eats 1 cup at each meal. At the end of the day, she has had her 4 total servings. But *at each meal, her portion was 2 servings*—that's how much she decided to eat.

The second woman prefers to have a big meal in the evening, so she saves up all her vegetable servings till then. At dinner, she eats 2 cups of cooked vegetables. At the end of her day, she has eaten the same 4 servings of vegetables as the first woman. But *her portion for the meal was 4 servings*. That's how much *she* decided to eat.

A serving of vegetables was the same for both women, but the portions they chose were quite different.

I'M ALREADY OVERWHELMED!

Is that what you're thinking? If so, don't worry. You can find seven-day meal plans for your calorie target in Part 3 of this book. Meal plans are an easy way for you to change your diet immediately, before you've completely gotten the hang of how to do it yourself. This book contains dozens of customized meal plans. There's a meal plan for you! And there is information about meal planning in Chapter 9. So fear not.

MY DASH DIET FOR WEIGHT LOSS PROGRAM

Using what you've learned in this chapter, fill in the blanks below:

1. My calorie target is: _____.
2. My daily servings targets in each food group (from Table 4.3) are: _____.

Vegetable	Fruit	Grain	Dairy	Meat	Nuts/Seeds/Legumes	Added Fat	Sweets

5

The Food Groups:
Going Hi-Lo-Slo

IN THIS CHAPTER we look at the "nuts and bolts" of your eating plan: the DASH food groups. You'll learn what counts as a serving. And I provide you with a Hi-Lo-Slo "index" for each food group so you can easily see which foods are better suited to your weight-loss program and which to limit or avoid.

VEGETABLE

Vegetables are rich in important minerals and vitamins, and contain lots of fiber that is important for weight loss because it makes you feel fuller on fewer calories. There are more vegetables in the DASH Diet than you'll find in the typical American diet—or in many other weight-loss diets, for that matter. This is because we know that vegetables contain a lot of key nutrients that help improve our health. The table below shows how many servings of vegetables you should eat every day to lose weight and get healthier as you do so.

How many servings of vegetables should you eat every day?							
Calorie Target							
	1,200	1,400	1,600	1,800	2,000	2,200	2,400	2,600
Servings	4	4	4	4	4	4	5	5

Enter the number of servings of vegetables you need to eat every day: _____

HOW MUCH IS 1 SERVING OF VEGETABLES?

1 cup raw leafy vegetables, lightly packed (spinach and romaine, red leaf, and green leaf lettuces, etc.)

½ cup nonleafy raw vegetables (carrots, broccoli, peas, peppers)

½ cup cooked vegetables (spinach, kale, broccoli, cauliflower, carrots)

¾ cup vegetable juice

½ medium potato or ¼ cup mashed potato

10 french fries

½ cup tomato sauce

Vegetables are also right at the top of my list of Hi-Lo-Slo foods. They are *high in volume* because they have such a high water content; they are naturally *low in calories*; and they take time to chew and swallow so they are relatively *slow to eat*. In the table below, emphasize the vegetables in the "Choose" column to maximize your weight loss. And try to use a variety of vegetables. Don't meet your vegetable servings target every day by eating only broccoli or only carrots. First, that will get very boring. Second, different vegetables have different vitamins and nutrients. To get the full health benefit of the DASH Diet, choose a variety of vegetables.

HI-LO-SLO VEGETABLE CHOICE INDEX

Almost all vegetables are excellent Hi-Lo-Slo choices. But there are some to limit or avoid.

Choose	Limit	Avoid
Raw vegetables and leafy greens	Potatoes	French fries
Frozen vegetables	Avocados	Frozen vegetables in cream or cheese sauce
Vegetables roasted with little added fat or oil, or steamed		Deep-fried vegetables, including tempura

Potatoes deserve a special mention if you are trying to lose weight. Be careful to limit potatoes in all forms, and especially avoid french fries and potato chips. That's because potato consumption is linked to overweight and obesity. Think about it this way: In a recent study published in the *New England Journal of Medicine,* a team of investigators from Harvard University analyzed the connection between the types of foods people ate and how their weight changed over a period of many years. The analysis included over 120,000 people, so it was a very sizeable study. In their analysis, they reported their findings as the change in weight that would occur over a four-year period if people ate one serving of each food every day. They found that for every one serving of vegetables per day, people lost 0.2 pounds every four years. Not so for the potato. For every serving per day of plain potato that was eaten (baked, mashed, and so on), people gained 1.3 pounds every four years. For potato chips, they gained 1.7 pounds per four years. And for America's favorite form of potato, the french fry, they gained 3.4 pounds every four years. Over a period of years, those gains certainly add up. So de-emphasize potatoes while you are trying to lose weight. ***What about baked potato chips?*** Potato chips may be America's go-to snack, but when it comes to your health they are best left on the shelf. While baked chips might be lower in fat and calories (120 calories for 15 baked chips—1 serving—versus 160 calories for 15 fried chips), they don't offer much in the way of nutrition. If you are looking for a snack, pretzels, snack crackers, and even pita chips are a better option.

Selection Suggestions, Preparation Pointers

To take full advantage of the potential for vegetables to support your weight-loss efforts, it's important to make the right decisions when choosing and preparing them.

Vegetables are naturally low in calories, so avoid adding unwanted calories during cooking. Use only a minimum of fat if you are sautéing. And of course, skip the heavy sauces.

It doesn't matter whether you microwave, boil, roast, or bake them—vegetables keep 80 percent of their nutrients during the cooking process. In general, though, you should cook vegetables only until crisp-tender, with just enough water to create steam but not so little you burn the cooking container. Crisp-tender vegetables take longer

|||||||||||||||||||||||||||||||

DASH FAQ

My parents didn't much care for fruits and vegetables, so I didn't grow up eating them at home. As an adult, I don't feel confident coming up with ways to increase how much produce I eat in my diet. Do you have any suggestions?
—Doris, Dartmouth, MA

Please see the answer to FAQ 3 in Section V,
Frequently Asked Questions.

to eat, too. When cooking on the stovetop, use only a small amount of water and keep a tight-fitting lid on the pot so the vegetables cook quickly.

If you like them that way, the best way to serve most vegetables is raw. A vegetable salad is the perfect Hi-Lo-Slo preparation, especially when served with a low-calorie dressing. A vegetable salad is an excellent delivery system for limited amounts of the foods you like that are not so Hi-Lo-Slo, such as meat. An example of this is to enjoy grilled lean beef on top of a bed of greens.

DASH In Action

1. **Find out how many servings of vegetables you need to eat every day.**
2. **Learn what a serving of vegetables is.**

■ FRUIT

Like vegetables, fruits are *high in volume* because they have such a high water content; they are naturally *low in calories*; and they are relatively *slow to eat*. In other words, they are top-notch Hi-Lo-Slo foods.

Refer to the table below for how many servings of fruit to eat every day based on your total calorie target.

How many servings of fruit should you eat every day?								
Calorie Target								
	1,200	**1,400**	**1,600**	**1,800**	**2,000**	**2,200**	**2,400**	**2,600**
Servings	3	4	4	4	4	5	5	5

Enter the number of servings of fruits you need to eat every day:

_____

HOW MUCH IS 1 SERVING OF FRUIT?

1 medium apple, orange, peach, pear
½ grapefruit or ½ medium (7-inch) banana
¾ cup 100% fruit juice
½ cup chopped fresh, canned, or frozen fruits
¼ cup dried fruits (apricots, cranberries, currants, dates, figs,
    peaches, prunes, raisins)

If you're trying to lose weight, another reason to eat lots of fruits is that most are high in fiber. High-fiber foods help you lose weight because they make you feel fuller on fewer calories. That's because the fiber stays in your digestive system longer than the contents of other foods. Whole fruit has more fiber than fruit juice, even 100% fruit juice.

Of course, fruits are also high in vitamins and minerals that are essential for good health, which means if your weight-loss diet is high in fruit, you are going to get healthier as you lose weight. And they offer

HI-LO-SLO FRUIT CHOICE INDEX

Refer to this list for which fruits fare better on the Hi-Lo-Slo index.

Choose	Limit	Avoid
Any fresh fruits	Fruit juice	Canned fruits in heavy syrup
Frozen fruits (no syrup)	Dried fruit	Frozen fruits in syrup
Canned fruit in natural juice (no added sugar)		

us a low-calorie and healthy way of satisfying a craving for something sweet. For all these reasons, the DASH Diet recommends more fruit servings than most Americans eat. There are more fruits in DASH than in most other weight-loss diets, too.

There are two exceptions: *Fruit juice* is on my "Limit" Hi-Lo-Slo index because it's not Slo—it's easy to consume a lot of it very fast, which can make the calories add up. It also does not have all the nutrients and fiber you'd get from whole fruit. I recommend that you not have more than one DASH serving of fruit juice per day (6 ounces). If you usually drink more than this per day, consider diluting ¾ cup juice with ¾ cup water. That way, you can drink 12 ounces but still limit your fruit juice to one 6-ounce serving. Get your other fruit servings from whole fruit.

Dried fruits are also in the "Limit" category because they aren't Lo or Slo. Think about it this way: Raisins are just grapes with the water removed. If you count the number of raisins in one DASH serving (¼ cup), you'll count about seventy-five. And it wouldn't take you long to eat those seventy-five raisins. Now imagine seventy-five grapes. Same calories as the raisins. But it would take you longer to eat them, and you'd certainly feel more full after you ate them. So enjoy dried fruit, but in moderation.

Selection Suggestions, Preparation Pointers

Making the right choices when selecting and preparing fruit to eat will ensure these foods will support your weight-loss goals.

"Mix it up" is the best guideline when choosing fruits to include in your diet. Focus mostly on fruits in the "Choose" column of the Hi-Lo-Slo index when making your selections. I recommend fresh fruit because it tastes a bit better, contains slightly more healthy nutrients, and takes a bit longer to eat because it is in its natural state. But frozen and canned fruit can be an important part of any weight-loss diet so long as you select products without sugar added. Look for products packed "in their own juices" or "in water."

It's easy to work fruit into Hi-Lo-Slo recipes and meals. One way to do this is with lots of fruit on top of a low-fat yogurt or whole-grain cereal—whether for breakfast or a snack. Here are some other ideas:

- Make a quick smoothie in the blender by pureeing peaches and/or nectarines, a touch of your favorite fruit juice, crushed ice, and a light sprinkling of nutmeg. Add "lite" vanilla yogurt for creaminess if you want. The thicker it is, the more Slo it will be to eat.
- Serve fruit wedges with chunks of low-fat cheese and whole-wheat crackers—apples are a great choice for this.
- Toss grapefruit and/or orange sections in a fresh crunchy salad of mixed greens—the sweet citrus and crisp lettuce are a surprisingly delicious combination.
- Grill fruit skewers over medium-hot coals for a fun-to-eat and tasty barbecue treat.
- Make frozen fruit kabobs using pineapple chunks, bananas, grapes, and berries. Or just freeze grapes and berries for a refreshing treat.
- Fruit salad in seconds: Drain mandarin orange slices and empty into a bowl. Add sliced banana, sliced apple, and some blueberries or raisins.
- Make juice cubes by pouring 100 percent fruit juice into an ice cube tray and freezing. Sucking on these is a Slo treat to satisfy your sweet tooth.

||||||||||||||||||||||||||||

DASH FAQ

**I don't have a clue about how to buy
and store fruit. Any suggestions?**

**Please see the answer to FAQ 4 in Section V,
Frequently Asked Questions.**

DASH In Action

1. **Find out how many servings of fruit you need to eat every day.**
2. **Learn what a serving of fruit is.**

■ WHOLE GRAIN (BREADS, CEREALS, RICE, AND PASTA)

Whole grains are important sources of fiber, minerals, and vitamins. When you're eating the DASH Diet for Weight Loss, you eat more grain servings every day than from any other food group. We realize that most grain products are made from refined wheat or other grains (that is, not whole grain). Refined grain products are allowed in the DASH Diet. But, because whole grains offer so many more nutrients, we encourage you to really emphasize whole-grain products in your diet.

Because grain foods come in so many different varieties (breakfast cereal, bread, rolls, crackers, rice, and so on), this is the trickiest food group to master. So we're going to provide a more detailed description of grain foods and instructions for estimating grain servings. And because there can be so many selections within a category of grain foods (think crackers or bread), this is one category where you need to know a bit about food labels so you can make wise choices. So we introduce food label reading in this section as well.

Refer to the table below for how many servings of grains to eat every day based on your total calorie target.

How many servings of grain should you eat every day?							
Calorie Target							
	1,200	1,400	1,600	1,800	2,000	2,200	2,400	2,600
Servings	5	5	6	6½	7	8	9	10

Enter the number of servings of grains you need to eat every day:

_____

HOW MUCH IS 1 SERVING OF GRAIN?

One 1-ounce slice whole-wheat, whole-grain, or white bread
½ small (about 3-inch) bagel
1 ounce cold cereal such as bran flakes or shredded wheat
    (see "Cold Cereal" section below for more details)
1 ounce uncooked oatmeal (cooks to about ¾ cup)
½ cup cooked rice or pasta (measure this out a few times till
    you get good at estimating what ½ cup looks like on a
    plate)
2 graham cracker rectangles, 4 saltine crackers

||||||||||||||||||||||||||||||

DASH FAQ

**I've heard that carbs are "fattening." How, then,
can they be part of a weight-loss program?**
—SAMUEL, ORLANDO, FL

**Please see the answer to FAQ 5 in Section V,
Frequently Asked Questions.**

Estimating Servings of Bread Products

As you can see in Figure 5.1, bread products come in all kinds of sizes
and shapes. Being able to roughly estimate the number of DASH servings in a piece of bread or a bagel is important. For example, let's say
your DASH goal is 6 servings of grain foods each day. If you have a
sandwich for lunch on two slices of bread as shown in the upper left

Figure 5.1 Bread products come in all shapes and sizes.

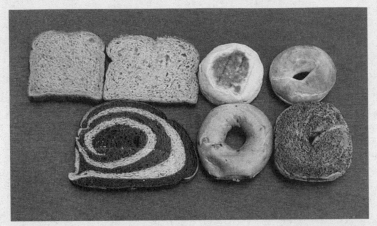

One DASH grain serving equals one 1-ounce slice of bread. But which slice? The slice in the upper left equals 1 serving. Going clockwise from there, the next slice is 1½ servings; the English muffin is 2 servings; the small bagel is also 2 servings. The two bagels on the bottom row are each 4 servings. And the large, free-form slice of bread is 2 servings.

of the figure, you have eaten 2 grain servings, and you have 4 servings left for the rest of the day. But if your lunch sandwich was prepared on a large bagel, that's 4 servings, so you have only 2 servings left for the day. So take a good look at this figure to learn how to estimate servings in bread products.

Today a slice from a typical loaf is either 1 ounce or 1½ ounces. A good rule of thumb is that if your slice of bread is square, it is 1 ounce; if it is more rectangular, it is 1½ ounces. If you are unsure, you can always check the Nutrition Facts Panel on the side of the package. It will tell you how many slices are in a serving and how many ounces that is. Eating a sandwich made with two slices of bread that are 1½ ounces each but thinking they are really only 1 ounce is the difference of an entire grain serving and about 80 calories.

Cold Cereal

For cold cereals, we recommend you always check the food label to understand what a serving is. That's because these cereals are very different in their forms (flakes, puffs, O's, biscuits) and their volumes. In DASH, 1 serving of cold cereal is 1 ounce (about 30 grams). Here we show the labels for a puffed rice cereal and a granola-type cereal. You can see that 1 DASH serving of puffed rice is about 1¼ cups (that's about 1 ounce). But for the granola, 1.9 ounces only fills ½ cup. So 1 DASH serving (1 ounce) of granola cereal would be about ¼ cup!

Puffed rice

Nutrition Facts
Serving Size   1¼ Cups (33g)

Granola cereal

Nutrition Facts
Serving Size   1/2 cup (55g/1.9 oz.)
Servings Per Container About 7

Our advice is to read the labels on cereal boxes, see how much cereal is 1 ounce (a DASH serving), then teach yourself what that amount of cereal looks like in your bowl. Let's say you're going to have the granola cereal. Measure out ½ cup (if you are planning to eat 2 servings of grain) and put it in your cereal bowl. Now you know what the amount you plan to eat looks like. After measuring it out for a couple days, you'll be able to just pour it into your bowl without the measuring cup.

Some cereal labels will require a little arithmetic. For some, what is called a "serving" on the label might be 1½ ounces or even 2 ounces. You just need to remember that a DASH serving is 1 ounce (about 30 grams). If the label says your favorite Granny's Great Bran Flakes is 2 ounces per 1 cup, then 1 DASH serving is ½ cup (1 ounce). The good news is most people eat only two or three types of breakfast cereal. So you should have to learn this only a couple of times for your different cereals.

Here are a few additional pointers for selecting a breakfast cereal:

- Granola-type cereals tend to be higher in calories.
- Avoid cereals that have the words "sugar" or "frosted" in their name.
- Pick cereals that are whole grain (see Guide to Recognizing Whole-Grain Foods).

Snacks: Crackers and Pretzels

Grain-based snacks are another potentially confusing type of grain product. Think how many different varieties of chips, crackers, and pretzels you can find in the snack aisle at the grocery. And they differ in fat content, calories, and whether they are made from whole grain. How do you choose? Like all grain products, we encourage you to choose snacks that are made from whole grain and low in fat. Snacks are one of the main grocery items where marketers spend their money trying to convince you to buy their product. Don't be fooled! Be sure to familiarize yourself with how to recognize a grain product that is whole grain and low in fat so you are sure to choose a snack that is going to be consistent with the DASH Diet for Weight Loss program. We describe how to use food labels to choose whole-grain and low-fat products below.

Pasta

Look for whole-grain pasta. It's a healthy choice. Pasta comes in many shapes and sizes. The best way to learn how to recognize what your portion of pasta looks like is to measure it out. Let's say you plan on 1 cup of cooked pasta to meet two of your DASH grain servings (½ cup of cooked pasta equals 1 DASH serving of grain). Measure out 1 cup and put that amount on your plate. Once you feel comfortable that you know how much to serve yourself, you can stop measuring.

Sometimes it can be helpful to measure out the amount of pasta you will need before you cook it. That way, you won't waste any and you won't have extra pasta that you might be tempted to eat. Here's a handy trick that works for spaghetti. A bundle of spaghetti or linguine

Figure 5.2

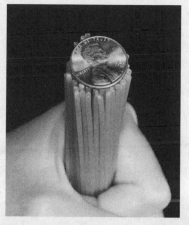

A bundle of spaghetti as big as a penny will yield 2 DASH servings of cooked pasta.

as big around as a penny will yield about 2 DASH servings (1 cup) after it's cooked. And one-half of a 16-ounce box of spaghetti will yield 8 servings (4 cups).

As I have said, I recommend whole-grain products that are low in fat. Whole grains that are low in fat are Hi-Lo-Slo foods because they are *high* in volume (usually), *low* in calories, and tend to be *slow* to eat. They are also high in fiber, which helps us feel fuller on fewer calories.

The whole grains that register highest on my Hi-Lo-Slo index are

HI-LO-SLO GRAIN PRODUCT CHOICE INDEX

Refer to this list for which grain products fare better on the Hi-Lo-Slo index.

Choose	Limit	Avoid
Whole-grain breads and cereals	White breads and cereals made with refined grains	Prebuttered garlic breads
Whole-grain pasta	Refined grain pastas	Crackers (refined flour)
Brown rice and quinoa	White rice	Pastas in cream sauces

crusty whole-grain breads, crunchy bran-type cereals, whole-wheat pasta, and brown rice.

Selection Suggestions, Preparation Pointers

Whole grains are a rich source of Hi-Lo-Slo foods. So long as you choose right, these healthy carbohydrates will fit well into your weight-loss goals.

Many people, when first seeing the amounts of grains they are expected to eat while following the DASH Diet for Weight Loss, are surprised that they are allowed so many servings. The important thing to note here is that serving sizes are small. As I mentioned about cold cereal and pasta, it is a good idea to measure out "loose" products such as cereals, rice, and pasta the first few times you serve them to yourself. Pour them into different bowls and see what they look like on your usual dinner plate. You might find that you are often eating as many as two to three servings of grains in one side of rice or bowl of cereal! And one bagel can have as many as 4 grain servings. So while it is recommended that you eat more servings from the grain category than any other category, it is particularly important to pay attention to your portions when it comes to grains.

Try to make as many as possible of the grains you eat whole grains that are low in fat—that includes breads, pasta, rice, crackers, pretzels, and cereals. Try to limit baked goods made from refined flour—things like croissants, muffins, donuts, cookies, and other processed grain products.

Here are some pointers that will help you choose a product that is whole-grain.

Guide to Recognizing Whole-Grain Foods

- See where the whole grain falls in the ingredient list (usually at the bottom of the food label). Choose products where the first ingredient on the food label contains the word "whole" (or one of the other "whole grain" terms shown in Table 5.1 below).

- When you see a product where the whole grain is the third or fourth ingredient on the list, this means there might be only a tiny amount of whole grains in the product.
- Don't be duped by claims on the box that say "Made with Whole Grain!"—this can mean any amount of whole grain.

Figure 5.3 Whole-grain food labels

MADE FROM: UNBROMATED UNBLEACHED ENRICHED WHEAT FLOUR (FLOUR, NIACIN, REDUCED IRON, THIAMINE MONONITRATE [VITAMIN B1], RIBOFLAVIN [VITAMIN B2], FOLIC ACID), WATER, RYE FLOUR, WHEAT GLUTEN, RYE MEAL, YEAST, CONTAINS 2 PERCENT OR LESS OF: SOYBEAN OIL, SALT, CARAMEL COLOR, CARAWAY SEEDS, COCOA PROCESSED WITH ALKALI (DUTCHED), CALCIUM PROPIONATE AND SORBIC ACID TO RETARD SPOILAGE, MONO AND DIGLYCERIDES, WHEAT FLOUR, MALTED BARLEY FLOUR, DEXTROSE, SUGAR, LACTIC ACID, DEHYDRATED ONIONS, DEHYDRATED GARLIC AND ENZYMES.

If the first item listed on the ingredient list isn't a whole grain, then the product isn't whole grain. The label above is from a box of rye crackers. Because the crackers are dark in color, many people would mistake them for a whole-grain product. But the first ingredient is enriched wheat flour, not whole-wheat flour. *This is not a whole-grain product.*

The next label is from another package of crackers. Its first ingredient is clearly labeled "whole grain wheat." So *this is a whole-grain product.*

INGREDIENTS: WHOLE GRAIN SOFT WHITE WINTER WHEAT, SOYBEAN OIL, SALT.
CONTAINS: WHEAT.

Watch the fat content, too: In addition to choosing whole-grain products, the products you choose should be low in fat. This is because, per gram, fat has more calories than any other nutrient. There are 9 calories in 1 gram of fat, while protein and carbohydrate both

Table 5.1	
Terms That Mean "Whole Grain"	
Here is a list of terms you will see on food labels. If the first ingredient in the ingredient list is in the left column, the product is truly "whole grain." If it's in the right column, it's not.	
Indicates a whole-grain ingredient or food product	**Is most likely not whole-grain ingredient or product**
Wild rice	Wheat flour
Whole-grain corn	Wheat
Whole-grain barley or pearled barley	Unbleached wheat flour
Whole wheat	Stone-ground wheat (if whole grain, label description should be "stone-ground whole wheat")
Whole spelt	Rye flour or rye
Whole rye	Rice flour
Whole oats or oatmeal	Rice
Wheat berries	Pumpernickel
Triticale	Multigrain (this simply means it's composed of various grains, not necessarily whole)
Sorghum	Enriched flour
Quinoa	Degerminated cornmeal
Millet	Cornmeal
Bulgur or cracked wheat	Corn flour
Buckwheat	
Brown rice	

have 4 calories per gram. By choosing whole-grain products that are low in fat, we know that the product will be relatively low in calories. Here are some pointers that will help you choose a product that is low in fat.

GUIDE TO RECOGNIZING GRAIN PRODUCTS THAT ARE LOW IN FAT
- Find the number given for Calories from Fat on the Nutrition Facts panel.
- Divide the Calories from Fat by the total Calories in the product.

Figure 5.4 Choosing low-fat products

Nutrition Facts

Serving Size   1 Cup (59g/2.1 oz.)
Servings Per Container   About 12

Amount Per Serving	Cereal	Cereal with ½ Cup Vitamins A&D Fat Free Milk
Calories	190	230
Calories from Fat	10	10

Divide Calories from Fat by Calories

10/190 = 0.053

Total Calories from Fat is
0.053 or about 5%

	% Daily Value**	
Total Fat 1g*	2%	2%
Saturated Fat 0g	0%	0%
Trans Fat 0g		
Polyunsaturated Fat 0.5g		
Monounsaturated Fat 0g		
Cholesterol 0mg	0%	0%
Sodium 250mg	10%	13%
Potassium 320mg	9%	15%
Total Carbohydrate 46g	15%	17%
Dietary Fiber 7g	29%	29%
Sugars 17g		
Other Carbohydrate 22g		
Protein 5g		

To ensure the grain products you are choosing are low in fat you should practice this quick calculation. Divide the Calories from Fat by the total Calories. That percentage should be less than 30 percent.

- You should choose products where the number of calories from fat that you calculate is less than 30 percent (about one-third) of the total Calories.
- Don't be duped by claims on the package that the product is "Trans Fat Free!" The product can still be high in fat and contain a lot of unhealthy saturated fat.

When enjoying grain-based foods, go easy on high-calorie spreads, sauces, and toppings. This includes spreads such as butter and jam on bread and toast, creamy pasta sauces over spaghetti, and sugar on cereal.

DASH In Action

1. **Find out how many servings of whole grains you need to eat every day.**
2. **Find out what a serving of whole grains is.**

■ DAIRY (MILK, CHEESE, YOGURT)

"But I thought dairy foods are fattening." That's what many people say when I explain the importance of dairy for good health. It tells me why a lot of folks who are trying to lose weight assume they've got to cut dairy out of their diets. As a result, the typical "dieter"—especially women—tend to not eat nearly enough calcium. But calcium is an important part of a healthy diet, and dairy is the most efficient and convenient way to get it. But there is much more to dairy than just calcium. It is also a rich source of protein, phosphorus, and other important nutrients.

There is a simple way to enjoy dairy foods while losing weight: emphasize low-fat and nonfat dairy products—yogurt, cheese, and milk. These products have all the nutritional value of full-fat dairy products, minus the fat and calories.

How many servings of dairy products should you eat every day?							
Calorie Target							
1,200	1,400	1,600	1,800	2,000	2,200	2,400	2,600
Servings 2	2	2	2½	2½	3	3	3

Enter the number of servings of dairy you need to eat every day:

_____

Which dairy foods fit best into the Hi-Lo-Slo category? At the top of my list are nonfat (skim) milk, nonfat yogurt, and cottage cheese made with skim milk. Not as high on my list are hard cheeses, even when

HOW MUCH IS 1 SERVING OF DAIRY PRODUCTS?

1 cup milk
⅓ cup nonfat dry milk powder
½ cup low-fat cottage cheese
1½ ounces low-fat cheese
1 cup low-fat or nonfat yogurt, fruit flavored or plain*
½ cup low-fat or nonfat frozen yogurt

* A note about yogurt: Most of the yogurt "cups" you buy in the supermarkets now are 6 fluid ounces or other sizes. In the DASH Diet, 1 serving of yogurt is 8 fluid ounces (1 standard cup measure). Because we recommend using yogurt in dips and smoothies as well as for eating by itself, it is a good idea to buy the larger tub of yogurt and portion it into 8-ounce servings.

HI-LO-SLO DAIRY CHOICE INDEX

Refer to this list for which dairy products fare better on the Hi-Lo-Slo index.

Choose	Limit	Avoid
Low-fat and nonfat milk	Low fat and nonfat frozen yogurt	Whole milk
Low-fat and reduced-fat cheeses		Full-fat cheese
Low-fat and nonfat yogurt		Ice cream
Low-fat cottage cheese		

made with skim milk. That's because it's hard to feel full and satisfied on small amounts of these low-volume foods. It's also easy to lose track of servings and overeat cheese.

ARE YOU PUTTING BUTTER IN YOUR COFFEE?

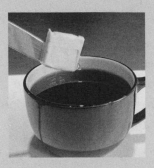

Even "little" changes can make a difference over time. Here's an example.

Let's say you have one large cup of coffee every day—like a Starbucks grande or a Dunkin' Donuts medium. And you add some kind of dairy to it. The average person adds about ½ cup of dairy to a coffee that size. Whether it's nonfat milk or whole milk or light cream, how much difference can that half cup make? The table below shows how many calories are in that 4 ounces of dairy over the course of one month, depending on what you add.

What You Add	Calories in a Month
Nonfat Milk	1,300
Whole Milk	2,400
Light Cream	7,100

And the amount of butterfat that you add by using light cream is like adding almost 7⅔ sticks of butter (almost 2 pounds) to your coffee every month!

So if you switch from light cream to nonfat milk for your one grande per day, you'll lose 1½ pounds per month from just that one change.

LASTING IMPRESSIONS

In the interviews I did with successful weight losers as I was writing this book, I spoke with T.T., a 44-year-old engineer. A week after our interview, he sent me this e-mail:

Dr. Moore,
There was one thing I forgot to mention last week. I've always remembered your story about what you add to your coffee. I was always a cream/two sugars guy. But after hearing you describe how much butter I was adding to my coffee, I gave it up instantly. Gross. It was one of those things that really had an impact, and it made me change to being a "Black with 2 Equal" coffee drinker.

If you don't like the nonfat version of milk, yogurt, or cheese, try "downshifting." Start by dropping down to 2% milk and to reduced-fat cheese. After a week or two, consider downshifting again to 1% or nonfat. It's true that consuming dairy products in their "whole-fat" form is not a good idea if you are trying to lose weight, but reduced-fat dairy products—especially ones at the top of my Hi-Lo-Slo index—will fit in well to your DASH Diet for Weight Loss program.

Selection Suggestions, Preparation Pointers

If you're like most Americans, you don't get enough healthy dairy in your diet. Here are some ideas for getting the right number of servings of low-calorie dairy into your day. At breakfast:

- Eat cereal with 1 serving or more of nonfat or 1% milk.
- Make oatmeal with nonfat or 1% milk instead of water.
- Spread low-fat or nonfat ricotta cheese and honey or fruit preserves on toast.

- Try nonfat yogurt jazzed up with wheat germ, granola, or crunchy cereal.

At lunch:

- Eat nonfat yogurt.
- Top sandwiches with a slice of low-fat cheese.
- Finish lunch with an ice-cold glass of nonfat or 1% milk.
- Make "creamy" soup with nonfat or 1% milk.

At snack time:

- Instead of coffee or tea, sip on hot cocoa made with nonfat or 1% milk.
- Munch on fresh vegetables with a dip made from nonfat yogurt.
- Try a smoothie made with nonfat yogurt and your favorite fruit.

At dinner:

- Add low-fat or nonfat cheese to casseroles or meatloaf.
- Top vegetables with a sprinkle of low-fat cheese.

|||||||||||||||||||||||||||||||

DASH FAQ

What advice can you give someone who knows how important dairy is to a complete weight-loss program, but who is lactose intolerant?
—Henry, Atlanta, GA

Please see the answer to FAQ 6 in Section V, Frequently Asked Questions.

Dessert time:

- Enjoy pudding made with nonfat or 1% milk.
- Enjoy nonfat yogurt or cottage cheese mixed with fresh fruit.

DASH In Action

1. **Find out how many servings of dairy you need to eat every day.**
2. **Learn what a serving of dairy is.**

■ MEAT, FISH, POULTRY, AND EGGS

Meat, fish, and poultry—referred to collectively as "meat"—are sources of high-quality protein and important vitamins and minerals. Eggs are included in this group because they are also good sources of high-quality protein and can occasionally be substituted for meat.

Meat is a concentrated source of saturated fat and doesn't fare well on my Hi-Lo-Slo index—it is low in volume, high in calories, and often quick to eat, especially when prepared by fast-food outlets. That's not to say I recommend you completely cut meat out of your diet. In fact, that's one of the reasons the DASH Diet for Weight Loss gets such high marks—there are no foods that are out of bounds.

How many servings of meat, fish, and poultry should you eat every day?								
Calorie Target								
	1,200	1,400	1,600	1,800	2,000	2,200	2,400	2,600
Servings	1½	1½	1½	1½	1½	2	2	2½

Enter the number of servings of meat/fish/poultry you can eat each day: _____

HOW MUCH IS 1 SERVING OF MEAT/FISH/POULTRY/EGGS?

3 ounces* cooked lean meat, such as beef, veal, or pork

3 ounces cooked fish or shellfish

3 ounces cooked skinless, white meat poultry, such as turkey, chicken

3 ounces low-fat deli meats

3 whole eggs or 6 egg whites

*Note: 3 ounces of cooked meat is about the size of a deck of cards.

HI-LO-SLO MEAT CHOICE INDEX

Refer to this list for which meat, fish, poultry, and eggs fare better on the Hi-Lo-Slo index.

Choose	Limit	Avoid
Lean cuts of beef, pork	Red meat	Highly processed meats such as bacon and hot dogs
Skinless chicken and turkey breast	Dark meat poultry	Poultry with the skin on
Lean deli meats such as turkey breast	Regular deli meats	Highly processed deli meats such as salami, bologna, and liverwurst
Fish		Fried chicken, beef, or fish
Whole eggs and egg whites	Egg yolks	

Americans tend to eat more red meat than poultry and fish. But both poultry and seafood contain less saturated fat than red meat. For weight loss, I recommend you eat more poultry and fish than red meat.

You can also substitute eggs in your diet for several servings of meat, so long as you follow the substitution guidelines below.

FITTING EGGS IN: THE THREE GOLDEN RULES

Eggs have been getting a bad rap for a couple of decades now because of concerns about cholesterol, but there is certainly a place for eggs in a healthy diet so long as sensible guidelines are observed. The three golden rules where it comes to eating eggs are moderation, sensible cooking techniques, and healthy additions.

- *Moderate your consumption:* Count three eggs as one serving of meat when figuring out your DASH nutritional goals for the day. Because of the relatively high cholesterol content, restrict your whole egg consumption to five per week. However, because an egg's cholesterol is all in the yolk, you can eat more than five eggs a week if you eat only the whites of the eggs (which make delicious omelets and scrambled eggs) or egg white products such as Egg Beaters.
- *Use sensible cooking techniques:* To cut the fat content in your egg recipes, use nonstick pans or nonstick cooking spray so you don't have to use butter. Another option is to poach or boil your eggs so you don't need to cook them in butter.
- *Add healthy foods to your egg recipes or meals:* Breakfast is the time to work some healthy ingredients into your egg recipes. The most Hi-Lo-Slo way is to fill your omelet with vegetables such as tomatoes, grated zucchini, and sweet peppers. Scrambled eggs made with milk are another way to include a nutrient-rich food in an egg recipe. Eaten with whole-grain toast and a banana or grapefruit, a breakfast omelet will give you a terrific jump on your DASH goals for the day.

Selection Suggestions, Preparation Pointers

Meat, fish, and poultry are concentrated sources of calories. Eating too much of these foods is generally not compatible with a weight-loss program. However, animal proteins can be part of your weight-loss program so long as you choose wisely when purchasing them and incorporate these foods into Hi-Lo-Slo meals and recipes.

Here are some selection suggestions.

- All fish is naturally low in saturated fat, so choose fish instead of poultry or beef at least twice each week.
- When buying meat, choose lean cuts. For beef, look for eye of round or top round. Ground beef should be 90% lean or greater. For veal, select shoulder, freshly ground veal, cutlets, or sirloin. Pork lovers should go with lean pork loin or tenderloin.
- Buy chicken and turkey without skin; if this isn't possible, remove the skin before cooking. White meat contains fewer calories and less saturated fat than dark meat. Try freshly ground turkey made from the breast.
- Limit deli meats to 1 serving (3 ounces) per week. Although convenient, deli meats tend to be highly processed and contain higher amounts of sodium. Choose meats in their natural form as often as possible.
- Limit goose and duck, as they are high in calories and saturated fat, even with the skin removed.
- Go meatless at least once a week, choosing a meat alternative such as legumes, beans, or a meat alternative (see the "Vegetarian" text box below and Chapter 10 for more about meatless eating).

Meat should not be the centerpiece of your meal. As far as possible, make it the accompaniment to lots of beautifully prepared vegetables and whole grains. On a Hi-Lo-Slo dinner plate, your meat should take up one-quarter of the plate; your vegetables and whole grain should occupy three-quarters. A small amount of grilled chicken surrounded by brown rice and a medley of broccoli, carrots, and green beans is an example of a Hi-Lo-Slo meal that includes animal protein. Another example is some strips of grilled sirloin atop a deep bed of healthy greens and other vegetables.

A hearty vegetable stew accented by chunks of lean lamb or a vegetable-rich stir-fry with a small amount of meat are two more ways to enjoy small amounts of meat along with other filling ingredients.

When preparing meat for these Hi-Lo-Slo meals, follow these guidelines:

- Seafood is lower in fat, but avoid fried fish covered in greasy batter or swimming in butter.
- Remove the skin from poultry. Taking the skin off a chicken breast reduces calories from about 195 to 140 and fat grams from 8 to 3.
- Cut the fat off meat. Trimming the fat off a 3-ounce piece of broiled sirloin steak lowers calories from 240 to 150 and fat grams from 15 to 6.
- Drain off the fat after cooking ground beef.
- Place meat on a rack when roasting, broiling, or braising so fat can drain away.
- Avoid fatty processed meats such as bologna, salami, hot dogs, sausages, and bacon.

DASH In Action

1. **Find out how many servings of meat you can have every day.**
2. **Learn what a serving of meat is.**

■ NUTS, SEEDS, AND LEGUMES

In the DASH Diet, we put nuts, seeds, and legumes into a single food group. All three offer important health benefits. They are concentrated sources of protein and fiber, and in the case of nuts and seeds, healthy

THE VEGETARIAN OPTION

"I'm a vegetarian. Can *I* eat this diet?" The answer is "Yes." Several years ago I developed a meatless version of the DASH Diet for Weight Loss. In addition to helping you lose weight, this vegetarian weight-loss plan will provide the same benefits as the regular version. That's because the proteins in the replacement foods (legumes and eggs, mostly) do much the same job that the animal proteins do.

I have not developed a vegan version of my diet because without dairy products, I cannot be sure the diet will improve health in the same ways. There are certain vitamins and minerals in dairy that provide important benefits related to bone and circulatory health. I am not saying that a vegan version of the DASH Diet doesn't provide all the same benefits as one with dairy in it does—I am just saying that I haven't seen proof either way.

It's easy to adapt the DASH Diet for Weight Loss to make it meatless. One way is to follow the vegetarian meal plans provided in Part 3. There are meatless meal plans for almost all calorie targets.

You can also structure your own meatless weight-loss diet by making appropriate substitutions. The key is knowing how much of the meat replacement counts as a serving of meat. These replacements are described in detail in Chapter 10.

Meat alternatives (count as 1 DASH serving of meat/fish/poultry)	3 ounces seitan 9 ounces tofu 4 ounces tempeh ½ cup dehydrated TVP (textured vegetable protein)

WHICH FOODS ARE IN THIS GROUP?

Nuts: almonds, Brazil nuts, cashews, chestnuts, hazelnuts, macadamia nuts, peanuts, pecans, pine nuts, pistachios, walnuts

Seeds: pumpkin, sesame, sunflower

Legumes: soybeans (the most nutritious legume and the most common legume crop in the world), black-eyed peas, chickpeas/garbanzo beans, lentils, and black, red, white, navy, and kidney beans. Legumes play an important part of the DASH Diet for vegetarians.

fats as well. But your "daily servings" number is low because even though nuts are packed with nutrition, they're also packed with calories. Nuts and seeds are sort of the opposite of Hi-Lo-Slo foods—they are Lo in volume, Hi in calories, and Fast to eat. It's easy to lose track of how many servings you eat and exceed your calorie limit for the day. That means that while you definitely want to include nuts and seeds in your diet, it's extra important to stick closely to the number of recommended servings.

How many servings of nuts, seeds, and legumes should you eat every day?							
Calorie Target							
1,200	1,400	1,600	1,800	2,000	2,200	2,400	2,600
Servings ¼	¼	¼	½	½	½	½	1

Enter the number of servings of nuts, seeds, and legumes you need to eat every day: _____

For most people, the recommendation for this food group is less than 1 serving per day. If your goal is ½ serving per day, you might prefer to have one full serving every other day.

Figure 5.5 This is 1 DASH serving of almonds (⅓ cup).

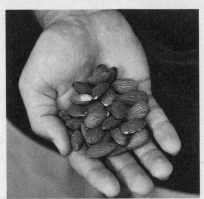

HOW MUCH IS 1 SERVING OF NUTS/SEEDS/LEGUMES?

In general:
⅓ cup nuts
2 tablespoons seeds
½ cup cooked dried beans/legumes

Specifically:
⅓ cup almonds, walnuts, peanuts, cashews, etc.
½ cup cooked beans such as kidney, pinto, and navy
½ cup cooked chickpeas and lentils
½ cup hummus
2 tablespoons peanut butter
2 tablespoons sesame seeds
2 tablespoons shelled unsalted sunflower seeds

Selection Suggestions, Preparation Pointers

Nuts and seeds are not Hi-Lo-Slo foods. They are concentrated sources of goodness—and calories. However, you can include them in

HI-LO-SLO NUTS/SEEDS/LEGUMES CHOICE INDEX

Refer this list for which nut, seed, and legume products fare better on the Hi-Lo-Slo index.

Choose	Limit	Avoid
Beans and legumes cooked without added fat or sweeteners	Nuts	Baked beans with added fat or sweeteners
	Hummus	Refried beans

your weight-loss diet so long as you follow Hi-Lo-Slo principles. That means eating them in moderation, and more important, incorporating them into Hi-Lo-Slo meals and recipes.

Nuts and seeds can be incorporated into recipes that are Hi-Lo-Slo. This is another instance where we include foods in the DASH Diet for Weight Loss that many weight-loss plans discourage you from eating.

Nuts: Toss nuts into stir-fries, salads, and pasta. Sprinkle chopped nuts on top of a bowl of soup or your favorite casserole or vegetable. Start your day with nuts on top of yogurt or oatmeal.

Seeds: Pumpkin seeds can be eaten raw or cooked in Hi-Lo-Slo dishes. They are delicious toasted and sprinkled, while hot, with low-sodium soy sauce and served on salads. Sunflower seeds can be sprinkled over salad or breakfast cereals.

Legumes: Legumes can be the main ingredient in a dish or liven up Hi-Lo-Slo dishes such as salads, soups, and casseroles. For example, you can toss chickpeas or kidney beans in a salad. Legumes can be used as a meat replacement, in

LEGUMES ARE NUTRITION SUPERSTARS

Legumes are naturally low in fat and a major source of complex carbohydrates, fiber, protein, and minerals such as potassium, magnesium, and zinc.

In vegetarian cultures or where meat is unavailable or too expensive—China and India, for example, the two most populous nations in the world—legumes are often the main source of protein.

In many cuisines, legumes are paired with grains for a well-rounded nutritional package. This is because the proteins in the legumes "complement" the protein in grain foods, thereby offering a more nutritious protein dish. Thus, the soybean is paired with rice in China; beans, lentils, and chickpeas with wheat and barley in Middle Eastern and Indian cuisines; and beans with corn in Mexican and Tex-Mex dishes.

which case you can increase how many servings of them you can eat.

DASH In Action

1. **Find out how many servings of nuts, seeds, and legumes you should eat every day.**
2. **Learn what a serving of nuts, seeds, and legumes is.**

■ ADDED FAT AND OIL

In the DASH Diet for Weight Loss, we encourage you to avoid foods that are inherently high in fat, such as high-fat cuts of meat or high-fat pastries. But the fats and oils that we ask you to count in your daily DASH servings are the fats you *add* to your foods when you eat them—things like butter, olive oil, and the oils in salad dressing. These might seem small in quantity, but the calories add up to be pretty big. To keep your calorie intake within your target number, it's important to address the added fat in your diet.

How many servings of added fat should you eat every day?								
	Calorie Target							
	1,200	**1,400**	**1,600**	**1,800**	**2,000**	**2,200**	**2,400**	**2,600**
Servings	½	½	1	1½	2	2½	3	3

Enter the number of servings of added fat you can eat every day: ________

Added fats and oils are by definition calorie-dense foods—the opposite of the Hi-Lo-Slo foods you want to emphasize in your diet. You can include them in your diet but in very limited amounts. I would like you to especially reduce the amount of butter that you use. Like all animal fats, butter contains what we call "saturated fat"—the kind that

HOW MUCH IS 1 SERVING OF ADDED FAT?

1 teaspoon soft margarine or butter
1 tablespoon regular mayonnaise or sour cream or
  2 tablespoons low-fat mayonnaise or sour cream
1 tablespoon salad dressing or 2 tablespoons "lite" salad
  dressing
1 teaspoon oil (olive, corn, canola, safflower, or other
  vegetable oils)

HI-LO-SLO ADDED FAT CHOICE INDEX

Refer to this list for which added fat products fare better on the Hi-Lo-Slo index.

Choose	Limit	Avoid
Low-fat versions of the following products: mayonnaise, salad dressing, sour cream	Olive oil	Butter
	Canola oil	Mayonnaise
	Trans-fat-free margarine	Whipped cream

raises cholesterol levels. Vegetable fats contain just as many calories as butter but don't raise your cholesterol. In fact, olive oil and canola oil can even improve your cholesterol level. So use vegetable oils, but to lose weight, use them sparingly.

||||||||||||||||||||||||||||||

DASH FAQ

When grocery shopping, it's always a good idea to choose foods that are low in fat if I'm trying to lose weight, right?

Please see the answer to FAQ 7 in Section V, Frequently Asked Questions.

WHAT ABOUT TRANS FATS?

One of the few foods I will tell you to cut out of your diet *completely* is trans fats.

In general, I recommend moderate amounts of polyunsaturated and monounsaturated fats such as canola and olive oil, which are heart healthy, and limited amounts of saturated fat because it can cause high cholesterol and heart disease.

I recommend you avoid trans fats completely because they are a synthetic substance that has been linked to serious health problems. Trans fats are created when oils are chemically changed from a liquid to a more solid fat, a process called "hydrogenation" because hydrogen is added. Studies have shown that trans fats increase "bad cholesterol" and lower "good cholesterol." Saturated fats, too, increase the "bad cholesterol," but unlike trans fats they don't lower "good cholesterol." More recent studies suggest trans fats may cause other health concerns. For instance, regularly eating foods high in trans fats may interfere with your body's ability to metabolize fats you need for the growth and functioning of vital organs such as your brain.

Foods that often contain trans fats include:

- Cookies and crackers
- Doughnuts
- Potato chips
- Peanut butters
- Nondairy creamers
- Deep-fried meat, fish, and chicken
- Salad dressings
- Some cereals
- Margarine

(*continued on next page*)

You can avoid trans fats by following these guidelines:

- Avoid products containing the words "partially hydroge-nated" on the ingredients label. And don't buy foods with any trans fats listed on the food label.
- When eating out, ask your server whether the restaurant fries or bakes using partially hydrogenated oils.

In addition it is important to:

- Keep your saturated fat intake low. Just because a food doesn't contain trans fats doesn't mean that you should eat one with saturated fat in it instead. Saturated fats are not just high in calories—they are associated with heart disease.
- Remember that polyunsaturated and monounsaturated fats are "good" fats, but even though they are heart healthy, they contain as many calories as other fats—about 9 calories per gram.

Selection Suggestions, Preparation Pointers

- Use half the salad dressing you typically do now. Pour it into a spoon (instead of straight out of the bottle) to control the amount you use.
- Try low-fat or nonfat salad dressing and mayonnaise.
- Use a small amount of a heart-healthy oil whenever a recipe calls for melted shortening or butter.
- When frying, stir-frying, or lining a baking pan, use vegetable oil sprays to cut down on how much oil you use.
- Make your own salad dressings and dips. Creamy dressings and dips can be made with plain low-fat yogurt instead of sour cream or mayonnaise.

DASH In Action

1. **Find out how many servings of added fat you can have every day.**
2. **Learn what a serving of added fat is.**

■ SWEETS

The DASH Diet for Weight Loss recommends far less sugar-sweetened food and beverages than the typical American diet. Sugary foods are high-density foods and not Hi-Lo-Slo, and they don't contain any important nutrients to benefit your health. Keep them to an absolute minimum if you're trying to lose weight.

To satisfy your desire for sweets, try sugar-free fruit-flavored gelatin or, best of all, frozen, canned, or fresh fruit for dessert. Fruit gives you the sweetness you crave and lots of vitamins, minerals, and fiber. Nonfat frozen yogurt is a sweet treat that counts as 1 DASH serving of dairy per ½ cup. Because they are so high in calories due to their sugar content and because they provide very little other nutritional benefit, I include regular soda and sugar-sweetened drinks like fruit punch as "sweets."

How many servings of sweets should you eat every day?							
Calorie Target							
1,200	1,400	1,600	1,800	2,000	2,200	2,400	2,600
Servings ½	½	½	½	½	1	1	1½

Enter the number of servings of sweets you can eat every day: _____

HOW MUCH IS 1 SERVING OF SWEETS?

¾ cup sugar-sweetened soda

1 tablespoon maple syrup

1 tablespoon sugar

1 tablespoon jelly, jam, or preserves

½ cup sugar-sweetened gelatin dessert

1 ounce jelly beans

¾ cup sugar-sweetened lemonade or fruit punch

3 pieces hard candy

½ cup sherbet

1 Popsicle

Selection Suggestions, Preparation Pointers

Since sweets are such a small part of the DASH Diet for Weight Loss, let's look at how to cut back on these foods, since many people who struggle with their weight tend to eat too much of them. Most important, limit yourself to the number of servings you should be eating and find healthier, low-calorie alternatives to high-calorie sweets.

One of the healthiest ways to satisfy your sweet tooth is with fruit, "Mother Nature's candy." You can do this at dessert time or as snacks.

You can complement these choices with low-calorie dairy items. As an example, you can get much of the taste and mouthfeel of an ice cream sundae by taking half a banana and some berries, adding one scoop of "lite" frozen yogurt, and topping it with low-calorie chocolate syrup and a tablespoon of crushed nuts. Not only will you satisfy your craving for something sweet, cold, crunchy, and flavorful, but you'll also get a serving of fruit, low-fat dairy, and nuts, all of which are important to the DASH Diet. Another idea for a sweet snack is creating a trail mix of mini pretzels, with a smaller amount of chocolate chips, dried fruit, and peanuts.

You don't have to go without sweet treats. You just need to find lower-calorie alternatives. And there's fun in finding out what these are.

DASH In Action

1. **Find out how many servings of sweets you can have every day.**
2. **Learn what a serving is.**

6

Challenging Foods: Snacks, Drinks, and Mixed Dishes

IT IS EASY to keep track of your servings when you're choosing from the major DASH food groups as I showed you in the previous chapter. But there are certain areas of our daily food choices that don't fit neatly into this format. These require attention so they don't become problem areas. We cover three main challenges in this chapter: snacks, drinks, and estimating what's in dishes that are composed of several different foods (what we call "mixed dishes"). We also briefly discuss ways to cope when eating out, either in restaurants or at someone else's house.

SNACKING SMART

The DASH Diet for Weight Loss is a satisfying diet of whole foods. It isn't a "starvation diet" that is impossible to stick to in the long term and that has you feeling hungry all the time. But if you find yourself with a rumble in your stomach between meals, or if you enjoy taking a break with a snack at certain times of the day, then you need to learn to "snack smart." Snacking smart means finding snacks that are Hi-Lo-Slo and keeping track so you don't go over your calorie target for the day.

Making a habit of smart snacking can also get you out of the habit of hitting the vending machine or the candy aisle of a convenience store when you get an urge for something to munch on.

The following are some excellent alternative snacks:

- Whole fresh fruit or canned fruits packed in their own juice
- Unsalted pretzels mixed with a small amount of nuts and dried fruit
- Graham crackers and other reduced-fat crackers
- Sugar-free gelatin
- Low-fat or nonfat yogurt
- Air-popped popcorn, plain, with no added salt
- Raw vegetables with a low-fat dip (such as my "Dill"icious Dill Dip)

Most of these snacks also provide you with needed servings of DASH foods, especially fruits, vegetables, low-fat dairy, and whole grains.

One of the keys to healthy snacking is making sure you have access to these foods when you want them. That means planning ahead. It's a good idea to include Hi-Lo-Slo snacks on your shopping list. Make sure you stock up so you're not caught short with nowhere to go other than that vending machine.

Refer to Table 6.1 for calorie contents of some common snack foods. For weight loss, stick with the lower-calorie selections.

Make Your Own 100-Calorie Snacks

Making your own 100-calorie Hi-Lo-Slo snacks can provide you with personalized and delicious ways of snacking smart. It's also cost-effective—the do-it-yourself approach to snacking is much less

Table 6.1

Calories and Number of DASH Servings in Common Snacks

Item	Calories	DASH servings
Snack Foods		
Pretzels, 1 oz.	100–120	1 grain
Granola bar, 1.5-2 ounces	150–200	1–2 grain
Fat-free granola bar 1.5 ounces	100	1 grain
Popcorn, air-popped, 3 cups	110	1 grain
Frozen Yogurt, ½ cup		
Frozen yogurt, low-fat	145	1 dairy
Frozen yogurt, nonfat soft serve	100–150	1 dairy
Yogurt, per 8 fl. oz. cup		
Yogurt, low-fat, plain	120–160	1 dairy
Yogurt, low-fat, fruit on the bottom	200–250	1 dairy
Yogurt, nonfat, plain	110–130	1 dairy
Yogurt, nonfat, fruit on the bottom	180–200	1 dairy
Gelatin Dessert, 1 snack cup		
Sugar-free gelatin	10	*Sugar free gelatin does not contain enough nutrients to count toward your servings in any of the DASH food categories.
Regular gelatin	70	1 sweet
Fruits and Vegetables		
Apple, 1 medium	50	1 fruit
Banana, 1 medium, 7-inch	105	2 fruit
Cantaloupe, ½ cup	25	1 fruit
Carrots, ½ cup baby carrots or carrot sticks	25	1 vegetable
Celery, ½ cup sticks	10	1 vegetable
Cherries, sweet, pitted, ½ cup	50	1 fruit
Grapefruit, ½	40	1 fruit
Grapes, ½ cup	50	1 fruit
Honeydew melon, ½ cup	25	1 fruit

Item	Calories	DASH servings
Fruits and Vegetables (*cont.*)		
Orange, 1 medium	60	1 fruit
Peach, 1 medium	35	1 fruit
Pear, 1 medium	80	1 fruit
Pineapple chunks, ½ cup	40	1 fruit
Plum, 1 medium	30	1 fruit
Strawberries, sliced, ½ cup	25	1 fruit
Watermelon chunks, ½ cup	25	1 fruit
Canned pineapple in 100% juice, ½ cup	75	1 fruit
Canned fruit cocktail in its own juices, ½ cup	40	1 fruit

expensive than the commercial 100-calorie snack packs we see in grocery stores.

Here are some ideas:

- 1 rice cake spread with 2 teaspoons almond butter or natural peanut butter
- 1 cup sliced bananas and fresh berries
- 20 unsalted pretzel sticks, 1 reduced-fat string cheese stick, celery sticks (all you can eat)
- 1 medium apple with 1 ounce low-fat cheese
- 1 cup fresh fruit salad sprinkled with 1 tablespoon slivered almonds
- ½ of a reduced-fat string cheese stick and 4 whole-wheat snack crackers
- ½ medium banana sprinkled with 2 tablespoons shredded coconut
- 3 cups unsalted air-popped popcorn
- 1 cup strawberries with ⅓ cup plain nonfat yogurt
- All-you-can-eat green veggie sticks (cucumbers, bell peppers, celery) with 1 tablespoon "lite" dressing for dipping
- ½ cup unsweetened toasted oat cereal with ¼ cup blueberries and ½ cup nonfat milk
- 1 hard-boiled egg with 1 slice melba toast

Don't obsess about making your snacks exactly 100 calories. Here are some guidelines on how to get close enough: Start by finding the calorie values for your chosen snacks. You may be able to get this information off the box if you bought the product already packaged. Figure out what weights of the snack correspond to 50 calories and to 100 calories. Once you've calculated that, weigh out the quantity using a kitchen scale. You can figure out what quantities of the product to mix and match with other items—cereal with fruit, pretzels with cheese, and so on. There you go—your own 100-calorie snack! Once you get the hang of what a 100-calorie snack looks like, you can eyeball it in the future.

LIQUID CALORIES: A REAL PROBLEM

"I watch my food intake, but I don't really count what I drink."

If that sounds like you, you're not alone. When it comes to weight control, many people don't pay nearly enough attention to the beverages they consume. Maybe you think that sugar-sweetened sodas are the villain here. You'd be right, but only partially so. Whether a soda or a glass of cold milk, there is one big problem that's true of all beverages: Calories in liquid form aren't sensed by our brains the same way calories in food are. So you can drink a lot of calories at a meal and still feel hungry for food. A scientific study found that people eat the same amount of food regardless of whether their dinner beverage contained calories or not. It's as though calories in drinks are invisible—until they reappear around your waist. So watching how many calories you consume in beverages is really important for weight loss. Given the fact that the average American consumes 20 percent of their calories in beverage form, you have an opportunity to improve your health if you replace the empty calories in the beverages you drink with more nutritious ones. And in addition to improving your health, reducing your consumption of high-calorie beverages will enable you to lose weight more successfully.

But back to sugar-sweetened sodas. This is a real challenge to America's waistline. The average teenager drinks two and a half cans of soda (almost 1 quart) per day. That's about 330 calories! And it's not just teenagers. Young adults (20 to 39 years old) drink about the same amount. And calories aren't the only problem with soda. Soda contains no nutrients or food value. Yet it displaces healthy beverages like milk and 100% fruit juice from the diet—drinks that *do* contain valuable nutrients. So soda adds calories and reduces intake of healthy nutrients. When trying to improve health and lose weight, there is truly no worse combination.

The most important thing to know when choosing beverages is which ones will help promote good health and weight loss and which ones are likely to stand in the way of your health and weight-loss goals. Here is a quick guide to what to drink if you want to lose weight. I have divided common beverage choices into Recommended (with a special discussion of diet soda), Conditionally Recommended, Okay in Moderation, and Avoid.

Recommended

Plain water: Water is essential for health and contains no calories. And if you drink two glasses of water before a meal, you will feel full sooner and eat less. For variety, try sparkling water with a wedge of lemon or lime.

Coffee and tea: These are fine if you don't load them up with sugar and cream. If you do need "additives," try nonfat milk and artificial sweeteners like Splenda and Equal.

Vegetable juice: While not calorie-free, vegetable juice is low in calories and packed with nutrition. A 6-ounce glass (¾ cup—that's 1 DASH serving of vegetables) of tomato or other vegetable juice contains about 35 calories, compared to about 85 calories for 6 ounces of orange or apple juice. But if you are watching your blood pressure, watch out for the salt content of vegetable juice and select ones that are salt-free or reduced-salt.

Nonfat milk: Dairy products are an important part of the DASH Diet, and drinking milk is a great way to meet your daily dairy food goal. While it's true that milk has calories, you can get all the nutritional value of milk and fewer calories by drinking the nonfat version. An 8-ounce glass (1 DASH dairy serving) of nonfat milk contains about 90 calories versus 150 calories in whole milk.

Conditionally Recommended

Diet soda: Most nutrition experts don't promote diet soda, but for people concerned about their weight, diet sodas are a fact of life. And we think they are okay in moderation. They contain zero calories— a good thing. And they are not associated with weight gain in large studies, as sugar-sweetened sodas are. They do contain artificial sweeteners (mostly aspartame), and some research (mostly in animals) has suggested a link between artificial sweeteners and cancer. But no large studies in humans have shown that risk. So our conditional recommendation is that you can include diet sodas in your diet, but we would prefer that you not use them as your major form of fluid. If you need to carry a bottle of something with you through the day, water is a better choice.

Okay in Moderation

100% fruit juice: Real fruit juice is loaded with nutrients. But it is also fairly high in calories per ounce. Although 6 ounces (¾ cup) of 100% fruit juice counts as 1 DASH serving of fruit, juice doesn't contain all the same nutrients and fiber of the whole fruit—think of the difference between an apple and apple juice. We recommend that you not drink more than ¾ cup of fruit juice per day. Try drinking 100% juice watered down by half. After a week you will wonder how you ever drank the undiluted version.

Alcoholic beverages: If consumed in excess, alcohol can add a lot of calories and compromise your weight-loss efforts. In addition to offering no nutritional value, alcohol can also lower your resolve to eat right and may lead to overeating. Alcoholic beverages do not fit into any DASH food group, so all the calories you consume in alcohol must

CALORIES IN A "DRINK"

5 fl. oz. wine	120 calories
12 fl. oz. "lite" beer	100–120 calories
12 fl. oz. "heavy" beer	150 calories
1½ fl. oz. hard liquor	115 calories
8 fl. oz. Margarita	370 calories
8 fl. oz. Long Island Iced Tea	268 calories
8 fl. oz. vodka tonic (1.5 ounces vodka and 6.5 ounces regular tonic water)	169 calories

be added onto your daily calories from food. If you going to drink alcohol, limit it to no more than one or two drinks, and just a few days per week. More than that just adds too many calories and will sabotage your weight-loss efforts.

To help you moderate your alcohol consumption, try the following tips:

- Drink a glass of water in between alcoholic drinks.
- Do not use a straw; often, using a straw will increase drinking speed.
- Choose lower-calorie drinks like wine and "lite" beer over high-calorie beverages like Margaritas, Long Island Iced Tea, and daiquiris.
- In order to keep track of the amount you consume, do not refill your glass until it is completely empty.
- Consider diet tonic water or calorie-free sodas as mixers with hard liquor.

If you struggle with your weight, it will be a challenge to fit alcohol into a calorie-appropriate eating plan. A couple of glasses of wine once a week may not be the undoing of your weight-loss efforts, but you should proceed with caution for the reasons described.

Specialty coffee drinks: Coffee may not have any calories, but specialty coffee drinks do—big-time! Depending on the version of the drink you choose, that Frappuccino from Starbucks can have as many calories as a McDonald's Big Mac (or more).

You can keep the fat and calorie content of "gourmet" coffee drinks down by doing the following:

- Order a smaller size.
- Request nonfat milk.
- Ask the counter person about lower-calorie options—and order one.
- Order a regular coffee!

Here's a list of some specialty drinks from Starbucks. See how many calories you can save by choosing a "Tall" rather than a "Grande" and by choosing nonfat instead of the whole-milk version:

Table 6.2		
Calorie Content of Some Popular Coffee Drinks Made with Nonfat Versus Whole Milk		
	Calories in a "Tall" (12 oz.) with Nonfat Milk	Calories in a "Grande" (16 oz.) with Whole Milk
Cappuccino	60	140
Caffe Latte	100	220
Caffe Mocha	170	290
Caramel Macchiato	140	270
Skinny Flavored Latte	100	210
Skinny Cinnamon Dolce Latte	100	210

Avoid

Regular soda: You have already gotten the message that we don't like sugar-sweetened soda. It is high in calories and contains no healthy nutrients. Study after study has shown that drinking regular soda causes weight gain. So if you are serious about losing weight,

Figure 6.1

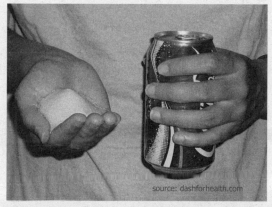

source: dashforhealth.com

One 12-ounce can of soda contains 9 teaspoons of sugar.
And not much else.

regular soda has to go. Use one of the better beverages discussed as Recommended. And if you are tempted to slip back to regular soda, try this experiment: Every 12-ounce can of soda contains 9 teaspoons of sugar (that's about a handful). So instead of popping open that can, pour 9 teaspoons of sugar into a bowl, grab a spoon, and dig in. Wash it down with 12 ounces of water. You will have just consumed the basics of a can of sugar-sweetened soda. You say you usually drink a 20-ounce bottle? The experiment for you is 14 teaspoons of sugar!

Sugar-sweetened fruit drinks and cocktails: Soda is not the only culprit where it comes to high-calorie drinks. Some drinks masquerading as "fruit beverages" are in fact mostly sugar and water. These are drinks with names like "grape drink" or "cranberry cocktail." Always check the labels on beverages with names like this to see what percent of the drink is real fruit juice. They can be as low as 15 percent juice. Sugar-sweetened tea drinks fall into this category, too.

Sports drinks: Unless you exercise for long periods in hot temperatures, you really don't need the electrolytes and other "benefits" of sports drinks that, compared to water, are much higher in calories. Water works just fine.

MIXED DISHES

How do you judge the number of food group servings when they are mixed together in a recipe—such as lasagna or stew? It's relatively easy to estimate serving sizes of foods on their own. Using the tables we provided in Chapters 4 and 5, you can estimate what a serving is of brown rice, carrots, salmon, or an apple. But it's a different challenge when foods are combined in one dish—what nutritionists call "mixed dishes." This is even more of a challenge when you are eating out or someone else has prepared the meal for you.

Our advice on this is to relax and do the best you can! Often you will have to guesstimate the number of servings in the meals you order in restaurants or are offered at other people's homes. The good news is that you learned a whole lot about serving sizes in the previous chapter, so this will be a lot easier for you than it was before you picked up this book. Here's how you might guesstimate serving amounts in the case of three different types of mixed dishes.

Dishes with Cheese, Such as Lasagna, Pizza, and Macaroni and Cheese

Dishes made with cheese are usually part cheese and part grain product—bread in the case of pizza, pasta in the case of lasagna or

---

DASH FAQ

I love pizza. Is it totally out of bounds on my weight-loss diet?

Please see the answer to FAQ 8 in Section V, Frequently Asked Questions.

macaroni and cheese. Cheese is hard to estimate because it melts and spreads, so you'll have to eyeball a bit. But a safe bet for a half-cup of pasta or lasagna is about ¼ dairy serving and ¾ grain serving. Depending on the thickness of the crust, the amount of the cheese, and the size of the slice, pizza can really vary. An average slice of cheese pizza from a large (16-inch) pie is about 2 servings of grain and 1 serving of dairy, so that is a good starting point. Adjust down for smaller slices, thinner crust, and less cheese. Adjust up for extra cheese, thicker crust, and larger slices.

Dishes with Meat, Such as Stews, Chili, and Stir-Fries

Dishes that are a mixture of vegetables and meat in a sauce are a little bit easier than dishes with cheese. The first thing to assess is the ratio of meat to vegetables. Do they seem about even? Are there more vegetables than meat? More meat than vegetables? If you are preparing the meal yourself, you'll know the exact proportions. If not, you'll have to guess. In general, estimating that there is ½ serving of meat and ½ serving of vegetables in a half-cup portion is safe.

Soups

Soup is a near-perfect example of a Hi-Lo-Slo food if you choose correctly. Broth-based soups that are made with lean meats and vegetables and are reduced in sodium are a great choice. They tend to have about ½ serving of meat and ½ serving of vegetables per cup. Adding frozen vegetables to your soup can boost the veggie content.

Cream-based soups generally have about the same ½ serving of meat and ½ of vegetables, but are loaded with added fat and calories.

When Eating Out

You can also avoid getting into too much trouble when eating out or dining at someone else's home by following these guidelines. Most important: Follow my guidelines for ordering meals in restaurants (see

Chapter 23, Learn How to Dine Out and Still Maintain Weight-Loss Goals).

For any mixed dishes that contain a high-fat item like meat or cheese, politely ask your server to request that the kitchen go easy on that item and increase the vegetables and whole grains around it. For example, if you order meat lasagna, ask your server to provide you with a half-portion and double up on the size of the salad. For example, for a chicken stir-fry, request that the kitchen halve the amount of chicken in the dish and double the amount of vegetables; also ask for brown rice instead of white. But it's true that sometimes, no matter how politely you ask, the chef cannot make your requested change to the dish. In which case, you may have to make another selection or simply eat less of the item (taking half of it home is a healthy and economical option).

And starting with a salad or a broth-based soup (two Hi-Lo-Slo selections), so you are less likely to overeat in the more calorie-dense areas of the meal, is always a good idea.

When Eating at Someone Else's Home

It's important to show good judgment when making special food requests at someone else's home. This is especially true when your host is making her "special recipe" or it is a festive occasion with celebratory foods.

That said, honesty is the best policy and it is often easiest to simply inform your host you are watching what you eat. Then, from whatever is being offered, ask for lots of what you know fits well into your DASH Diet for Weight Loss program—vegetables and whole grains, especially—and less of what you are trying to limit, such as meat, heavy sauces, potatoes, rich condiments, and the like. And don't forget to compliment your host enthusiastically on all the food!

7

What About Salt?

WE HAVE ALL HEARD that eating too much salt can be bad for us. But I haven't said much about salt yet in this book. Where does the DASH Diet for Weight Loss stand on salt intake?

There is strong scientific evidence that excessive salt intake raises blood pressure and makes the treatment of high blood pressure more difficult. Some people with congestive heart failure (heart disease) also need to reduce their salt intake. So the medical recommendation is that the 100 million Americans who either have high blood pressure or blood pressure in the higher part of the normal range (what we call "pre-hypertension") and those with congestive heart failure should reduce their salt intake.

What about the rest of us who don't have those medical concerns? What should we do about salt intake? My recommendation, and the recommendation of most physicians, is that all of us would be better off if we would reduce how much salt we eat, whether we have a health concern or not. The amount of salt that we *need* each day is a small percentage of what we typically eat. We could all cut back a lot on our salt intake and remain perfectly healthy.

Here is a little background on salt and how we can cut back. Americans eat about two teaspoons of salt each day. Obviously that doesn't all come from the salt shaker. In fact, only about 10 percent of the salt that we eat each day comes from the salt we add during cooking plus what we add at the table from the salt shaker. The vast majority of the salt in the American diet is hidden in the processed foods we eat—pizza, crackers, canned soup, deli meats, and more. There is even a lot of salt in some foods where we wouldn't expect it, like bread. Cutting back on high-salt processed foods is the key to cutting back on salt.

How much do we have to cut back? The current recommendation from medical organizations is that we should be eating less than one teaspoon of salt per day. So how do we get from our current two teaspoons to less than half that? Well here's the good news: If you begin following the recommendations of the DASH Diet for Weight Loss, you're already almost there.

That's because the DASH Diet recommends lots of fruits and vegetables and dairy foods. And it includes far fewer processed foods—things like chips and crackers and processed meats. So all you have to do is learn how to select low-salt versions of the processed foods you still eat.

WHAT IF I DON'T EAT ENOUGH SALT?

It's almost impossible to eat less salt than you need. This is because our "need" is very small and there is so much salt in almost all the foods we eat. Think about it this way: The current medical recommendations for how much salt we should eat still provide about seven times more salt than we need each day.

Before I give you suggestions for how to pick the right processed foods, I need to tell you about the difference between salt and sodium. They are not the same thing. Salt is what we buy at the store and add to our food. Salt is made up of two minerals: sodium and chloride. And it is the sodium in salt that causes the health problems. That's why food labels show us an item's sodium content, not its salt content. So when you start looking at food labels, it's sodium you'll be looking for.

SODIUM AND FOOD LABELS

Learn how to read the Nutrition Facts label on food packaging so that when you are choosing processed foods, you know how to make lower sodium choices. Try to pick foods that contain less than 5% of the recommended Daily Value.

The one time you can pick a food item with more than 5% of the Daily Value for sodium is if that item is a meal equivalent (for ex-

Figure 7.1 Checking sodium on a food label

Nutrition Facts

Serving Size (15g)
Servings Per Container 22

Amount Per Serving	
Calories 60	Calories from Fat 15

	% Daily Value*
Total Fat 1.5g	**2%**
Saturated Fat 0g	**0%**
Trans Fat 0g	
Cholesterol 0mg	**0%**
Sodium 210mg	**9%**
Total Carbohydrate 11g	**4%**
Dietary Fiber 1g	**4%**
Sugars 0g	**0%**
Protein 2g	
IRON	4%

*Percent Daily Values are based on a 2,000 calorie diet. Your daily values may be higher or lower depending on your calorie needs.

Here is a food label from mini wheat crackers. One serving is about ten crackers. The calories look pretty good (60 per serving). But look at the sodium: 9%! That's well above the 5% limit.

What do these "daily values" mean? A 5% daily value means that if you eat one serving of this food, you will get 5% of your total daily recommended amount of sodium. If you eat two servings, you'd get 10%. So if you eat two servings (20 mini crackers) of these stoned wheat crackers, you'd be eating 18% of your recommended sodium intake for the whole day. Not a good choice.

ample, a frozen dinner or pizza). Those items can have up to 20% of your Daily Value for sodium. Otherwise, stick with items that are less than 5%.

Some other tips include:

- Look for products that say "sodium-free," "very low sodium," "low-sodium," "light in sodium," "reduced or less sodium," or "unsalted." Because the government has implemented strict rules to govern such claims, you can be assured these are not false.
- Buy fresh or plain frozen vegetables. Canned vegetables are okay if labeled "no salt added." Or rinse canned vegetables, as this washes away the extra sodium in these products.
- Use fresh poultry, fish, and lean meats rather than canned or processed versions. Use herbs, spices, and salt-free seasoning blends in cooking and at the table instead of salt.
- Choose convenience foods that are low in sodium. Cut back on frozen dinners, mixed dishes like pizza, packaged mixes, canned soups or broths, and salad dressings, all of which often have a lot of sodium.
- When available, buy low- or reduced-sodium or no-salt-added versions of foods such as canned soup, dried soup mixes, bouillon, canned vegetables and vegetable juices, low-fat cheeses, condiments such as ketchup and soy sauce, crackers and baked goods, processed lean meats, and snack foods such as chips, pretzels, and nuts.

Here is a tip for cooking with less salt. You get a much greater taste of salt when the salt is on the surface of the food than when it is mixed throughout. So if you are making a stew and the recipe calls for two teaspoons of salt, cut that in half and add just a little to the finished stew on your plate. That surface salt will hit your taste buds and you'll never miss the extra salt that you didn't add during cooking.

After reducing sodium in your diet, food may taste bland to you for a period of time. But here's the good news: Your taste buds will soon adapt to this lower salt way of eating. It takes only a week or so. Most people who cut back on salt say that the foods they used to love now taste too salty. If you don't want to cut back all at once, do it gradually. Reduce the amount of salt in your diet little by little so you slowly get used to your less-salty food. A couple of practical tips are to reduce the amount required by half, or mix half of the regular salted version of a food with the no-salt version. Over time, slowly switch to the lower salt or no-salt version.

Just as we learn to like the taste of salt, so we need to gradually unlearn it. Our health depends on it.

8

The Importance of
Food Tracking

IN THE PREVIOUS chapters, we stressed how important it is for you to learn how many DASH servings you should be eating each day and how much food constitutes a DASH serving. But of course the real point of all this—to lose weight—is achieved only if you actually follow the DASH recommendations. That's the hard part.

So here's a technique to help you follow those recommendations. It has been proven to work in many studies of weight loss. It's called "food tracking" (or food diaries or food logs). Basically, you write down everything you eat on a day-by-day basis. That's it. It's so simple that most people don't believe it can work and they don't even try. But it does work.

Here's one example of a study that tested food tracking. Several of the original DASH study investigators enrolled 1,685 people in a six-month weight-loss trial. The study subjects were taught the DASH Diet, had group sessions, were given exercise advice, and were asked to keep track of their food intake on a food diary form every day. On

"COULDN'T HAVE DONE IT WITHOUT FOOD TRACKING"

That's a quote from one of the successful weight losers in our DASH program. M.L. is a 44-year-old woman who had unsuccessfully tried several other weight-loss plans. But she lost 24 pounds on the DASH Diet. When we asked her what allowed her to be successful, she said there were several things. First, she liked the diet itself because it allowed a variety of foods and wasn't boring. Second, she said that keeping track of what she ate every day, especially in the first couple of months, was key. It helped her learn her recommended DASH servings and how much food equals 1 serving. And it helped her stay focused on what she should be eating. "After a while, I stopped recording my food every day. But if I felt myself starting to slip off the DASH Diet, I'd start the food tracking again and that got me back on track."

average, the group lost 13 pounds in six months. People who exercised more lost more weight (no surprise there). But people who kept more daily food diaries lost more weight than those who didn't. The people who kept no food diaries lost an average of about 8 pounds. The people who kept food diaries every day lost almost 18 pounds on average. Food tracking definitely works.

Keeping a log like this will help you in several ways. Most important, self-tracking is a good motivation tool that makes you more accountable for your actions. Also, putting something down in black and white reinforces your efforts, and makes it more "real." Finally, keeping a food log can help identify problem areas.

There is a sample Food and Exercise Log in Figure 8.1 on page 102. You can photocopy and use this one, or you can make your own. Just be sure the form will allow you to record both individual food items and DASH servings. After a while, keeping track of DASH servings will become easier and that's really what you need to be keeping track

Figure 8.1 Food and Exercise Log

	DASH Servings								Notes: (i.e., emotions, exercise, calories)
	Fruit	Veg	Grain	Dairy	Meat	N/S/L*	Fat	Sweet	
Breakfast	☐	☐	☐	☐	☐	☐	☐	☐	
	☐	☐	☐	☐	☐	☐	☐	☐	
	☐	☐	☐	☐	☐	☐	☐	☐	
	☐	☐	☐	☐	☐	☐	☐	☐	
	☐	☐	☐	☐	☐	☐	☐	☐	
Breakfast Total:	___	___	___	___	___	___	___	___	
	Fruit	Veg	Grain	Dairy	Meat	N/S/L*	Fat	Sweet	
Snack	☐	☐	☐	☐	☐	☐	☐	☐	
	☐	☐	☐	☐	☐	☐	☐	☐	
	☐	☐	☐	☐	☐	☐	☐	☐	
Snack Total:	___	___	___	___	___	___	___	___	
	Fruit	Veg	Grain	Dairy	Meat	N/S/L*	Fat	Sweet	
Lunch	☐	☐	☐	☐	☐	☐	☐	☐	
	☐	☐	☐	☐	☐	☐	☐	☐	
	☐	☐	☐	☐	☐	☐	☐	☐	
	☐	☐	☐	☐	☐	☐	☐	☐	
	☐	☐	☐	☐	☐	☐	☐	☐	
Lunch Total:	___	___	___	___	___	___	___	___	
	Fruit	Veg	Grain	Dairy	Meat	N/S/L*	Fat	Sweet	
Snack	☐	☐	☐	☐	☐	☐	☐	☐	
	☐	☐	☐	☐	☐	☐	☐	☐	
Snack Total:	___	___	___	___	___	___	___	___	
	Fruit	Veg	Grain	Dairy	Meat	N/S/L*	Fat	Sweet	
Dinner	☐	☐	☐	☐	☐	☐	☐	☐	
	☐	☐	☐	☐	☐	☐	☐	☐	
	☐	☐	☐	☐	☐	☐	☐	☐	
	☐	☐	☐	☐	☐	☐	☐	☐	
	☐	☐	☐	☐	☐	☐	☐	☐	
Dinner Total:	___	___	___	___	___	___	___	___	
	Fruit	Veg	Grain	Dairy	Meat	N/S/L*	Fat	Sweet	
Snack	☐	☐	☐	☐	☐	☐	☐	☐	
	☐	☐	☐	☐	☐	☐	☐	☐	
Snack Total:	___	___	___	___	___	___	___	___	
Daily Total:	☐	☐	☐	☐	☐	☐	☐	☐	

*Nuts, seeds, and legumes

TIPS FOR KEEPING YOUR FOOD LOG

Be honest—you'll only be fooling yourself: If you aren't honest, the journal won't be helpful.

Write down everything: This includes that handful of potato chips you had on the way out the door to the health club and the sip of juice taken just before leaving for work.

Be timely: Write things down as you eat them. Don't wait until the end of the day.

Be detailed, not vague: If you had fries with your dinner, don't write down "potatoes." The fact that they were fried is significant. This also goes for items like salad dressings. There are many dressings that are not only high in calories, but in fat as well.

of so you can stay on the DASH Diet. I have also made a version of this food log available for a download on my DASH for Health website, www.dashforhealth.com/foodlog.php.

Here's one more thing to pay attention to on your food log. If you are trying to manage your weight, you should be aware of issues such as when and why you eat foods that compromise your efforts to manage your weight.

Self-tracking can make us feel uncomfortable because it can be hard to admit that we succumbed to temptation or made the wrong choice of what to eat. However, when we face up to the decisions we've made, it is easier to change them. And that's what makes self-tracking such a successful tool for weight loss.

9

Is Meal Planning the Answer for You?

OVER THE YEARS, I have developed numerous resources for the thousands of participants in the weight-loss and health program I run. Meal plans are among the most effective resources that I offer. Sometimes known as "menu plans" or "eating plans," meal plans are a written list of what you will eat at mealtimes and for snacks. Meal plans take a lot of the work out of figuring out what and how much to eat, which can be very helpful in the early stage of eating the DASH Diet for Weight Loss. You will find all of the meal plans in Part 3.

WHY MEAL PLANNING WORKS

There are several reasons why meal planning can be helpful if you're following the DASH Diet for Weight Loss.

First of all, meal planning helps you avoid impulse eating. One of the biggest challenges of sticking to a weight-loss diet is impulse eating. We're much more likely to eat impulsively when there's nothing healthy around. Having food on hand to make a low-calorie meal quickly—and healthy snacks, too, if you're ravenous while you're making dinner—will help you avoid impulse eating. It also helps if you have meals frozen ahead of time that you can eat in emergency situations.

The variety that meal planning provides helps you stick to your weight-loss goals. You can plan a variety of meals instead of relying on the "same old, same old." Enjoying the food you're eating as part of your diet makes it more likely you will stick to your weight-loss goals.

Meal planning decreases the need for excessive eating out or ordering in. Without something to eat waiting at home at the end of the day, it's easy to decide to eat out or pick up something to take home. Unfortunately, not many restaurants go out of their way to help folks trying to manage their weight. Having quick-to-prepare meals waiting at home helps you steer clear of large restaurant portions that are high in fat and calories.

There are other reasons why so many people I've worked with like meal plans:

- Save time and money
- Ensure you get all the important nutrients you need
- Reduce visits to the grocery store (and cut down on impulse purchases)
- Avoid wasting food
- Cut down on packaged or restaurant and take-out meals that are often high in calories, fat, and sodium
- Reduce the need to spend the money on eating out
- Cut down on stressing about what to cook for dinner

MEAL PLANNING: HERE'S HOW

It's easy to get started with the DASH Diet for Weight Loss meal plans. To find the meal plan that's right for you, just use your calorie target number to find the corresponding plan in Part 3. There is a meal plan in this book for everyone: men and women, vegetarians and meat eat-

MEAL PLANS TEACH, TOO

L.A. is a 64-year-old retired teacher who lives in the Midwest.

I knew the DASH Diet would be a healthy way for me to eat, but I had a lot of trouble getting started on the diet and counting my food servings. When I switched over to following your meal plans, everything began to fall into place. The meal plans automatically gave me the right number of servings in each food group. But they also helped teach me how to recognize a serving of vegetables, a serving of rice, and so forth. So for me, the meal plans helped me get started in the program but also learn what I needed to be doing when I stopped eating the meal plans and began cooking for myself.

ers. Just be sure to find the meal plan that's right for your calorie target number.

If you are on the line between two different calorie targets, choose the lower-calorie meal plan. For example, if our calculator indicates you should be eating 1,700 calories per day, follow the meal plan for 1,600 calories, not the one for 1,800 calories.

We all have different likes and dislikes, so we encourage you to substitute meals and snacks when planning your meals. For example, if you don't like the look of Day 7's dinner, but you love the option for Day 4, feel free to eat Day 4's dinner twice during the week. The same goes for breakfasts, lunches, and snacks. And don't feel pressured to follow these meal plans down to the very last grain of brown rice. You are far more likely to stick to a diet of foods you like, so use the plans as a guide to help you choose a menu that suits your preferences. Don't be afraid to try some of the vegetarian options if you are a meat eater, and there are plenty of meat-free options for vegetarians on the meat-eater plans.

Now you've identified the meal plan you should be eating as part of your long-term, healthy weight-loss program. Here are your next steps.

Create a Shopping List

First, look at the ingredient lists to see all you will need for your week's meals. Create a list to take with you to the store. Sunday is a good day to do grocery shopping, especially if you can set aside some time for prep work afterward.

Prepare Some of the Ingredients Ahead of Time

While you're making dinner after grocery shopping, do some food prep so your meal preparation during the week is much easier and quicker. Make it an event—put in a movie you can watch while you're preparing the recipes, or tune into that day's "Big Game." Some examples of what you might do:

- Roast a whole bunch of vegetables at one time, store them in the fridge, and then heat them up just before eating.
- Shred low-fat cheeses for recipes and store in plastic bags.
- Chop vegetables for the stir-fry and veggie pizza, and store in food storage bags in the amounts you'll use for each recipe.
- Make homemade dressing for salads.

Put Your Plan into Action

Take a few minutes in the morning to think about what you'll be having for dinner. Take anything out of the freezer that needs to be thawed. And if you think you are likely to walk in the door hungry, plan to have your afternoon snack waiting for you to munch on while you prepare your dinner.

So you see, while meal planning takes commitment, effort, and organization, with some basic information it is easily done. Most important, it takes the daily pressure off of you to come up with healthy ways to eat, because you've planned and done a lot of the work ahead of time.

Meal planning empowers you to take more control of your life. After all, sometimes it can feel like our lives are out of control—the demands of work, friends, and family can make life feel chaotic. Eating poorly can contribute to that out-of-control feeling. It can be nerve racking to resolve to manage your weight but not have a plan for what to eat. Taking control of what you eat can add structure to your life and help develop a foundation for a healthier, more balanced way of living with less anxiety.

10

Vegetarians, This Diet Is for You, Too

THE DASH DIET for Weight Loss is not a vegetarian diet, but if it weren't for vegetarians, the diet wouldn't exist.

Let me explain. Much of the evidence that prompted the original DASH research was based on vegetarians. We knew that vegetarians tended to have lower blood pressure than the average meat eater. So the DASH researchers tried to design a diet that would offer the blood pressure benefits of the vegetarian diet. But we wanted the diet to be one that the "average American" would be willing to eat, so we included a limited amount of meat. And that's how the DASH Diet was born. As I have described earlier, now we know that the DASH Diet offers far more benefits than just lowering blood pressure. And so you see, the DASH Diet and vegetarians go back a long way!

But since the carefully constructed DASH Diet for Weight Loss contains some daily servings of meat, is it possible for you to follow the program if you're a vegetarian? Absolutely, so long as you are an ovo-lacto-, ovo-, lacto-, or pesco-vegetarian. Ovo-lacto-vegetarians are the most common type of vegetarian—they do not eat meat but do consume dairy and eggs. Several years ago I developed an ovo-lacto version of the DASH Diet for Weight Loss. Not only is this a diet appropriate for those already practicing a vegetarian lifestyle, but also for any of you who would like to experiment with going meatless for a period of time to see how it suits you—try one day a week to start.

HOW TO MAKE THIS DIET VEGETARIAN

So how does it work? The key is to replace the meat/fish/poultry servings in DASH with other protein-rich foods like legumes, eggs, nuts, and seeds. You can also use products like tofu, tempeh, seitan, and texturized vegetable protein (TVP) as alternative protein sources.

MEAT ALTERNATIVES

Several plant-based products can be used as substitutes for meat in recipes. Unlike beans or nuts, these products somewhat mimic the texture and mouthfeel of meat. Some of the most common meat alternatives are:

Tofu: a versatile high-protein meat alternative made from soybeans and water. It takes on the flavors used in cooking through marinades, sauces, and spices, so it's a perfect fit in most any recipe. Tofu is also high in calcium, has no cholesterol, and is low in calories and cost. You'll find tofu in the produce section of most grocery stores and in Asian and specialty markets. Tofu comes in different textures and densities—soft tofu is best for dips and smoothies, while firm and extra firm tofu are great for slicing (sandwiches), frying (vegetable stir-fries, stews, and soups), and crumbling (filling for lasagna and casseroles and making a spreadable tofu sandwich spread).

Tempeh: a close relative of tofu, made by fermenting and partially cooking soybeans prior to pressing them into a cake-like
form. It is chock-full of protein and fiber as it contains the ac-
tual soybean plus added grains such as barley, quinoa, millet,
or brown rice. Because of the spices, fermentation, and grains
added to the soybeans, tempeh has a nutty flavor and texture. It's a great addition to a meatless meal.

TVP, short for textured vegetable protein: made from defatted
soy flour and dried to resemble flakes. You can also find TVP in
larger chunks that are great for stews. Like tofu, it is flavorless
and takes on the flavors added, such as in a stew, casserole,
tomato sauce, or chili. Not only is TVP high in protein, it has a
high fiber content, giving it a boost over meat. To use, simply
add equal parts of boiling water to the TVP to reconstitute it,
then use freely in recipes instead of meat.

Seitan. also known as "wheat meat" because it tastes so similar to meat when it's cooked. Seitan is the gluten (protein)
derived from wheat flour. Its protein content is one of the
highest among meat substitutes, and it can be used in place
of meat in most dishes. Often even meat eaters are amazed at
how closely it resembles meat.

Here is how you replace meat servings with nonmeat choices.
For 1 serving of meat, fish, or poultry you can substitute one of the
following:

- 3 whole eggs (even those of you with high cholesterol can safely
  enjoy up to 7 whole eggs per week)
- 6 egg whites
- 9 ounces firm tofu

- 3 ounces seitan
- 4 ounces tempeh
- ½ cup dry texturized vegetable protein (TVP), measured before you add water
- ½ cup cooked legumes

All of the above alternatives provide about the same amount of protein as one serving of meat/fish/poultry except for legumes, which contain only about a third of the protein of the other items on this list. These items do differ a bit in calorie content. Keep that in mind as you decide which to eat and how often (see Table 10.1).

Vegetarians eating the DASH Diet can also select high-protein items in other food groups. For example, in the "grains" category, quinoa, amaranth, oats, teff, wild rice, buckwheat, and wheat berries are excellent protein sources. Greek yogurt provides twice the protein per serving compared to regular yogurt (be sure to get the fat-free or low-fat varieties). In the DASH "vegetable" category, spinach, broccoli, and peas are the richest sources of protein. So vegetarians can find all the protein they need in several DASH food groups. We recommend that you eat a range of those foods every day. As an example, have a couple of eggs (or egg whites) for breakfast, red bean chili for lunch, and tofu

Table 10.1		
Serving size and calories for meat alternatives:		
	Size of 1 DASH serving	**Calories per serving**
Meat/fish	3 ounces	140–220
Tofu (firm)	9 ounces	180
Tempeh	4 ounces	215
TVP*	½ cup (dehydrated)	160
Whole eggs	3	210
Egg whites	6	100
Seitan	3 ounces	120
Legumes	½ cup (cooked)	110–120

* Texturized Vegetable Protein

or seitan in a stir-fry at night instead of relying on just one of these products for your protein source.

Don't forget that, if you are replacing meat with legumes, you should still consume your assigned DASH servings of nuts/seeds/legumes as well.

What about if you are a vegan? Vegans eat no meat, fish, poultry, dairy, eggs, or honey. If you apply the general principles of the DASH Diet for Weight Loss to your vegan eating plan, you will probably lose weight, since vegan foods tend to be lower in overall fat and calories. But a vegan version of the DASH Diet has never been tested, so I cannot promise you that you will experience all the same health benefits.

VEGETARIAN MEAL PLANS

The DASH Diet for Weight Loss offers vegetarian meal plans to help you develop a meat-free way of eating that is balanced and filled with a variety of delicious, low-calorie choices. We have created vegetarian meal plans for every calorie target, and that means there's a vegetarian meal plan for you. The Vegetarian Meal Plans are Section II in Part 3.

Meal planning may be especially helpful if you're new to vegetarian eating. It will help you plan meals and shop for items you may not be used to searching for. For more on meal planning, refer to Chapter 9.

WHY VEGETARIANS ARE LESS LIKELY TO BE OVERWEIGHT OR OBESE

A well-balanced vegetarian diet is rich in vegetables, fruit, whole grains, and legumes and low in fat. The main meals are comprised largely of bean or soy dishes, vegetables, and whole grains.

It's true that meat—and red meat in particular—contains much more high-calorie saturated fat than a lot of other foods. However, it's not *just* because they don't eat meat that vegetarians are less likely to be overweight or obese. People who have chosen a vegetarian diet tend to pay attention to other areas of their health. They often exercise more and don't smoke. Just as important, if they have been practicing a vegetarian diet for some time, they will have developed skills and knowledge about how to eat a vegetarian diet that is both meat-free *and* lower in calories than the regular American diet.

AVOIDING POTENTIAL PITFALLS OF SWITCHING TO VEGETARIANISM

Simply eliminating meat from your diet won't make you lose weight. It comes as a surprise to many people that a poor vegetarian diet can actually be higher in calories than one with meat in it. So if you are a vegetarian trying to lose weight, or are thinking of becoming a vegetarian—or even if you are a "flexitarian" (switching back and forth between a meat-free diet and one with meat in it)—pay attention to the potential pitfalls of such a lifestyle. Learning to eat meat-free and low-calorie are separate skills that need to be mastered.

People who switch to a vegetarian diet without the right preparation or knowledge run the same risks as others who try to lose weight through other diets. These include eating a diet even higher in calories and fat than the one they were eating before, while even lower in essential nutrition. That's because if you're new to vegetarianism, you may not know how to cook and shop for healthy, low-calorie meat-free dishes, or how to order when eating out.

Even the lead dietitian in my weight-loss and health program fell into this trap when she became a vegetarian. All she did was omit the meat from her eating plan. That got boring and limiting, so she started making high-fat, cheese-filled casseroles to make her diet more satisfying and to ensure she got enough protein in her diet. Bad move! When her cholesterol rose 30 points, she got serious about learning how to choose a balanced diet made up of appropriate foods.

And let's face it, America is not very vegetarian-friendly, and Americans in general tend to be unadventurous eaters. Many who give up meat simply revert to eating a diet that is virtually the same as the one they were eating before—just without the meat. Cheesy pizza and casseroles, bowls of pasta with heavy sauces, plates of mashed potatoes and gravy and french fries—these are all readily available vegetarian options that we are familiar with and know how to prepare and order when eating out. They are also high in saturated fat and calories.

Then there is the tendency to want to replace the satisfaction we got from eating the meat on our plate with fatty alternatives such as cheese and cream. Plus many of us think that if we're not eating a meal with meat in it, we get a free pass to eat larger portions.

These tendencies are compounded by the fact that Americans tend to be quite fussy eaters. There's a theory that because we are such a wealthy culture where food is so cheap, we haven't had to experiment with less-expensive "weird" foods. So even when someone takes the big step of "going vegetarian," they may not be willing to try foods such as tofu, TVP, tempeh, or even soy milk, which are staples of delicious, low-calorie vegetarian meals around the world.

Here are some additional recommendations on how to avoid pitfalls when eating a vegetarian diet.

BE ADVENTUROUS

Eating a vegetarian diet presents a wonderful opportunity to try foods you may not have thought about eating. Tofu gets an undeservedly bad rap from people who don't know how to cook it, and there are plenty of ways to enjoy this low-calorie, highly nutritious food. There may be common vegetables that are not at the top of your list of favorite foods, but you can rediscover these as you begin your journey into this way of eating. Sautéed spinach with garlic and a bit of olive oil adds punch to your plate. Roasted Brussels sprouts and butternut squash or sweet potatoes make a dynamic duo. Try making healthy stir-fry dishes, curries served over brown rice, and veggie and low-fat bean burritos with mushrooms and soy cheese. You are limited only by your sense of adventure.

PRACTICE PERFECT PORTION CONTROL

Even if you're eating meat-free, portion control is key to weight loss. People sometimes have a tendency to eat too much of something when they know it's healthy and relatively low in calories. Remember that all food has calories and that just because a meal is vegetarian doesn't mean you are free to overindulge. Keep an eye on portion sizes and try not to interpret eating meat-free as a free-for-all.

GO EASY ON THE CHEESE

Cheese is one of the main sources of calories and saturated fat in the American diet. Just think about it—we put parmesan cheese on pasta already floating in creamy cheese sauces and atop lettuces adorned with fat-laden salad dressing! A pizza chain introduced a pizza that has cheese stuffed into the crust! Many people switching to meat-free diets overdo their cheese intake. Cheese is a dense source of calories—a little of it contains a lot. Make sure you stay within your DASH limits on your cheese intake, and wherever possible, opt for low-fat or nonfat choices.

EXERCISE SALAD BAR SENSE

Salad is one of the most widely available choices for vegetarians—it's an easy go-to when eating out or traveling. You can find a well-stocked salad bar in many grocery stores and restaurants, and if you make the right selections, you can assemble a meat-free meal that is also low in fat and calories. However, there are calorie minefields in a salad bar, and choosing unwisely can mean you end up eating a meal that's even higher in calories than the one you might have eaten with meat in it.

Here are some navigation tips for when you're next at a salad bar:

- Start by piling your plate with "green" food. Watercress, arugula, romaine lettuce, kale, and spinach are excellent sources of calcium, iron, and vitamins C and A.
- Move on to the other vegetables and legumes. Pile on colorful veggies like tomatoes, cucumbers, jicama, beans and peas (kidney beans and chickpeas are favorites at the salad bar), cabbage,

bell peppers, broccoli, cauliflower, corn, beets, artichoke hearts (not oil-packed), hearts of palm, carrots, and more. Add color, flavor, fiber, and texture with minimal calories. Avoid vegetables drenched in oil or creamy sauces.

- Watch out for the pots of creamy, calorie-laden stuff, such as pasta and potato salads, egg salad, coleslaw, and just about anything that is creamy and white. Foods that are white are usually blended with high-calorie cream cheese, sour cream, or mayonnaise.

- Steer clear of crunchy extras at the end of the line! Croutons, chow mein noodles, crispy wonton strips, banana chips, sunflower seeds, and sugar-coated raisins or cranberries. Two to four tablespoons of just one "crunchy" food can add 40 to 100 calories. A sprinkle of cheese, a handful of croutons, and a spoonful of raisins and sunflower seeds may seem virtually harmless, but that innocent salad is now a diet disaster packed with too many calories. While dried fruit and sunflower seeds are healthy, for weight loss use them in small and limited amounts.

- Grains are an important part of the DASH Diet, but the breads offered at the salad bar usually aren't the whole-grain varieties that DASH recommends. Cornbread is common, but one little cornbread square with a pat of butter adds over 200 calories to your "healthy" salad. Since cornbread is made from a whole grain (corn) and is already high in fat, skip the added pat of butter. Your best bet is the whole-grain pita; dip it in your fat-free salad dressing! Also avoid the croutons that are typically drenched in fat and pack up to 100 calories in a half-cup.

- Most salad bars now feature many choices of flavorful low-calorie salad dressings. Try a variety of vinegar flavors without the oil. Raspberry, balsamic, rice, champagne, fruit, sherry, or white wine vinegar can add a splash of flavor to any vegetable, fruit, or pasta salad. Even creamy salad dressings now come in low-calorie versions. Instead of putting dressing on top of your salad, leave it on the side and dip your vegetables or fork into it. You'd be amazed at how much less dressing you eat that way.

Worried that cutting meat out of your diet will narrow your choices? It's quite the contrary. You can use a vegetarian meal plan to practice weight management *and* expand your nutritional horizons. Your world will open up with variety and taste. If you are already a vegetarian, you have a head start on healthy eating, and with the reminders in this chapter, are even better positioned to make the most of your considered nutrition decision.

How Much You Move

EARLY IN THE BOOK, we discussed how weight management works—the balance between calories in (how much you eat) and calories out (how many calories you burn through activity). And to lose weight, you need to reduce calories in or increase calories out or, better yet, do both. In the last section, we talked about reducing calories in. The eating plan I've shown you decreases your daily *calories in* by 500 calories, which will cause you to lose 1 pound per week. We talked about the right number of DASH servings for you and how to select the Hi-Lo-Slo foods in the DASH food groups that are particularly valuable for weight loss.

Now we are turning to *calories out*. How can you increase your activity to maximize your weight loss?

THE IMPORTANCE OF EXERCISE

Increasing how much physical activity you do is an extremely important part of any weight-loss program. It is important for a number of health reasons. Physical activity:

Burns calories: I just explained this but it bears repeating: Physical activity is fundamental to the DASH Diet for Weight Loss because it burns calories.

Boosts metabolism: The more muscle on our bodies, the faster our metabolism and the more calories we burn. As we get older, we naturally start to lose muscle mass, which causes our metabolism to slow down. A vicious cycle occurs: The less muscle we have, the slower our metabolism is, and the slower our metabolism, the more likely it is that we'll gain weight. Physical activity is the key to breaking this cycle. Regular physical activity means you build muscle, which in turn means your metabolism will speed up. The beauty of this is that more muscle speeds up our metabolism even when we are at rest, not just when we're working out.

Increases strength: It is important to maintain muscle strength. Even if we don't need strength to do a lot of heavy work, having strong muscles allows us to do even routine daily activities more easily. It also helps us avoid injuries.

IMPROVED FITNESS MEANS BETTER HEALTH

Being physically fit is good for you. Most of us know that. Sometimes it's surprising to learn just *how* good it is for us. Exercise is so powerful that people who start exercising improve their health *even if they don't lose any weight.* Exercise:

- reduces risk of heart disease and stroke;
- reduces risk of developing diabetes;
- reduces risk of some types of cancer;
- improves sexual function;
- increases your chance of living longer;
- improves your mood.

|||||||||||||||||||||||||||||||

DASH FAQ

**Any ideas for squeezing exercise
into my crazy schedule?**

**Please see the answer to FAQ 9 in Section V,
Frequently Asked Questions.**

The effect of exercise on mood deserves special mention. Most of us know the feeling of well-being we experience after we are physically active. Scientists are learning just how powerfully exercise affects our minds. A recent study demonstrated that people who did as little as twenty minutes of physical activity a week reported less psychological distress than folks who did no exercise at all. Those who participated in sports or exercised every day had even better mental health. The kinds of activities reported by participants were wide ranging and included sports, walking, vigorous housework, and yard work. I think this mood effect of exercise is especially important for people who are trying to lose weight. Staying positive and feeling good about yourself are so important in keeping you motivated on your diet. So exercise really offers powerful benefits for a weight loser.

All signs point to you becoming more active! So how to get started?

11

Walking Your Way
to Weight Loss

IF YOU AREN'T exercising now, you're not alone—fewer than 16 percent of Americans exercise every day. That being the case, it's probably a good idea to start slowly to avoid getting discouraged and to prevent injury. If you have medical conditions that exercise might aggravate, such as heart trouble or arthritis, you might want to talk to your doctor before starting an exercise program. The advice we give here is generally safe, but your doctor, who knows the details of your medical condition, is the best source of advice for you.

For people who haven't exercised for some time, or who are very overweight, I generally recommend starting with a walking program. Walking is a terrific calorie-burning activity because

- It doesn't require any special equipment.
- It doesn't cost anything.
- You can do it almost anywhere!

These are three different walking programs depending on your fitness level.

Beginner's Walking Program			
Follow this if you are elderly, very overweight, or very out of shape.			
Week	How far? (miles)	How long? (minutes)	How often? (# times/week)
1	¼	10–15	2–3
2	½	12–15	2–3
3–4	¾–1	20–25	3
5–6	1–1½	20–30	3–4
7–8	1½–2	27–36	3–4
9–10	2–2½	35–44	4
11–12	2½–3	43–51	4
13–14	2½–3	40–48	4
15+	3–3½	48–56	4–5

Moderate-Intensity Walking Program			
Follow this if you are somewhat fit.			
Week	How far? (miles)	How long? (minutes)	How often? (# times/week)
1	½–1	8–15	2–3
2	1½	23	2–3
3–4	1½–2	21–26	3
5–6	2–2½	29–39	3–4
7–8	2½–3	35–42	3–4
9–10	2½–3	34–41	3–4
11–12	2½–3	33–39	4
13–14	3–3½	39–46	4–5
15+	3½–4	46–52	4–5

(continued on next page)

Advanced Walking Program			
Follow this if you are regularly active.			
Week	How far? (miles)	How long? (minutes)	How often? (# times/week)
1	½–1	6–12	2–3
2	1½	18	2–3
3–4	1½–2	18–24	3
5–6	2–2½	24–30	3–4
7–8	2½–3	30–36	3–4
9–10	3–3½	36–42	3–4
11–12	3–3½	33–40	4
13–14	3½–4	42–48	4–5
15+	3½–4	40–44	4–5

WORDS TO THE WISE WALKER

If the shoes don't fit, you're gonna quit. Buy a good pair of shoes that fit right. Several companies now make shoes designed specially for walking, though a good pair of running sneakers or cross trainers should work just fine. Don't go out on a long walk in your new shoes right away. Wear them around the house for a day or so to break them in. Good socks are also a must to prevent blisters.

Dress for success. If you're planning to dress for very cold weather, be sure it is easy for you to remove an item or two as you warm up.

Know where you're going. You don't have to walk the same route every time, but be familiar with where you're going to be going on any given day. Will it be the high school track? A municipal bike/walking path? Local woodlands? Scout out some good sites.

Make a date and go steady. Mark your walking days and times on your home calendar and stick to them. Remember that your walking program is a priority.

Have a contingency plan. If the weather is bad, make sure you have a backup plan. One idea is to do several laps around the local mall. Look into whether there is a mall-walking program near where you live.

Get a friend involved. You are more likely to stick with an exercise program if you don't want to let someone down. Find a friend who also wants to make exercise a part of his or her life. Plus, walking is a great way to get away from the distractions of home, and talking while walking is a great way to socialize!

Ease in. Don't try to start too fast. If you overdo it, you're more likely to quit. Follow the schedules in the programs above.

Keep track. Record your walking excursions on your Food and Exercise Log, or keep a monthly walking diary.

Table 11.1			
Heavier people burn more calories as they walk.			
Walking faster also burns more calories per mile.			
Calories burned per 1 mile at:	Weight		
	150 pounds	200 pounds	250 pounds
3 mph	75	100	125
4 mph	85	115	140
6 mph (jog)	115	150	190

Walking for exercise is a great "step" toward burning extra calories. How many calories are you burning? It depends on how much you weigh; it takes more energy to move more weight.

You burn a few more calories per mile if you walk faster, but the main advantage of walking faster is that you cover more distance in whatever time you have. For example, let's say the 200-pounder in the table above goes out for a one-hour walk. At three miles per hour, she walks three miles and burns 300 calories. At four miles per hour, she walks four miles and burns 460 calories.

12

Ramping Up Your Fitness Program

THERE ARE MANY fitness activities that will help you burn those extra calories. Walking is just one of them. There's also aerobic dance, cardio machines, yoga, strength training with weights, Rollerblading, biking, and many more. When you are ready to move beyond walking or you just want to add a new activity for variety, there are lots to choose from.

First decide whether you want to do your exercising at home or in a gym. If at home, you will need some equipment. For strength training, you will need some weights (such as dumbbells) or some elastic bands to create resistance that you work against. These are mostly useful for exercising your arms, shoulders, and chest. There are a number of leg exercises that you can do without fancy equipment. For example, put your back against a wall and bend your knees till you are in a sitting position (but without a chair). You'll definitely feel the strain in your thigh muscles.

The other main muscle group to exercise is your core, the muscles of your abdomen, sides, and back. There are many exercises for your core that you can do with an inflatable exercise ball. If you want to do more cardiovascular exercise, there are exercise videos you can work out to. Or purchase a piece of cardio equipment such as a stationary bike, treadmill, or elliptical trainer.

If you prefer to work out at a gym, you can take advantage of their equipment. And organized classes, such as aerobics or bike spinning, can be a great workout and fun, too. The other advantage of a gym is that you can take a lesson or two from a personal trainer. A good trainer can assess your current fitness, listen to your goals, and give you a workout program that fits your situation. Even if you want to do most of your work at home, it could be a good idea to get started with some personal trainer sessions.

Here are some tips to help you make exercise a habit.

- Choose an activity you enjoy.
- Tailor your program to your own fitness level.
- Set realistic goals.
- Give your body a chance to adjust to your new routine.
- Don't get discouraged if you don't see immediate results.
- Find a partner for a little motivation and socialization.
- Build some rest days into your exercise schedule.
- Listen to your body. Don't overdo it.
- Try to do something every day; a little bit of exercise is better than none at all.

STRENGTH TRAINING

In discussing exercise for weight loss, we have usually advised that the best way to burn calories is to engage in cardiovascular exercise—the kind of exercise that gets your heart and lungs pumping and burns a lot of calories while you're doing it. More recently, we've included strength training as an aid to weight loss. It's true: Strength training with weights benefits people trying to lose weight for a couple of very important reasons.

First, the more muscular you are, the more efficient your body is at burning calories. I described this earlier when explaining the relationship between body muscle and metabolism. Even just sitting there at your desk, you burn more calories if you are more muscular. Second, being stronger makes it easier to do your cardiovascular exercise and even the types of tasks you encounter in daily life. You will have more energy, won't get tired so easily, and will be less prone to injury.

A full discussion of strength training is beyond what we can do in this book, but here are a couple of suggestions on how to start a strength training program.

Where to Begin

Start by deciding where you are most comfortable—at a gym or working out at home. While a local fitness center or gym can offer the biggest variety of equipment, many people cannot afford to join a fitness center or don't feel comfortable exercising in public.

How Often Should I Strength-Train?

It only takes twenty-five to thirty minutes of strength training two or three times a week to get results. The workouts should be spaced two or three days apart to allow your body sufficient rest. Do your aerobic

---

‖‖‖‖‖‖‖‖‖‖‖‖‖‖‖‖‖‖‖‖‖‖‖‖‖‖‖

DASH FAQ

Won't exercising make me even hungrier and by doing so, make me eat more than I should?

Please see the answer to FAQ 10 in Section V, Frequently Asked Questions.

work on the days you don't do strength training. It is important to be consistent with workouts, so schedule them into your daily routine.

Reps and Sets

Rep is short for "repetition"—the number of times you make a particular motion, such as lifting a dumbbell over your head or doing a sit-up. A *set* is a series of reps—the number of reps you do before your muscles fatigue and you take a break. One set could be five, ten, or twelve repetitions. A good way to start is to pick the amount of weight that allows you to perform two or three sets of twelve to fifteen reps for each exercise. When in doubt, use less weight and do more reps.

Obviously, when you are performing fewer reps, you'll have to increase your weight in order to stress the muscles enough to continue to strengthen them. When you go back to the higher reps, you'll have to decrease your weight a bit. You may find you are lifting more than you previously did.

Stretching

Stretching the muscle you've just worked after you complete each set ensures suppleness with your strength. Doing a complete total body stretch at the end of every strength-training session assists in injury prevention and increases flexibility.

13

Increasing Lifestyle Exercise

LIFESTYLE EXERCISE is the physical activity you perform in the normal course of a day. Common forms of lifestyle exercise include household chores, yard work, walking or biking to work or public transportation, playing with the kids, and almost anything that involves moving more than you would if you were sitting on the couch watching television.

A major study published in the *Journal of the American Medical Association* proved that lifestyle exercise was as effective as a structured workout program at helping participants improve their heart health, lower their blood pressure, and lose weight. The report stated that you only need to do thirty minutes of lifestyle exercise a day to receive these important health benefits—and you can break this up into three ten-minute blocks of time.

The problem is that many people avoid lifestyle exercise. Either they take advantage of modern technology to do the work for them or they simply choose to not do anything at all. If that's you and you want to lose weight, now is the time to change.

Here are some ways to increase how much lifestyle exercise you get.

AT WORK

- Hold a meeting with a colleague during a short walk instead of in an office or conference room.
- Stand and stretch instead of staying seated while talking on the phone.
- Walk to a colleague's office instead of calling them or sending an e-mail.
- Take a walk at lunchtime.
- Get off the bus or subway a couple of stops before you get to work or home and walk the remaining distance.
- Walk around the terminal while waiting for a flight to leave when traveling.
- With time to spare on a business trip, explore an unfamiliar city on foot or take advantage of your hotel gym.

AT HOME

- Do household chores yourself instead of hiring someone to do them.
- Do your own yard work: rake leaves, weed, pick up trash, clear brush, and mow grass (with a push-mower, not a ride-on model!).
- Take frequent walks to get your muscles moving. Consider a ten-minute walk after breakfast or before dinner, and take longer walks twice a day on weekends.
- Ride a bike to the local convenience store when you run out of a single household item.
- Walk your dog frequently and take him/her to the park to play.
- When you go to the supermarket, leave your car at the far end of the parking lot, then carry your groceries back to the car if you can.

Your ultimate goal is to move more. Unless you're swimming or biking, this means taking more steps as you progress through your day. If you are a person who is motivated by being able to beat your own personal best, a great way to keep track of how much you walk every day is with a pedometer. Pedometers are relatively inexpensive (you can get a good one for under $30), easy to use (just clip it to your belt, pants, or skirt), and give pretty accurate recordings of the number of steps you take. Experts agree that to be healthy we need to take about 10,000 steps a day, whereas most Americans take about 3,000 steps a day.

INTRODUCING THE (ROUGHLY) 100-CALORIE WORKOUT

It's easy to burn an extra 100 calories. I have developed seven workouts to help you do just this. Most of these workouts require no fancy equipment and you don't have to go to the gym to do them. You can make them part of your daily life. In many cases, you don't even have to change clothes—a different pair of shoes is usually all you need. (These calorie estimates are for a 150-pound person.)

Walk for 15 minutes: Instead of driving everywhere, make a point of walking. If you walk briskly, you can cover a mile in fifteen minutes. Walk to public transportation. Park on the far side of the lot at work, the grocery store, or mall. Walk after lunch at work. You don't have to do it all at once. By the end of the day, if you've walked a mile, you've burned 100 calories!

Climb stairs for 10 minutes: Always try to take the stairs at work instead of the elevator. At lunchtime, you can use the stairs like a gym. Get a 10-minute workout by going up and down. You can ramp up the effort by increasing your pace or by carrying a backpack filled with books.

(continued on next page)

Go dancing for 20 minutes: You don't have to go clubbing until the wee hours to dance (although, why not?); you can do it in your living room or kitchen while you're at home. If your significant other or kids want to join in, even better. If not, it's their loss! (Unfortunately, the razzing you'll get for this does not burn any calories.)

Do yard work for 20 minutes: Why pay someone else to do things in the yard when you can do them yourself—and get a workout while you're doing it! Raking, clearing brush, and small projects that involve digging can be a great workout. Less intensive activities such as planting flowers and edging flowerbeds also burn calories.

Cycle for 10 minutes: If you can, bike to work. Otherwise, get a bike rack for your car and take your bike to work for a brisk lunchtime ride. If none of this is convenient, make a point of taking a ten-minute ride at about 15 miles per hour before you head out the door for work, or when you get home. (Using a stationary bike for ten minutes gives about the same workout.)

Do housework for 20 minutes: The same principle applies to housework as it does to yard work—channel your inner cheapskate! Vacuuming, mopping, and scrubbing are all good ways to burn calories.

Jump rope for 10 minutes: A jump rope is a handy and portable item you can keep at home or bring to work with you. Get it out during your lunch break at work to jump rope for ten minutes and you'll feel your heart going and your lungs pumping in no time. At home, jump rope while watching TV instead of sitting on the couch.

Sure, it's easier to be inactive, and that explains why so many of us are overweight and suffering from inactivity-related conditions, many of them life threatening. But by making small adjustments to your daily schedule and doing short workouts, you can change—and prolong—your life. It's not always easy to find the time to do any of these things. In fact, it's a lot easier to find excuses not to do them. But if you make the effort to try a couple of these, you will be amazed at how much better you will feel—and how much better you will look.

"WHAT'S THE PERFECT EXERCISE FOR ME?"

I hear this question a lot. Out of all the different kinds of exercise out there, from lifestyle exercise to working out at the gym to yoga classes to competing at sports to long-distance running, there is definitely one that's the best for you. It's *any exercise you will do regularly!*

That's right: Any exercise you do consistently is a "perfect" form of exercise. That's because most people simply don't exercise enough, and unless your job involves vigorous physical activity, chances are you don't either. Studies tell us only one in five Americans exercises regularly. So it doesn't matter whether you play mixed doubles tennis, do tai chi, or walk with a work colleague at lunchtime five times a week; so long as you're doing more exercise than you were, then you're doing right by the DASH Diet for Weight Loss.

So if your principle for selecting food is Hi-Lo-Slo, your guideline for exercise should be, "Just go, go, *go!*"

Building Your Skillpower

LOSING WEIGHT on the DASH Diet for Weight Loss is simple to understand. That doesn't mean it's going to be *easy to do*. It's not easy to change habits. And eating habits are some of the most deeply ingrained habits we have. To change these habits will take practice and perseverance.

After all, temptations and triggers are everywhere. What about if your spouse or kids insist on having donuts in the house? When the local fast-food restaurant on the way home from work seems a much more attractive alternative than going to the gym? Or when you sit down on the couch with a quart of ice cream because you are bored or stressed out?

In the face of all the challenges before you, how is it possible to maintain your commitment and adhere to the program?

Willpower isn't enough. What is needed to bridge the gap between knowledge and results is what I call skillpower. Skillpower is part inspiration, part perspiration—a combination of practical knowledge and self-motivation.

Over the past decade, countless people who are using the DASH Diet to lose weight have told me what works and what doesn't. Their feedback is built into this section.

14

Create Realistic Goals
You Can Reach

ONE OF THE KEYS to achieving your weight-management objectives is effective goal setting. If you are reading this book, your goal is weight loss and maintaining that lower weight. Let's focus, then, on the behaviors, efforts, and actions that will ultimately help you reach and stick to these weight-management goals. All too often we give short shrift to this process. Setting unrealistic, unreachable goals leads to failure and discouragement. But setting realistic, achievable goals leads to success. So it's worth spending a minute to explain what we mean by effective goal setting.

I recommend a goal-setting strategy that is SMART:

Specific,
Measurable,
Action-oriented,
Realistic, and
Timed

We know that goals with these attributes are more likely to be achieved.

Here's a goal that's not SMART: "I'm never going to eat chocolate again for the rest of my life." It's not realistic, not specific, not a very real time frame (the rest of your life?!), and not action-oriented (it says what you are not going to do, not what you *will* do). Or, "I'm going to go to the gym every day." Not realistic and not timed.

Let's look at a goal that is SMART: "In the next week, I will go for a twenty-minute walk at lunchtime four times."

> *Specific:* Walk, not something general like "get more exercise." At lunchtime.
> *Measurable:* Twenty minutes. Four times. Both measurable.
> *Action-oriented:* It says what you will do, not what you won't, or what you'll stop.
> *Realistic:* The length of the walk and the frequency are realistic.
> *Timed:* This commitment will last for one week.

How about one that's eating-related? Let's say you want to stop eating ice cream after dinner. "I will set up a snack of three cups of air-popped popcorn sprinkled with cinnamon sugar. Then tonight, when I get those ice cream cravings, I will enjoy that snack instead."

> *Specific:* Prepare the snack. Eat it instead of ice cream.
> *Measurable:* You'll know by the end of the night if you've succeeded.
> *Action-oriented:* It says what you will do (prepare and eat the snack), not just that you will not eat the ice cream.
> *Realistic:* It's just one night. Sometimes that's a good way to start. The popcorn is a sweet alternative to the sweet ice cream, so it is a more realistic swap than, say, carrot sticks.
> *Timed:* One night.

THE IMPORTANCE OF "REALISTIC"

Sometimes the thought of making a change can seem overwhelming. "I'll never be able to do this," we sometimes think to ourselves. That's why it helps to make our goals more manageable. If you know you have to follow your resolution only for today, then it will feel more doable. And when you wake up tomorrow, all you have to worry about is getting through another day. That's why "one day at a time" is a useful time frame for behavior change, and has become the catchphrase for many twelve-step programs. At times, even though we set SMART goals, trying to make more than a couple of changes at a time is overwhelming. Back up, pick one or two areas you can make significant change in, and achieve some success with those. Don't reach for an overwhelming number of goals all at once.

An important note: "One day at a time" doesn't mean not planning ahead. One of the key components of making successful change is to plan ahead. For example, make sure you have healthy foods available to help you meet your DASH goals, or make plans to meet an exercise partner.

REWARD YOURSELF

Give yourself a reward when you reach a goal. For example, if your goal was to eat the popcorn instead of ice cream—and you did—get yourself something you've been wanting (except ice cream; make the reward unrelated to food). You can even build the reward into the goal. "If I walk at lunch four days this week, I'm going to splurge for that manicure [or golf shoes]." It's important to celebrate your successes the same way you celebrate the accomplishments of others.

A SETBACK DOESN'T MEAN ALL IS LOST

If you fail to accomplish your goals, it doesn't mean you're a failure. You are not back to square one. The knowledge you have gained has

IMPORTANT PRINCIPLES OF AN EFFECTIVE REWARD SYSTEM

- Reward behavior, not outcome. Reward yourself for behavior changes that are likely to lead to weight loss. Do not reward yourself for how much weight you lose.
- The reward must be valuable to you, no matter what anyone else thinks.
- Reward yourself immediately, or as soon as possible after, the desired behavior occurs. Delaying the reward reduces its effectiveness as a behavior modifier.
- The reward must come after the behavior, not in anticipation of it.
- Never give yourself the reward if you didn't earn it.
- Each time you earn a reward, take the time to congratulate yourself.

not evaporated into the atmosphere. It is yours and you can choose to reapply it. No one can take away what you have learned!

It would be great if you could completely change your eating and exercise patterns and never experience a setback again in your life. This is unrealistic. Relapses are normal. You should be happy with "three steps forward, one step back" progress. Make gradual improvements so that sometime in the not-so-distant future, you will have adopted enough healthy behaviors—and perhaps shed enough unhealthy ones!—so that you can be proud and satisfied with your success. But the real success is to maintain those patterns for life.

GOAL-SETTING EXERCISE

Like any other skill, goal setting needs to be learned. It is not easy to set a really good goal. It requires practice to be successful. Try it out now. Refer to your Personal DASH In Action Plan to start working on goal setting for your weight-management efforts.

Personal DASH In Action Plan

Now is the time to get into action and plan ahead. Use this form anytime you're setting new goals. First, pick one behavior you'd like to change. Now set a goal that addresses it. Remember to focus on your behavior and on a short-term goal. When phrasing your goal, use the words "I will . . ." It's more powerful!

You can set these goals for exercise, to improve your diet, or for behaviors such as making food-tracking records.

For my short-term goal, *I WILL*

_____

_____

_____

_____

Remember, your goal should be specific, measurable, action-oriented, realistic, and timed.

15

Use Your Tools

I PROVIDE A VARIETY of tools for you in this book. These tools have been tried and tested over the last decade by the many thousands of members of my weight-loss and health program and have been found to be extremely useful.

Your most effective tool is the Food and Exercise Log located in Chapter 8. Keeping a log helps in a couple of ways: It is a good motivation tool that makes you feel more accountable for your actions, and putting everything down in black and white reinforces your efforts. Reinforcing your record keeping with a tool such as a pedometer to track your physical activity can enhance your self-monitoring efforts.

When you are trying to manage your weight, it really helps to keep track of more than just the raw numbers; you should pay attention to such issues as *when* and *why* you eat foods that compromise your efforts to manage your weight. You can do this by adding comments to the Notes column on your Food and Exercise Log and review it at the end of every day to see if there are any undesirable patterns that you could try to break. You can find the Food and Exercise Log in Chap-

---

DASH FAQ

What are the advantages of using a pedometer?

**Please see the answer to FAQ 11 in Section V,
Frequently Asked Questions.**

---

ter 8, or you can download it from my website at: www.dashforhealth
.com/foodlog.php.

The DASH Diet for Weight Loss meal plans are tools, too. You can find these in Part 3. The meal plan is an effective tool for weight loss for several reasons:

- You don't have to decide everything you will eat in a day. The meal plan does that for you.
- It teaches you about food groups and serving sizes.
- It enables you to plan ahead for healthy, Hi-Lo-Slo meals.
- You avoid the "same old thing" at the dinner table.
- It includes healthy recipes.
- It helps you eat out less.
- It includes a variety of meals.

Of course, to get the most out of your tools you have to take them out of the toolbox. Use them—they're yours.

16

Employ Visualization Techniques

IF YOU HAVE TRIED to lose weight many times before and not succeeded, then you are like millions of Americans before you, and you may feel success is beyond your grasp. But I know you *can* learn and change. To literally believe you can succeed, you can use "visualization techniques" as part of your DASH Diet for Weight Loss program.

Visualization is the process of holding and concentrating on an image in your head of how you want something to be. In doing so, it becomes a reality.

To visualize eating lower-calorie foods, hold a picture in your mind of a "healthy you," one slimmer and in prime physical condition, eating lots of Hi-Lo-Slo foods and feeling more vibrant and dynamic. The clearer and more vivid your image, the better. If you have a picture of yourself when you were at a healthier and more desirable weight, use that to establish your visualization.

People who practice visualization techniques find that after not too long, they will move closer to their weight-loss and health goals. Over time, exercise becomes more appealing, and high-calorie, fatty, and salty foods will be less tempting.

Visualization *works*. The more you imagine something as a reality, the more likely you will behave in ways that match that reality. Its more enthusiastic proponents are professional athletes. With millions and millions of dollars riding on pro sports, athletes wouldn't be doing it if it wasn't effective!

Why does visualization work? No one quite knows. But like prayer,

THREE VISUALIZATION EXERCISES TO LOSE WEIGHT AND GET HEALTHIER

Exercise One: Positive Imagery

Start by getting in the right frame of mind to begin your visualization session.

- Sit quietly and comfortably.
- Start breathing deeply.
- Close your eyes. Keep them closed during your visualization. Keep your belly relaxed. Let the relaxation spread from your belly into your legs and upper body.

Visualize yourself standing in front of a full-length mirror, a noticeably slimmer you looking back. Picture yourself stepping into the mirror, becoming one with that image, and actually transforming into that slimmer you. Feel yourself slimmer, your clothes hanging more loosely from your body.

Exercise Two: Affirmation

Start by using the relaxation technique in Exercise One.

Now imagine this scene:

I am walking on the beach, feeling slim and attractive. I feel the sun on my skin and smell the ocean air. It feels fantastic to be so healthy and full of energy thanks to how slim I am. I hear the sound of the waves and the seagulls overhead. People are looking at me and commenting on how slim and healthy I look. It feels great to be alive and to be enjoying the gift of this slimmer, healthier body. I am more confident, healthy, and serene.

Whenever you sit down to eat, take a couple of minutes to go through Exercise One or Two. Either will help reinforce your desire and commitment to eat in a healthier way.

Exercise Three: Fight a Craving

Again, start by using the relaxation technique in Exercise One.

Imagine a situation in which you are vulnerable to overeating or craving a food that doesn't fit with your nutrition goals. For example, you are at home alone with a tub of ice cream left over from a party. Imagine opening the container, looking at the ice cream, and smelling it. Let the craving develop, and don't fight it. Now visualize stuffing the tub of ice cream into the trash. Or visualize yourself putting it away, out of sight. Doing this will make it more likely you will follow this course of action the next time such a situation arises.

If you have a problem resisting cravings, practice this visualization three times a day for a few minutes each time.

meditation, and hypnosis, it seems visualization works by sending a message to the subconscious. The mind is a powerful thing!

Once you have developed a clear vision of your healthy self, you need to tell yourself that this is the healthy person you are *now, today*! You need to phrase your visualizations in the present. Say *I am,* not

I will (after all, haven't you been saying *I will* for years?), because the subconscious mind understands the present better than anything. The more you visualize your goal and repeat your affirmation—preferably out loud—the more likely you will succeed.

By practicing visualization, obstacles in the way of your weight-loss goals become a lot easier to overcome. You have a clear picture in your mind about what you want and how to achieve it. In this way, you will truly believe you can succeed.

17

Practice Conscious Eating

CONSCIOUS EATING is being aware of *what* you're eating and *why* you're eating, and not eating any more when you're full. Practicing conscious eating is a key to weight loss.

Trouble is, most of us tend to eat unconsciously. We eat while we work, drive, walk, talk, make shopping lists, watch TV, read, and do other assorted activities. When was the last time you just *ate,* paying attention to the experience of actually tasting the food?

Conscious eating helps you in several ways. First of all, it is an opportunity to relax for one of the few times in our busy lives. And if you are trying to lose weight, conscious eating helps you slow down the pace at which you eat. This is an added dimension to the Slo component of my recommendation to eat Hi-Lo-Slo foods. In addition to choosing foods that are slow to eat, it's important that you take it upon yourself to *eat more slowly.*

Many people who struggle with their weight eat too fast. As a result, they overeat before the fullness signal in their brains is triggered, which takes about fifteen minutes. We all know the feeling of wolfing down a meal and feeling stuffed because we just ate much more than

CONSCIOUS EATING HELPS MARRIAGE

Another message from T.T.—

Dear Dr. Moore,
I had gotten into the habit of watching the news while munching on a bag of potato chips every evening as my wife got dinner ready. I remember when you first talked about "conscious eating," I said to myself, "Huh? Potato chips have taste?" I realized that I was eating the chips and never really paying attention. That motivated me to pay more attention to what I was eating. My wife began putting my napkin on top of my dinner plate as a reminder for me to really pay attention to what I was eating. It took a full month for me to really develop conscious eating as a "habit." Now I do it regularly. It has really helped me enjoy my food more but also understand when I have had enough. And my wife likes it, too. Now that I am tasting food, I compliment her more often on how good her cooking is. So conscious eating even benefits my marriage!

our bodies actually needed. When we groan and complain, "I didn't mean to eat that much," what we really mean to say is, "I didn't mean to eat that *fast.*"

The reverse applies, too. Most of us also know the feeling of eating just a small amount, pausing for a few minutes, and realizing that the small amount we initially ate filled us up and we no longer are hungry for the rest of our meal! A good example of this is when we are at a restaurant and eat some bread and a salad. We realize as we wait for our main course that . . . we're full! Conscious eating is a way of taking advantage of our fullness signal.

So eat consciously. Remember to *savor* each bite of food, considering carefully the flavor and texture of what you are chewing. Chew

FEEL FULLER ON LESS FOOD

It takes fifteen minutes or more for your brain to get the message your body has been fed. If you slow down how fast you eat, this will allow fullness signals to begin to develop by the end of the meal. The following are some other ways to achieve a feeling of satiety on fewer calories:

- Eating lots of vegetables can also make you feel fuller.
- Drink a warm beverage during your meal; it makes you feel fuller.
- Eat foods that require more chewing, such as raw vegetables.
- Put your fork down between bites.
- Pace your eating to the slowest eater at the table.

each mouthful of food at least ten times to appreciate it completely. This process helps you eat more slowly, which helps you eat less.

You can also use conscious eating before a meal to decide if you are really hungry, and during a meal to decide if you've had enough. When was the last time you were truly, physically hungry? Do you ever eat just because it's breakfast, lunch, or dinnertime? How about if you're serving food to others? Or do you eat just because there's food around?

Sometimes we eat for emotional reasons as well. Anger, fear, anxiety, stress, hurt feelings, boredom, and loneliness are all negative emotions that can lead people to eat when they're not hungry. Positive emotions can be triggers as well. Ever eat when you're celebrating, or just plain happy? Well, none of these situations or emotions has anything to do with hunger.

To avoid eating when you're not hungry, get in the habit of asking yourself the following question beforehand: *Am I hungry, physically really hungry?*

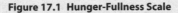

Figure 17.1 Hunger-Fullness Scale

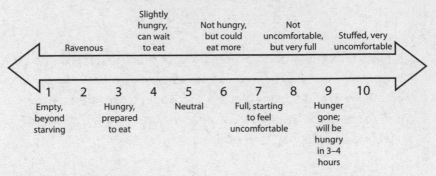

To answer this question, refer to Figure 17.1, the Hunger-Fullness Scale. At 5 you are at neutral—neither hungry nor full. If you don't eat, you get hungrier, your position on the scale going to 4 and then to 3, and so on. The opposite applies when you eat as you transition through the higher numbers on the right-hand side of the scale. At 6 you are satisfied, but may want to keep eating. At 7 you are "full." If you keep eating, you become overly full.

The key is to be conscious of where you are on this scale whenever you are ready to put food into your mouth. Your goal when eating is to eat slowly and stop when you reach the point of satisfaction, which is 6.

When deciding whether or not to eat in the first place, don't eat unless you are hungry. If you were to keep track, you would be surprised at how often you eat when you're not hungry.

Conscious eating makes the eating experience more satisfying. You gain a fuller appreciation of the food you put in your mouth. This is especially important at a time when cutting calories can make you feel deprived.

18

Ask for Support

I'VE LEARNED OVER the past decade from the men and women in my weight-loss and health program that it's crucial to get support if you are trying to make positive change in your life.

Support is available from many sources, including family, friends, and colleagues. The more places you get support from, the more likely you will achieve your goals.

FAMILY AND FRIENDS

Your family and friends are the ones whose support you may need most. Start off by asking your friends and family to respect your desire to change your eating plans. Have a family meeting to describe and discuss what you are trying to achieve. Maybe others in your family would want to make the same changes. If they don't, tell them how much you will appreciate their encouragement as you make this big change. You'll be surprised how supportive they will be.

It's great if your family is willing to help. But you may not want them looking over your shoulder all the time. Talk to your family about how they can be most helpful—positive reinforcement is usually more welcome than being constantly corrected.

Some other ideas:

- Hang your Food and Exercise Log (found in Chapter 8) somewhere prominent so that you and everyone else can be reminded of your goals.
- Put money in a fund every time you make a choice that is likely to help you achieve your weight-loss goal, and then when you reach a certain goal, reward yourself and your family with a non-food-related treat. That helps everybody in your house win when you win.
- If your family chooses to keep eating their same old way, clear a shelf in the pantry and an area in the fridge where you can keep

---

SUCCEEDING TOGETHER

B.W. is a 53-year-old factory supervisor who started the DASH Diet in 2005. He was the only one in his household trying to follow DASH. Although he made some improvements in his eating habits, he failed to lose any weight for two years. In 2007, his wife's doctor told her that she had high blood pressure and should start the DASH Diet. Working together, he and his wife stopped buying the high-calorie sweets and snacks that had been their big temptation in the past. And they started emphasizing larger servings of fruits and vegetables with their home meals. B.W. has lost 35 pounds and his wife has lost 25, and they have kept the weight off for three years. B.W. said:

Following the DASH Diet became a lot easier when we made our entire household a DASH-friendly zone. Even my two teenage sons eat the DASH Diet. It's nice to know that we're teaching them habits that will keep them healthy for years to come.

your particular food items. Make it a house rule that all junk food be kept in a different area.

AT THE OFFICE

You may be closest to family and friends, but you probably spend more time with people you work with. It's important that you let your colleagues know you are making some changes in your life. It might surprise you how many are considering doing the same thing. The same way you did with your family and friends, you can approach your workmates individually and tell them in a friendly and nonconfrontational way of your intentions to lose weight and improve your health. Let them know how much you will appreciate their help and encouragement. It may take you a while and some diplomacy, but see if you can get the support of your workmates on the following goals:

- Can we make the office a "junk food–free" zone?
- Can we have business lunches at restaurants that offer healthy choices, and especially a good salad bar?
- I'm going to start taking the stairs if it's just a couple of floors. Would you like to join me?

||||||||||||||||||||||||||||||

DASH FAQ

What's your recommendation for dealing with people who try to tempt me into eating foods that aren't on my eating plan?

Please see the answer to FAQ 12 in Section V, Frequently Asked Questions.

19

Conquer Emotional Eating

DO YOU REACH for the ice cream or potato chips when you're not even hungry, usually in response to how you're feeling? If so, you might be a victim of "emotional eating."

Emotional eating takes place when you eat large quantities of food—usually "comfort" or junk foods that are high in fat and calories—not because you are actually hungry but because you are using the food to cope with certain feelings. Overcoming emotional eating is an important skill.

WHY WE EMOTIONALLY OVEREAT

Some experts believe that much of the overeating in our society is caused by emotions we can't deal with. Sometimes we don't even recognize the connection between how we feel and why we are eating. Weight gain isn't the only negative consequence of overeating. Gorging on foods that don't fit into a healthy lifestyle can edge out healthier foods and deprives you of nutrients you need to be healthy and fight chronic disease.

Why do so many of us practice emotional eating? We learn early in life that food can temporarily make us feel better. As we get older, we may revert to using food to help us cope with emotional distress. Emotional eating may become a mechanism that gets in the way of learning more mature coping skills.

IDENTIFYING EMOTIONAL TRIGGERS

There is a long list of feelings that can trigger overeating: depression, loneliness, anger, anxiety, boredom, frustration, stress, relationship problems, and low self-esteem. Do you eat in response to any of these feelings? Then you are probably an emotional eater and will benefit from learning strategies to manage your emotional problems without heading to the fridge or vending machine.

First, though, you need to be able to recognize emotional triggers. To identify your own triggers, on your DASH Food and Exercise Log jot down what you are feeling when you eat—especially when you overeat. These notes should include emotions, stressors, and situations that make you want to reach for food. It won't be long before you begin to identify patterns associated with your overeating.

People with serious emotional eating patterns should see a counselor to identify and treat the emotional disorder. But I can give you a few suggestions to help break the connection between emotions and overeating.

DISTRACTION IN ACTION

When you are tempted to reach for food and you know you're not hungry, instead try one of the following activities:

- Call a friend.
- Read a book.
- Write a letter.
- Answer an e-mail.
- Take a luxurious bath.

- Call a friend and talk about your cravings (often they just go away).
- Go for a walk.
- Do some sit-ups or stretch out those stiff muscles.
- Do a small house project you've been avoiding, or wash the car.
- Drink a large glass of water.
- Chew a piece of sugarless gum.

Any activity that takes your mind off your negative feelings can be used as a substitute for overeating.

Meditation: An effective way to connect with underlying feelings, and to understand that overeating isn't the answer.

Relaxation exercises: Help you deal with stress and anxiety that makes you want to overeat.

Individual or group counseling: Provide you with support so you understand you aren't the only person dealing with such feelings, and that if other people can establish coping mechanisms, so can you.

There are degrees of emotional eating. There's probably no one who hasn't eaten something when they've been bored or lonely and not hungry at all. But for some people, emotional eating may be a chronic and very serious problem leading to obesity. How do you know if you have a serious problem? Here are some signs:

You eat large amounts of food when not physically hungry.

You eat very quickly and don't pay attention to the taste or texture of the food.

You hide food because you are embarrassed at how much you are eating.

You eat until you are uncomfortably full.

If these describe you, then seek the counsel of a professional who can help you. Your family doctor can provide a referral to a professional who specializes in disordered eating.

20

Stave Off Cravings

EARLY ON in this section, I recommended that you remove items from your pantry or fridge that don't fit with your DASH Diet for Weight Loss goals. No matter how rigorous you are at this "spring cleaning," most people trying to manage their weight will still face situations when they are tempted to eat more than they should at home, or to eat things they shouldn't. How can you "stave the crave"?

Tune out the tube: Television is one of the most powerful triggers for people, especially the commercials for fast food and other munchies. One of the most effective ways to prevent TV-inspired snacking is to *watch less TV*. Most people watch too much TV anyway, so here's just another reason to turn it off! If there is a TV program you just have to watch, mute the commercials since they tend to be filled with urgings to eat high-fat, high-sodium, and high-calorie foods.

Another challenge with watching TV is that it provides a huge opportunity for unconscious eating. You sit down with a bag of chips or cookies, and before you know it, you have eaten the whole bag. Cutting back on TV watching is a good way to break this cycle. Read a book or play a board game with your family members. Better yet, go for a walk or reserve TV watching for when you are exercising on a treadmill or stationary bike. You'll be burning calories instead of consuming them!

Suck it up: Choose a beverage to satisfy your craving instead of something solid to eat. For many folks, anything that satisfies the urge to get something in their mouths works. Others swear by a warm beverage. A decaffeinated tea or low-calorie hot chocolate may fit the bill. Avoid alcohol, which is high in calories and can cause problems with sleep as well as blunt your commitment to avoid snacks!

Brush and floss: We're all supposed to brush our teeth and floss at least twice each day. Right after eating a healthy meal, brush and floss your teeth very thoroughly. This is known to lessen cravings to eat.

Practice conscious eating: When you get the urge to snack, ask yourself, *Am I really hungry or is there something else going on?* This strategy is known as conscious eating. Refer to Chapter 17 on the subject.

Idle hands are a snacker's playground: Avoid the kind of boredom or inactivity that can lead to urges to eat when you shouldn't. Pick a task that keeps your hands busy and your mind off the munchies. It helps to make a list of things you enjoy doing at night and refer to that list when you feel a snack attack coming on.

Chew on it: Chewing gum can keep snack urges at bay. Choose a sugarless brand.

Don't keep undesirables at home: If it's not there, you can't eat it! If you can't resist temptation, get rid of tempting foods.

Sack out: You can't eat while you're sleeping. At night, go to bed instead of reaching for something to eat. Avoid caffeinated beverages late in the day.

Eat healthy snacks: If you are going to snack, snack on healthy items. Try to think of a healthy snack that is like the unhealthy snack you crave and keep the healthy variety on hand. Your healthy snack will come closer to satisfying your craving if it is similar in texture to your craved food. You often crave cold and creamy ice cream? A very cold nonfat yogurt has a similar mouthfeel and might do the trick. Or instead of potato chips, try a measured portion of rice cakes or popcorn. Whatever your usual craving, plan ahead and have a healthy option available. Learn how to "snack healthily."

Don't let yourself get too hungry at night: It's important to eat enough during the day so you don't lose control at night and go to town on high-calorie snacks. Make sure you eat your full allowance of DASH foods during the day. Eat a Hi-Lo-Slo dinner with high-fiber items, as this is more filling. If you aren't ravenous when dinnertime approaches and if you eat a Hi-Lo-Slo dinner, you might find that the cravings are less urgent.

21

Learn How to Go
Grocery Shopping

HOW MANY TIMES have you returned from the grocery store and realized you've bought a whole lot of what you don't need—and neglected to buy much of what you *do* need?

Learning how to go grocery shopping seems so elementary. Yet many of us need guidance in this area of skillpower. It's especially important for those who struggle with their weight. And it's fundamental to meal planning, as we saw earlier.

Let's look at what I call the Four Essential Principles of Food Shopping. These principles will make your trips to the grocery store more efficient, and in doing so, support your goals of losing weight and getting healthy.

1. DON'T SHOP HUNGRY.

This is a simple yet important tip. If you go to the grocery store hungry, you may very well make impulse purchases that don't fit into your weight-loss program. At the very least, have a healthy and substantial snack before you go into the store—a couple of pieces of fruit and a large glass of water will take the edge off. Alternatively, do your grocery shopping after your evening meal, and make it an opportunity to get some exercise too by parking a good distance from the store entrance.

2. GO WITH A LIST.

Another obvious principle that so many people ignore. Shopping lists help you to be more efficient. Take a shopping list with you and stick to it.

3. STICK TO THE PERIMETER.

Avoiding aisles you've been down already can help you speed through the store and leave with a variety of healthy and Hi-Lo-Slo foods for you and your family. Most Hi-Lo-Slo foods are found around the perimeter of the store. On one side of the store you'll find fresh fruits and vegetables. Usually along the back wall are the meat section and the dairy department, followed by the bakery. It is in these sections that we recommend you spend most of your time and money. The center aisles are where you'll find the processed foods like snacks, cookies, and sweets. You should spend less time (and money) there.

4. AVOID FREE SAMPLES.

You might think the ice cream section is treacherous, but some of the most dangerous parts of any grocery store are the ends of the middle aisles where friendly folks offer samples of tasty foods. If you eat everything that's offered, you could be consuming an entire meal's worth of calories. A polite "No thank you!" is the appropriate response when offered any free sample. This is another reason not to go grocery shopping when hungry.

22

Make Your Kitchen Weight-Loss Friendly

KEEPING A WELL-STOCKED kitchen is a key to eating healthy. That sounds obvious, but putting it into practice can be a challenge. I am going to provide you with a list of products you should keep in your pantry, refrigerator, and freezer.

First, here are some hints on how to keep that kitchen well stocked:

- Keep a list of essentials (such as the one below) and make sure to keep the items in stock at all times. Customize it so it suits your own likes, dislikes, and dietary restrictions.
- As soon as you use up an item, write it on your shopping list so you won't be caught out when you need to include it in a meal.
- If you have favorite items you use frequently, buy in multiples; that way you'll always have on hand what you need. Canned tomatoes are a good example—they can be used for healthy pasta sauces and chili and stews and can be stored for long periods of time. Buy a case at a time if you have the storage space. The same

goes for ingredients for your favorite recipes, so you can make them a few times.

- If an item you use a lot is on sale, don't buy just one. Check out your local grocery store flyers regularly and stock up on kitchen and pantry items when they are on sale.

With a well-stocked kitchen, you can regularly prepare Hi-Lo-Slo meals your family will love.

IN THE PANTRY
Brown rice
Quinoa
Whole-wheat pasta
Ready-to-eat whole-grain cereals (shredded wheat, toasted oat, bran flakes)
Oatmeal (whole oats or quick cooking, not instant)
100% whole-wheat bread (small slice) and pita pockets
Flour (unbleached and whole wheat)
Cornstarch or arrowroot
Baking powder (aluminum free) and baking soda
Beans (dried and/or canned)
Canned tuna (packed in water, not oil)
Canned tomatoes (preferably no-salt-added)
Unsweetened applesauce
Dried fruit and nuts
Vegetable oil spray
Olive and canola oils
Low-calorie salad dressings
Low-sodium chicken, beef, and/or vegetable broth
Salsa
Reduced-sodium tomato sauce
Brown sugar
Vinegar (balsamic and white wine)
Reduced-sodium ketchup, deli mustard, "lite" mayonnaise
Low-fat granola bars

Pretzels (unsalted)
Low-fat whole-wheat snack crackers

IN THE FRIDGE
Fresh fruit (a variety)
Fresh vegetables (a variety)
Fresh-pack salad greens
Onions
Garlic
Low-fat or nonfat milk
Low-fat and nonfat yogurt (a variety)
Low-fat cottage cheese
Low-fat cheese (a variety)
Reduced-fat string cheese (mozzarella) sticks
Trans-fat-free margarine
Eggs and/or egg substitute
Reduced-fat, low-sodium deli meat, such as sliced turkey breast
Natural peanut butter
Tortillas, whole-wheat or corn (can be frozen, too)
Bottled lemon juice
Reduced-sodium soy sauce and teriyaki sauce

IN THE FREEZER
Frozen vegetables (plain vegetables; no sauces or salt)
Frozen fruit (without added sugar; such as blueberries,
    strawberries, raspberries)
Lean meats (skinless chicken breasts, low-fat cuts of beef, pork)
Fish
Low-calorie frozen desserts (frozen juice bars, nonfat frozen
    yogurt)

23

Learn How to Dine Out and Still Maintain Weight-Loss Goals

I'M TRYING TO *follow the DASH Diet for Weight Loss. What should I order?*

That's what you should be asking yourself as you browse through a restaurant menu deciding what fits with your DASH food group servings for the day and with your weight-management goals.

To make their food offerings tastier and appealing to the modern American palate, most restaurants serve overly large portions and load them with salt, fat, and sugar. Many restaurants now offer some menu selections that are healthy, but how to tell which ones they are?

WORDS TO THE WISE

Let's start off with a primer on which words on menus generally refer to high-calorie items and which ones are for healthier choices.

Words That Describe Restaurant Dishes	
High-Calorie Words	Low-Calorie Words
Cooking Methods and Preparations	
Sautéed, meunière	Raw (vegetables)
Fried, Southern-fried	Baked, roasted
Breaded	Grilled, broiled
Au gratin, scalloped	Steamed, poached
Hash-browned	
Parmesan (as in veal or eggplant Parmesan)	
Melted cheese	
Sauces	
Alfredo, cheesy	Marinara
Cream, creamy, special sour cream, Newburg	Au jus, natural juices
Butter sauce	
Hollandaise, béarnaise	
Bordelaise, wine	
Gravy	
Texture and Appearance	
Luscious, rich	Crisp and crunchy (when describing fruits and vegetables)
Crisp and golden, golden fried	Lean
Other Words	
Cream soup, chowder, bisque	Heart healthy
Pot pie	

It's straightforward: Avoid the foods in the left column, try to choose the ones in the right column. Of course, you can always ask the waitstaff how a dish is prepared. A simple rule of thumb for controlling calories would be to avoid foods that are fried or have sauces made with cream or butter.

RESTAURANTS WILL RESPOND

Many restaurants have responded to consumer demand for healthier options. Those options are usually flagged on the menu. And even fast-food restaurants are becoming more willing to accommodate specific requests on food preparation. So if you have specific requests for lower-calorie fare, you can usually "have it your way." You just have to ask.

WHAT TO ASK FOR

If you'd like something specially prepared, all you need to do is politely ask your server to ask the kitchen. The kitchen won't always be able to accommodate your request, but it doesn't hurt to ask for food that will help you reach your weight-loss goals. I know a lot of people are reluctant to do this. Maybe they don't want to seem too pushy or demanding. Or maybe part of the reluctance is because if you ask if something can be made without the butter (for example), you're afraid they will say yes—and subconsciously you really want the butter! So be honest with yourself: It's time to skip the butter. And don't be afraid to ask.

Here are some requests you can make that will help you enjoy a lower calorie meal when eating out:

- Does the chef make a low-calorie special?
- I'd like the chef to put half the meat and twice the vegetables on my plate.
- I'd like the fish prepared with no oil and the sauce on the side, and instead of the sides listed, could I have it over greens with a low-fat dressing?
- In that sandwich, please put half the meat and twice the vegetables.
- I'll take the turkey burger, but hold the cheese and mayonnaise.
- We'd like to share an entree and have it plated that way by the chef. (There's often a small extra charge for this.)
- Before you bring my food out, could you put half my entree in a "to-go" container?
- I'd like the dressing on the side of my salad.
- No bread and butter at this table, please.
- Instead of the chicken entree, I'd like the chicken broiled and served on a salad.

- Can the chef make any vegetarian entrees? (But remember that a vegetarian choice on a menu is not necessarily the low-calorie choice. Vegetarian dishes may be made with cheese, cream, butter, or oil, or they may be fried.)
- I'll have the burrito, but instead of rice, would you please have the chef make it with extra vegetables and half the cheese? And if the chicken burrito is white meat I'll have that, otherwise just the beans is fine.
- With my sandwich, I'd like a small salad instead of french fries.
- I'd like my fish/chicken broiled instead of fried or sautéed.
- No thanks, we don't want to see the dessert menu.

TRYING TO MANAGE YOUR WEIGHT?
Take This Restaurant Quiz

I hope you've learned enough to be able to answer the following questions correctly.

1. It is possible to stick to your DASH Diet for Weight Loss program when eating out at a restaurant because:

 a. Most chefs and maître d's are eating the DASH Diet for Weight Loss.
 b. Most restaurant servers have read the book *The DASH Diet for Weight Loss*.
 c. Most restaurant managers read the articles in major medical journals attesting to the effectiveness of the DASH eating plan.
 d. The DASH Diet for Weight Loss is an eating plan based on common foods, and you can always ask the waiter to modify one of the menu selections so that it's more DASH-friendly for you.

2. Which of these menu descriptions represents a more low-calorie option?

   a. Alfredo
   b. Béarnaise
   c. Cream sauce
   d. Baked

3. Which of these is an effective way to reduce calories when you eat out?

   a. Skip the bread and butter.
   b. Have two appetizers instead of an appetizer and an entree for your meal.
   c. Share an entree with your dining companion.
   d. All of the above

4. Which of these statements is true?

   a. It's rude and presumptuous to politely ask the server if the chef will prepare a meal for you using low-calorie ingredients and preparation methods.
   b. It is impossible for chefs to change ingredients and preparation techniques.
   c. Restaurants are oblivious to their customers' desires to eat healthier.
   d. Restaurants are in the business of keeping their customers, and they will accommodate customers' wishes to eat healthier to the best of their abilities.

(continued on next page)

5. Which of these salad dressings is probably lowest in calories and saturated fat?

    a. Ranch
    b. French
    c. Thousand Island
    d. Vinaigrette

6. Which of these salad bar selections should you avoid if you are watching your weight?

    a. Green vegetables such as watercress, arugula, romaine lettuce, spinach, green beans, snow peas, and broccoli
    b. Other-color vegetables such as tomatoes, peas, cabbage, bell peppers, cauliflower, corn, red beets, hearts of palm, and carrots
    c. Small amounts of unsalted nuts
    d. Bacon bits, potato salad, and crispy chow mein noodles

7. Why is eating slowly an effective way of feeling full on fewer calories?

    a. Your eating companions will steal your food.
    b. Calories evaporate from food when it is put on a plate.
    c. Most restaurants have a strict policy prohibiting people from eating slowly.
    d. It takes 15 minutes for your brain's fullness signal to kick in, and if you gobble your food down, you'll have exceeded your calorie target by the time your brain tells your tummy you've eaten enough.

If you answered *d* to all these questions, congratulations. You are officially qualified to eat in restaurants without blowing your weight-loss goals.

As you can see, there are plenty of ways to make eating out an experience that is more in line with your weight-management goals. Don't be afraid to speak up.

FINALLY: CELEBRATE EVERY SUCCESS!

It's easy to be impatient or too hard on yourself. Instead, give yourself credit for mastering the skills in this section. Every skill you learn and practice is a move in the right direction, and you deserve to feel good about your hard work. Of course, the challenge is to celebrate in a way that fits with your greater goals. If food has been your way of rewarding yourself, you will want to explore other ways to feel good. It is very important to feel good because when you do, you'll be able to accomplish so much more for yourself.

Doing It for Life

AS SOMEONE in my DASH Diet for Weight Loss program once said, "If you do what you've always done, you'll get what you always got." I didn't realize at the time she was quoting Mark Twain, but she hit the nail right on the head. The same unwise eating practices will get you the same results—a waistline that keeps expanding. But when she made the comment, it was more about how, if you continue to practice healthy changes, then the benefits you receive will also continue. Put another way: If you lose weight on this program and you keep doing what you did to lose that weight—guess what?—you'll keep that weight off.

This is especially important news for folks who have lost weight on other programs but gained it all back when they couldn't stick to the diet permanently, maybe because the diet was too extreme or too limited in the foods that were allowed. Or maybe they just decided that it was not a healthy way to eat for the rest of their life.

One of the positive features of the DASH Diet for Weight Loss is that the diet is easy to keep up. The eating plan is made up of common foods, and the calorie targets aren't so restricted that you feel deprived all the time. *It is a diet you can follow for life.*

Not just that, but you have been provided with a large box of tools you can use that will help you stick to the program. These tools help you practice the behaviors necessary to follow the eating plan and exercise recommendations. The behaviors that you practice as part of the program will eventually become habits—in the very best sense of the word. You'll find yourself practicing portion control by counting servings, choosing Hi-Lo-Slo foods and avoiding calorie-dense items, eating slowly and stopping when you're full, and exercising regularly.

When these behaviors really become habits, you may be surprised that you are doing them without thinking about it!

At the same time, it is important to be vigilant so you can maintain your lower weight and continue with this healthier way of living. In my many conversations with the men and women enrolled in my DASH for Health program, what I've learned is that there are several steps you can take to make it much more likely you will enjoy continued success.

PRACTICE THE PRINCIPLES

The DASH Diet for Weight Loss is built on several important principles. It's important for you to keep these in mind. Memorize these principles. Write them down. Type them up and put them on your desk at work, the fridge at home, in your wallet—wherever you need to so they become part of your consciousness.

Here are those principles:

- Learn how many servings you should be eating each day in each DASH food group (see Chapter 5, The Food Groups—Going Hi-Lo-Slo).
- Learn what a serving is and what counts as a serving for different foods (see Table 4.4, Serving Sizes in the Eight DASH Food Groups).

- Choose Hi-Lo-Slo foods and make meals using Hi-Lo-Slo principles (see Part 3, Meal Plans).
- Be active (see Chapters 11, 12, and 13 for exercise advice).

BE POSITIVE AND MAKE IT FUN

I like to think that following the advice in this book offers you more than just better eating habits, and even more than losing weight. It offers you an opportunity for a healthier life. Embrace that opportunity. A slimmer, healthier you is someone who lives life more fully. The new you doesn't just sit on the couch watching TV, letting life pass you by. You are learning new and healthier ways to prepare food; trying new varieties of vegetables, fruits, and grains (and maybe growing your own vegetables); enjoying active vacations; maybe even helping others start an exercise program because you've seen how much exercise has helped you. Maybe you aren't doing *all* these things, but you are doing at least a couple of them. Your new way of living should be enjoyed to the maximum, so be positive and make it fun.

CONTROL YOUR ENVIRONMENT

We live in a toxic food environment. There are huge amounts of cheap food everywhere. If you struggle with your weight, that can make it exceedingly difficult to maintain any weight loss you achieve. The key is to not be a victim. Just because it doesn't cost extra to "supersize" a meal doesn't mean you should; just because the smell of cinnamon buns wafts through the food court at the mall doesn't mean you must go in and buy one; and just because the buffet is "all-you-can-eat" doesn't mean you have to. The most important thing to understand: *You are in control of what you eat.*

At the same time you resolve to not be a victim of the toxic food environment, it's important to control your own surroundings to the extent that it's possible. This includes your home and workplace. I have provided you with lots of advice on ways in which to create an environment that supports your weight-loss goals, whether it's at home or work.

BACK TO THE BASICS

Help can be found in your DASH Diet for Weight Loss program whenever you need it. It's especially important in the event you find yourself gaining weight back. So keep weighing yourself every week. If your weight increases by 2 or 3 pounds, it is time for you to pick back up on your program. That means going back to basics. Reacquaint yourself with the concept of Your First Three Steps that I introduced in Chapter 4 to help you figure out how much to eat. Resume the food tracking system to make you more aware of what you are eating (using

---

PERMANENT CHANGES

Dear Dr. Moore,
I just wanted to let you know that I have been following the DASH Diet for five years now. I lost 28 pounds in the first year and have kept the weight off. I had tried many diet plans before DASH. Sometimes I would lose some weight but always I regained it. What I learned with the DASH Diet is that a "diet" is not just something you do until you lose the weight and then you go back to what you did before. That's a sure way of repeating failure. With DASH, I learned that proper eating habits should last a lifetime. So I continue to try to follow what the DASH Diet teaches every day. Watch your food groups and watch your food servings. Now that is my new "habit." And I'm planning to stick with it for the rest of my life.

Thanks,
S.Q.

the Food and Exercise Log in Figure 8.1). And remind yourself which are the best Hi-Lo-Slo foods and food preparations (outlined in Chapter 5). You might consider doing this for a week or two every year, regardless of whether you gain back some weight. The DASH Diet for Weight Loss will always be here for you. It will always work—if you work it. So don't be afraid to go back to the basics.

ASPIRE TO PROGRESS, NOT PERFECTION

We all want to be as good as we can be. And we want to meet our goals. If you are reading this book, then one of your goals is to lose weight. But don't make weight loss an obsession. Don't beat yourself up if your goal was to lose 40 pounds and you've lost only 30. I'm not saying you should settle for 30. I *am* saying don't get discouraged. Because if you get discouraged, it becomes easy to say, "I've failed. What's the use?" And then you can slip back into your old ways and your old weight.

Instead, as you continue to strive to hit your goal, think about how far you've come. Losing even 10 percent of your starting weight means you have already gotten a lot of the health benefits of weight loss—things like better blood pressure and heart health. The exercise you are doing makes you more fit and gives you more energy. And the healthy foods of the DASH Diet are protecting you from a host of medical problems—from heart disease to diabetes to cancer. So don't get discouraged. Celebrate your success. You have made a lot of progress, even if you are not yet perfect.

And what happens when you do hit your goal? You were shooting to lose 40 pounds and you did it! What do you say to yourself then? I hope you will say:

When I started on the DASH Diet for Weight Loss, I just wanted to lose weight. But I've learned that healthy eating is about more than losing weight. It's what I need to do to stay healthy for the rest of my life. And exercising regularly isn't just about burning calories. It's about how I stay fit and energetic and feeling good every day. And following the DASH Diet—keeping track of my servings and food groups—all of that isn't just what I did temporarily to lose weight. It has now become my new "habit." I'm doing it for my health. I'm doing it because it makes me feel good about myself. And I'm doing it for life.

Frequently Asked Questions

MANY OF THE RECOMMENDATIONS I've made in this book are based on what I've learned from the 18,000 people who have enrolled in our DASH for Health online program. They have been generous in sharing what works—and what doesn't. Many of the inspirational stories given directly to me by these men and women are featured in this book.

Many of the folks in my DASH for Health program also send me questions. And not surprisingly, quite a few of them hit the same hot-button topics. Some of their questions have already been covered in the preceding chapters. This chapter covers many of the frequently asked questions on topics that didn't quite make it into the previous chapters, but which deserve coverage because they are of such concern to so many people.

FAQ 1:
Almost every week in the newspaper I read about a new study about how to lose weight. Often these studies contradict one another. What should I believe?

I sympathize with folks who are confused by the barrage of information that comes from the media—much of which contradicts itself. Part of the problem is that there's now such a thirst for health knowledge among Americans that newspaper, radio, and TV reporters feel obliged to report on the results of every study that might make people sit up and take notice. The kind of stories that seem to disprove commonly held beliefs and sensible health information are especially popular—so-called man-bites-dog stories.

The problem with creating a big story out of an individual scientific study is that any single study may be flawed because of how the research was organized or because of factors the researchers couldn't have predicted. That's why doctors rarely change their recommendations based on a single study. Doctors are sometimes criticized for being "behind the times" because we don't immediately respond to new research, but this conservative approach has very good reasons.

For those of you who are confused about what to believe, here are the main points I would urge you to remember:

- Don't place too much emphasis on the results of a single study.
- Beware of media reports that highlight "surprising" or "dramatic" results of a single small study, especially if it contradicts accepted health ideas.
- Get the whole story. Read through to the end of the article or listen to the whole report. Often, "dramatic" results are described first, but then the report concludes by saying something like, "Until further research is done, follow existing recommendations."
- Follow the advice of professionals (nutritionists and doctors) who follow accepted and safe dietary practices.

FAQ 2:
Could a weight-loss pill be right for me?
Perhaps. There are several prescription medications available through your doctor that have been approved by the FDA for short- or long-term use. Weight-loss drugs may be appropriate for you if (1) your

BMI is over 30 (the obese range) or if your BMI is over 27 and you also have hypertension/high blood pressure, diabetes, or elevated cholesterol; and (2) you are participating in a diet and exercise program. Medications can also help you keep weight off and give you a healthy "grace period" within which you can adopt the lifestyle changes you need to maintain the weight loss.

You should have this conversation with your physician. Your personal physician knows your entire medical situation and is the best person to help you decide what's best for you. Most drugs actually have a quite modest effect on weight loss. Most of the weight loss occurs during the first six months of treatment. As the makers of all prescription weight-loss drugs state, their products should be used as part of a total weight-loss program that includes a low-calorie diet and exercise. The bottom line: There are no miracle drugs. If you're not willing to change your lifestyle, these drugs won't benefit you, and at best, the positive results will be temporary.

What about weight-loss pills that you can buy over the counter without a prescription? None of these has really been proven to be of much benefit. Some have actually been shown to be dangerous and have been removed from the market. I don't recommend any of them.

As you make your own decision, use common sense. If something sounds too good to be true, it's probably false. And so-called natural herbal preparations are not recommended as part of a weight-loss program. These products have unpredictable amounts of active ingredients and have not been shown in studies to be effective or safe. Some may have harmful side effects.

FAQ 3:
My parents didn't much care for fruits and vegetables, so I didn't grow up eating them at home. As an adult, I don't feel confident coming up with ways to increase how much produce I eat in my diet. Do you have any suggestions?

Vegetables and fruits are premier Hi-Lo-Slo foods. Yet most people who struggle with their weight don't get enough of them. The average American eats only about three servings of vegetables and fruits *combined* each day. The following recommendations are from tips I've received from participants in the DASH for Health program. They will help you increase how many vegetables and fruits you eat to meet your DASH Diet for Weight Loss serving goals and make your diet richer in Hi-Lo-Slo foods that make you healthier as you lose weight.

START EARLY

At breakfast time consider packing an egg-white omelet with spinach, tomatoes, and zucchini. Or add a sliced banana, berries, or raisins to your cereal to give yourself a head start on fruit servings. Ditto for a half grapefruit or piece of melon. Note: 100% fruit or vegetable juice is a concentrated source of goodness—and calories, too. It's easy to consume these products quickly and exceed your calorie target for the day.

YOU *CAN* TAKE IT WITH YOU

Vegetables and fruits are portable and give you a quick boost of flavor and energy anytime. Pack an apple, an orange, or a bag of carrot sticks in your glove compartment, purse, or briefcase. Note: Dried fruits are portable, but they are a concentrated source of calories and so we recommend against consuming these products too often.

BELLY UP TO A BAR

Find a good salad bar in your neighborhood and close to where you work for when you don't feel like preparing something yourself. Learn to make appropriate selections. If your workplace has a canteen without a salad bar, get together with a few colleagues and ask your employer to install one. And make sure the salad bar items offer plenty of what you need—in particular, low-fat salad dressings and appropriate leafy green vegetables in place of iceberg lettuce.

SEE-FOOD DIET

Put vegetables and fruits where you can see them and within easy reach. Keep a bowl of fruit on the counter in the kitchen. Make sure fruits and vegetables are clearly visible when you open the refrigerator. Cut up your favorite vegetables and store them in resealable plastic bags. If you see it, you'll be more likely to eat it.

STOCK UP

Go shopping on the weekend and buy plenty of fresh, frozen, and canned vegetables and fruits to eat through the week.

WHEN YOU'RE ALL ALONE

Are you shooting for three vegetables with dinner? That much food preparation can be a challenge, especially if you're cooking just for yourself or if other household members aren't interested in eating the DASH Diet. Some tips for getting that third vegetable without a lot of extra trouble:

- Don't forget about salad. Even most side salads contain at least 2 DASH servings of vegetables.
- Keep family-size bags of frozen peas, beans, and carrots in your freezer, so you can microwave a handful for yourself at dinnertime.
- Check out our vegetable recipes in Part 4. Several of them are suitable for freezing and reheating.
- Make a big enough batch to freeze several individual servings to enjoy later—with almost no extra work!

NIGHT MOVES

At the end of the day, the microwave is a quick, convenient way to prepare vegetables that preserves their nutrient contents. Pop a potato into the microwave at dinnertime and top it with your favorite salsa for a quick meal. Add microwaved broccoli and corn to your tasty tater and you've got a colorful, tasty, and nutritious meal. For dessert, top a scoop of low-fat yogurt with fresh berries or sliced peaches.

FAQ 4:
I don't have a clue about how to buy and store fruit. Any suggestions?

I get this question a lot, so I consulted a couple of experts. Here is what they recommend when shopping for fresh produce:

- Look for fruits and vegetables that look fresh and not bruised, shriveled, moldy, or slimy. Don't buy anything that smells bad.
- Ask the produce manager to help you choose an item you're unfamiliar with. Ask for a taste, for handling and storing information, or for a recipe card.
- Most fruits and vegetables are not "stock-up" items. Buy only enough for use in the next few days. Keep frozen fruits and vegetables on hand for when you are out of fresh.
- Keep produce in the top of your cart, as putting heavy groceries on top of it will bruise the items. Some items that seem hardy, such as cauliflower, actually are very delicate and bruise easily.

When you get your produce home:

- Keep most of your produce in the crisper. It helps it last longer because of the slightly higher humidity level. Keep all cut fruits and vegetables in the refrigerator.
- Wash produce just before you use it. Don't wash produce when you put it away.

To ripen unripe fruits, such as peaches, plums, and avocados, place them in a ripening bowl or a loosely closed brown paper bag (not a plastic bag). The natural ripening gases they give off will help them continue to ripen. To speed up the process, place a ripe banana or apple in the bag with the unripe fruit.

FAQ 5:
I've heard that carbs are "fattening." How, then, can they be part of a weight-loss program?
I don't blame you if you're confused about the role of carbohydrates like grains in your diet. One minute carbs are the enemy and the next they're the best thing since, well . . . sliced bread. Carbohydrates are any food made up of sugars, starches, celluloses, and gums. Most of us know that carbohydrates are a prime source of quick energy for the human body. But people are often surprised that carbohydrates come in many different forms. Many of us are aware that potatoes and white bread and white pasta are carbs, but did you also know that fruits are carbs? And so are vegetables.

I hesitate to label any food "bad" or "good," so let's just say that if you're trying to lose weight while eating healthy, some carbs are better than others. "Better" carbs can be found in foods that contain fiber and other important nutrients. They include plant-based foods (fruits, vegetables, and whole grains) that are high in vitamins, minerals, and phytochemicals. And the carbohydrate that's in these plant-based foods is mostly in the form of complex carbohydrate. Complex carbohydrate is still basically sugar, but it is a number of sugar molecules connected together in chains (we call this starch). Because these chains need to be broken down into individual sugar molecules during the process of digestion, most complex carbohydrates release sugar into our bloodstream rather slowly. So our blood sugar rises less than if we had eaten sugar. The best sources of complex carbohydrates are beans, lentils, whole grains, and vegetables.

There are several reasons to choose carbs with high fiber content:

- The type of fiber found in carbs like oats, beans, and some fruits helps lower cholesterol.
- Fiber helps you feel fuller on fewer calories.

- Fibrous foods tend to take longer to eat, giving your fullness signal the chance to kick in.
- Fiber adds bulk to your diet and improves bowel function.

"Less desirable" carbs are ones that are based mostly on refined and processed grains and sugar. Common carbs that are less desirable are sugar, pasta made from refined grains, white rice, pastries, cake, chips, and cookies. Foods based on refined grains and starches, and also sugar, provide quick energy to your body, which you might need if you're participating in a sports event. However, the same way your blood sugar goes up quickly, it also comes down fast. This is known as "spiking and crashing" and leaves you feeling lethargic and hungry after your blood sugar goes back down.

Most important from the standpoint of a person who is trying to manage their weight, these simple carbs contain a whole lot of calories but very little in the way of important nutrients. Their high calorie count is usually because of the added sugar content in these products.

By making sure your diet contains lots of "better" carbs and very few "less desirable" carbs, you get the best of both worlds—a diet lower in calories but packed with good nutrition!

FAQ 6:
What advice can you give someone who knows how important dairy is to a complete weight-loss program but who is lactose intolerant?
Some people have trouble eating dairy products because they get an upset stomach—gas, stomach pains, or diarrhea. This is known as being lactose intolerant. The condition is especially prevalent in people of East Asian, African, and Middle Eastern descent.

If you have trouble digesting dairy products, try taking lactase enzyme pills or drops with dairy foods to make them more digestible. These items are available at drug and grocery stores. A number of companies manufacture lactase supplements. The most popular brand is Lactaid, but health food stores and pharmacy chains often offer their own versions. Typical tablets contain 3,000 lactase units, and the usual dose is one or two tablets taken before you consume dairy products. You might have to experiment to see how many tablets you need.

Here are some other tips for people who are lactose intolerant who still want to consume beneficial dairy products:

- Drink milk in smaller portions, for example, ½ cup instead of a full cup.
- Try natural aged or ripened cheeses such as swiss and cheddar. Not only do these cheeses contain little, if any, lactose, but they are an important source of calcium and other essential nutrients.
- Choose yogurts that carry the "live and active cultures" seal. These "friendly" cultures act like lactase since they break down the lactose in the digestive tract. Small (½-cup) servings of ice cream or frozen yogurt may not cause symptoms.
- Lactose-reduced and lactose-free milk and milk products are available in many grocery stores.

Despite the fact that some degree of lactose intolerance is pretty common in African Americans and in older people, we had very little problem with lactose intolerance symptoms in our participants in the original DASH study.

FAQ 7:
When grocery shopping, it's always a good idea to choose foods that are low in fat if I'm trying to lose weight, right?
Not necessarily. Many food items labeled "low-fat" or "fat-free" are actually packed with sugar for flavor. Because sugar is high in calories, this means those products are not suitable for someone trying to manage their weight. Many of these reduced-fat products can have as many calories per serving as regular products—and sometimes more!

For example, a fat-free fig cookie has 70 calories while the regular version has only 50 calories. A half-cup of premium nonfat frozen yogurt has 190 calories while the regular has just 180 calories. The reduced-fat version of a certain peanut butter has 190 calories per 2 tablespoons, which is the same amount as the regular fat version.

Unless we understand that low-fat foods aren't always low-calorie, we might make a habit of eating products that don't fit with our weight-management goals, and even worse, overindulge in them because we think they are low in calories. Some studies have shown that people tend to eat more of a food when they think it is "healthy."

Many foods marketed as low-fat or no-fat are the ones we tend to overindulge in. Cookies, ice cream, pie, cream sauces—an all-star team of diet-busting delicacies. When you are trying to lose weight, it's important to cut back on these categories of foods, and if and when you do purchase them, to make sure they are not just low in fat, but also low in calories.

The bottom line is "buyer beware." Something labeled as low-fat doesn't mean it is going to make you less fat!

FAQ 8:
I love pizza. Is it totally out of bounds on my weight-loss diet?

Pizza is one of the most common foods in the American diet. If you are going to eat pizza, portion control is particularly important. Instead of having an entire meal of only pizza, plan to have just one small slice of thin-crust pizza and eat it with a big salad and "lite" dressing on the side. That takes pizza from a potential gut-buster to a Hi-Lo-Slo meal.

As a comparison, take a look at the difference in fat and calories of these two meals:

> 3 slices of "meat lover's" pizza: 1,110 calories, 45g fat
> 1 slice veggie pizza (½ the cheese) and a side salad with low-fat
>   dressing: 350 calories, 7g fat

Here are some suggestions for how to feel fuller on less pizza:

- Eating lots of vegetables on the pizza can make you feel fuller.
- Eat foods along with your pizza that require more chewing, such as a salad of raw vegetables.
- Use a knife and fork to eat the slice instead of your hands.

- Put leftover pizza away before you are tempted to go back to the box.

WHAT YOU ORDER

When ordering pizza, be sure to follow a few simple guidelines: (1) reduce the amount of cheese on the pie; (2) avoid meat; (3) load up on vegetables; and (4) avoid stuffed crust or deep-dish pizza. If you're with friends and no one is interested in the low-fat option, order a small pizza to split with someone or take the other half to go.

WHAT YOU EAT WITH IT

Salad is your best bet for an accompaniment to your pizza. Avoid high-fat, high-calorie sides such as cheese sticks and chicken wings.

WHAT YOU WASH IT DOWN WITH

You can inadvertently jack up the calorie content of your pizza meal by washing it down with a large soda, which can contain up to 300 calories. If you must have soda with your pizza, make it a diet product. Better yet, drink water, juice mixed with sparkling water, or nonfat milk.

FAQ 9:
Any ideas for squeezing exercise into my crazy schedule?

When I ask people what it would take to make it easier for them to start an exercise program, I get the same answer over and over: "It's just so hard to find the time!" Work, families, and all the other things that slip into our busy schedules make finding the time for exercise really hard. Here are some suggestions to get you up and moving toward better health and fitness.

IDENTIFY TIME WASTERS

First, figure out just where your time is going. Many people use lack of time as a reason to not do something. How many times have you said, "I can't go to the gym because I don't have time"? But you may also be watching TV for an hour or two every night, answering e-mails or phone calls from friends, or just being a couch potato. It is helpful to look at your day and determine where your time goes. Make a list of the empty time in your day that you could fill with physically active pursuits. Then make a date with yourself to exercise during some of that empty time. Let's look at other ways to slip in a bit of activity.

CRUNCHING FOR TIME?

Many of us spend eight hours or more each day at work. How about fitting in some exercise during your workday? Look in your local yellow pages to see if there is a gym nearby—many employers are now even offering discounts on gym memberships! Sneaking in thirty to sixty minutes at lunch is a great way to get in your exercise, even if it is just a walk around the building or outside. Do children take up all of your exercise time? Then mix the two. Take a family walk, go for a bike ride, or even try in-line skating! All of these activities are great ways to get moving, and they teach children the importance of daily exercise.

RISE AND SHINE

Getting up thirty minutes earlier every morning is a great way to get in your exercise. Getting outside for a walk, jog, or bike ride when the air is cool, traffic is light, and the world is just waking up is good for you both physically and psychologically. And once you get started, exercise gives you more energy, so it is easier to climb out of bed and greet the day.

QUICKIES ANYWHERE

Remember the exercise rule: *Every step counts*. Park a little farther away and walk an extra 200 feet. Try not using the elevator—always use the stairs if you are going up only one or two floors or down less than three. If you are ten minutes early for your next meeting, walk around the building instead of waiting in an empty meeting room.

Fit fitness into empty time slots. When you're standing in a checkout line, go up on your tippy-toes, then back down again. Repeat ten times. Sure, people might look at you a little strangely—but maybe you'll make new friends. Sitting at your desk, put your hands on the arms of your chair, then lift your entire body up, hold two seconds, and release; repeat ten times. In the kitchen, do counter push-ups while dinner is simmering, performed just like a regular push-up, but using the counter instead of the floor.

FAQ 10:
Won't exercising make me even hungrier and, by doing so, make me eat more than I should?

Many people who are considering beginning an exercise program for weight loss think that it may be a double-edged sword: *Sure, I'll burn more calories, but won't I want to eat more all the time, too?*

In fact, most of the evidence suggests that exercising *decreases* appetite immediately afterward because it increases body temperature, which makes you less hungry.

It may be true that after your body temperature returns to normal after exercising, the result of burning all those calories is that you will want to replace them—and replace them fast. That's why it's always good to have a plan to eat healthy food after you exercise, which is a matter of having the right food around. Make sure you have healthy items such as fruit and yogurt at your disposal so that if and when you get post-exercise munchies, your first inclination isn't to pull into that fast-food joint for a "Double McGreasy" when you have an apple or banana in your car, or to go to the convenience store for a pint of ice cream when you know you have yogurt and tasty snack mix waiting at home.

FAQ 11:
What are the advantages of using a pedometer?

To stick with an exercise program, most people need individual tracking, feedback, and encouragement or close support.

A pedometer is a belt buckle–size device you wear on your hip that keeps track of how many steps you take. A pedometer has three main roles in a weight-loss program: It tracks you by continuously collecting current activity; it provides feedback by providing immediate information on your activity level; and it is an environmental cue by reminding you to be active. A good, accurate pedometer will cost $20 to $30 and upwards.

How do you use your pedometer to lose weight? Your first task is to establish a baseline. Wear your pedometer for a few days and figure out on average how many steps you take a day. Write down your total every night. Most adults take somewhere between 2,000 and 5,000 steps daily. Your goal should be 10,000 steps each day.

It is important to be sure you wear your pedometer properly. It should stay upright. If tilted, it's not accurate. The pedometer registers the up-and-down movements we make with each step. The best place to position your pedometer is on your waistband at your hipbone. If you're overweight and this is not possible, attach your pedometer at the side of your waist, directly beneath your armpit, or even on your backside.

FAQ 12:
What's your recommendation for dealing with people who try to tempt me into eating foods that aren't on my eating plan?

You may encounter special challenges from people around you who deliberately or inadvertently subvert your weight-loss attempts. I call these people "diet saboteurs." They bring you food as gifts, push food on you, or leave food around for you to find. They may try to undermine your efforts deliberately, but most of the time they probably do it without thinking. Here are some suggestions to resist a saboteur:

Create and practice a ready response for when saboteurs push food.
Stand in front of a mirror and act out the script with the ending
you choose. Remember, to handle saboteurs successfully, you
only have to say "no" one more time than they say "have some."
Being prepared to respond appropriately greatly increases your
chances of success. Here are a few lines you can use:

"No thanks. I've had enough."

"Oh, I love your cakes, but I have to take a rain check this
time."

"Losing weight is hard for me. Please help by not offering
food."

"That's so thoughtful of you. I wish I could have some,
but I've made a commitment to myself to eat healthier. I'll
have to pass."

"It looks wonderful, but I'm too full to eat another bite."

*Suggest nonfood activities if you have to spend time with a sabo-
teur.*

*Call ahead to inform the saboteur you won't be eating at his or
her home.* Better yet, invite the saboteur to your house or suggest a nonfood activity.

*Minimize contact with the saboteur, or avoid the saboteur en-
tirely.*

Retreat. If you can't influence the saboteur, remove yourself
from the situation. Leave the party, buffet, or holiday gathering and take a brisk walk.

Take the food but don't eat it. You can always give the food to
someone else or throw it away.

Be sure that you are not a saboteur yourself. We all have the
tendency to persuade guests to try foods that we have made.
Respect others' decisions to pass.

FAQ 13:

Should I be taking a vitamin supplement in order to be truly healthy?
The DASH Diet provides you with all the nutrients you need. I know not everyone starts out following the DASH Diet perfectly. By including a variety of fruits, vegetables, and whole grains in your diet every day, you are most likely doing just fine. But if you feel that you'd like to take a multivitamin supplement as added insurance, that's okay. Taking a multivitamin each day probably isn't necessary, but it won't hurt you. And extra vitamins or minerals as recommended in pregnancy, for older persons, or as recommended by your doctor are a good idea.

FAQ 14:

The DASH Diet encourages seafood. But I have read about chemicals in seafood. So what's the truth—is seafood good for us or not?
Fish and shellfish are an important part of a lower-calorie, healthy diet. They contain high-quality protein and other essential nutrients, are low in saturated fat, and contain omega-3 fatty acids. A balanced diet that includes a variety of fish and shellfish can improve heart health and ensure children's proper growth and development. So where's the problem? There are basically two problem chemicals and they are found in some specific kinds of fish. The chemicals are mercury and PCBs.

MERCURY

Nearly all fish and shellfish contain traces of mercury, which builds up from low levels of mercury in the water. For adults, these small amounts of mercury in seafood are not important. However, mercury may harm an unborn baby or young child's developing nervous system.

The risks from mercury depend on the level of mercury in the fish and how much fish you eat. By following three FDA recommendations for choosing and eating fish or shellfish, pregnant women, women who might become pregnant, nursing mothers, and young children can enjoy the benefits of eating fish and shellfish and minimize their exposure to the harmful effects of mercury. Follow these recommendations when feeding fish and shellfish to young children, but serve smaller portions.

1. Do not eat shark, swordfish, king mackerel, or tilefish (aka golden bass, golden snapper) because these particular fish contain high levels of mercury.
2. You can eat up to 12 ounces (4 DASH servings) per week of fish and shellfish that are lower in mercury. Shrimp, canned light tuna, salmon, pollock, and catfish tend to be lower in mercury. Additionally, the fish used to make fish sticks are commonly made from fish low in mercury (just make sure you bake the fish sticks instead of frying them).
3. Check local advisories for the safety of fish caught by family and friends in your nearby lakes, rivers, and coastal areas. If no advice is available, limit consumption to 6 ounces (2 DASH servings) per week.

If you do not fall into one of the categories of persons to whom the FDA's guidelines are directed, the dangers of harm from eating even those fish considered high in mercury is probably negligible. However, it is best to show caution and restrict your consumption of high-mercury fish to just once a week.

PCBs (POLYCHLORINATED BIPHENYLS)

PCBs have recently been found in salmon, which is otherwise one of the healthiest fish to eat because of the high levels of omega-3 fats in the species. And the PCB levels were higher in farm-raised salmon than those that lived in the wild. So should we now be avoiding salmon? Absolutely not.

The good news for salmon lovers and for those who want to get more healthy omega-3 fats in their diets is that the FDA says it is not necessary to reduce the amount of either farm-raised or wild salmon in your diet. Most farm-raised salmon are generally released into the wild to feed naturally after an initial period in the pen, which reduces the risk of toxins.

Despite these concerns, most kinds of fish can be eaten without cause for concern. The best way to reap the most health benefits from fish and seafood in our diets is to include a wide variety of different types of fish and stick to your recommended DASH servings when choosing portion size.

FAQ 15:
Any ideas for healthier, lower-calorie brown bag lunches?
Sure, packed lunches are great for kids—and they are a low-calorie, healthy way for us grown-ups to stick to our DASH Diet for Weight Loss goals, too. Here are some tips.

Papa's got a brand new bag. If you can't find your old elementary school lunchbox, not to worry—there are new hi-tech versions that will make a stylish accessory for the well-dressed businessperson. Buy a Thermos if you're into soups—a great Hi-Lo-Slo food.

Keep up with your ingredient list. Make sure you have a variety of Hi-Lo-Slo ingredients in your fridge and pantry that can be part of a variety of packed lunches, such as whole-wheat bread and the ingredients for sandwiches (including plenty of good lettuce, tomatoes, and cucumbers), low-fat mayo and mustard, yogurt, small containers of nonfat or 1% milk, small boxes of raisins, rice cakes, small bags of popcorn, etc. Of course, you should always have lots of fruit in your home for snacking, and this fruit can go in your lunchbox, too.

Plan ahead. If you find yourself too rushed to make a packed lunch before you head out the door to work, do a lot of it the night before. Assemble the components of your packed lunch and put them in the lunchbox you can keep in the fridge. To keep your sandwich from getting soggy overnight, put your bread, meat, and veggies in different bags and assemble the sandwich just before you eat it.

Don't forget fluids. Remember to pack something to drink. A small carton of nonfat milk will help you meet your DASH goals for dairy, and is the perfect accompaniment to most meals. If you're a soda-holic, make sure you choose a diet version (of course, water is always a great choice), and get your dairy from yogurt or a slice of low-fat cheese on your sandwich.

Slight indulgence. It's important to restrict fats and sweets in your diet, but as I've said many times before, nothing is completely out of bounds with the DASH Diet. If you know you want something sweet after a meal, pack a few chocolate kisses with your meal. Some food makers now market 100-calorie bags of cookies and crackers. If you have to have a bag of chips with your sandwich, go with a 1-ounce bag—and make sure your sandwich is particularly healthy and stuffed with fresh vegetables.

Be cool. Always put an ice pack in your lunchbox. Place the most perishable items on the ice pack or on a very cold container.

Waste not. Leftovers make great lunchbox items. When cooking the night before, make a little extra and place it directly in an airtight container in the fridge to be added to your packed lunch. Restaurant portions are huge, so when eating out, "doggy-bag" half your meal to put in your lunchbox. You get two meals for the price of one, and don't feel stuffed that night!

Emphasize fruit and dairy. We have found that people have a hard time hitting their daily DASH goals for fruit and dairy if they aren't at least halfway there by lunch. So try to add foods from those groups to your lunch choices. As a reminder, here are the DASH serving equivalents for these two challenging food groups:

Low-Fat Dairy (1 dairy serving each):
1 cup low-fat yogurt
1 cup nonfat or 1% milk
½ cup low-fat cottage cheese
1½ ounces low-fat cheese

Fruit (1 fruit serving each):
1 apple (tennis-ball size)
1 orange (tennis-ball size)
½ medium (7-inch) banana
½ grapefruit
¼ cup dried fruit
½ cup fruit salad
¾ cup fruit juice

Remember that packed lunches are anything but boring. In fact, variety can be the standard, not the exception, so long as you observe some basic guidelines and match your creativity with your nutritional preferences.

FAQ 16:
I do so well all week, but the weekend is always my undoing. Eating out with friends, staying up late, and going out for brunch on Sundays and I'm always right back where I started.
Ignoring your health goals on the weekend can undo much of the good you did for yourself during the week. It's a classic example of taking two steps forward, one step back.
Several studies show that weekends can be a nutritional minefield.

A 2003 study in the journal *Obesity Research* showed that American adults eat about 115 more calories on weekend days than on weekdays. That doesn't seem like much but translates to a 3½-pound weight gain per year!

Why is it some people have trouble sticking to their health goals on weekends? Some reasons are obvious, others less so. More important, what can you do about it?

I DESERVE IT!

I worked hard all week. I should allow myself an indulgence.

There are ways to reward yourself for a hard workweek that *support* your health goals instead of undermining them. Instead of a tub of ice cream, reward your labors with a massage, a movie, or a health-positive gift such as new exercise shoes. If you feel you have to treat yourself with food, make the trip into town for a small ice cream cone or a piece of expensive chocolate that you take the time to savor.

MY SCHEDULE'S ALL MESSED UP.

When everything's topsy-turvy, how can I be expected to stick to my routine?

Just because you don't have a work routine doesn't mean your health goals should suffer. Make a plan in advance for how you're going to keep up with your diet and exercise on the weekend. Instead of telling yourself, *I need to make sure I get some exercise this weekend,* take specific steps ahead of time. These might include scheduling a walk or hike with a friend, an appointment with a personal trainer, a bike ride along the river or lake with your spouse—the list goes on. Make sure your plan includes a time and place.

As for diet, plan for the meals you're going to eat at home. Even if you don't need a meal plan during the week, you should consider making one for the weekend if you expect you'll have trouble. Don't forget to shop for the ingredients ahead of time.

I WANT TO CHILL.

Let me relax on the weekend, take a break from my diet and exercise goals.

All of us need time to unwind, and if you work Monday to Friday, the weekend is a natural time to do it. It's important not to let "relaxing" turn into "vegetating." Take some time to chill out, but find ways to relax other than lying on the couch all day watching television. Most people find it more pleasant to relax after they've had some exercise, so consider scheduling your workout early in the day so you can afford some downtime later on.

Try also to use some of your weekend free time in support of your weight-loss goals. You can shop for and prepare food for the upcoming week, create meal plans, and make arrangements to exercise (call a friend or colleague to schedule a lunchtime walk, book a tennis court, or make an appointment with a personal trainer).

I'LL START AGAIN ON MONDAY.

What the heck, I'll go back to my health goals next week.

If you suspend your commitment to your health program from Friday evening to Monday morning, that's a whopping 36 percent of the week. Just because the weekend *feels* so short doesn't mean it is! Most important, the feelings of regret you experience on Monday morning after letting your health goals fall by the wayside are not worth the fleeting pleasures available. Behavioral experts advise us to "think it through." In other words, on Friday think how you'll feel the next morning or on Monday morning after replacing your nutrition and physical activity program with overeating and under-exercising. Conversely, remember how good it feels to wake up in the morning having stuck to your diet and fitness goals—you feel better physically and psychologically. Feeling like this reinforces your determination and reminds you that *you can do it!*

FAQ 17:

I've heard that skipping meals isn't a great idea when trying to lose weight. If I skip breakfast, doesn't that open up more calories for me to eat later at night when I prefer to snack?

It's perhaps not surprising that some people think simply eliminating a meal from their daily schedule is the easiest way to accomplish weight loss. With our busy lives, breakfast is often the meal people choose to cut from their daily intake.

In fact, the opposite is true, according to at least two studies published in the *Journal of the American Dietetic Association*. These studies have shown that eating a healthy breakfast is one of the indicators of a successful weight-management program. And the National Weight Control Registry has kept track of 10,000 participants who have lost weight and kept it off. Of those successful weight losers, 78 percent eat breakfast.

Why is breakfast so important for a person's weight-management program? There are a couple of reasons. First of all, healthy breakfasts tend to include whole-grain products like cereal or bread. And those foods are high in fiber, so you feel full. Breakfast is also a great place to get your fruit servings as fruit on your cereal or a glass of fruit juice.

The second reason is that eating breakfast makes it more likely you'll eat a healthy lunch. Skipping your morning meal can make you ravenous come lunchtime. Consequently, you may not just overeat but also indulge in food choices that don't fit with your weight-management goals. It's a myth, by the way, that a large breakfast makes you hungrier by midmorning—we all need to eat regularly during the day.

So . . . eat a healthy breakfast and lay the foundation for a healthy day.

FAQ 18:

I love sandwiches, so can you make any suggestions for making this portable meal lower in calories and healthier?

Here are a few tips for a healthier sandwich:

Trim the middle: Ask them to put half as much of the filling on as they usually do, whether it's meat or a meat salad such as tuna fish salad or chicken salad (and ask for low-fat versions of these items if they have them). Avoid processed meats such as salami and bologna.

Go with the grain: Ask for your sandwich on whole-wheat bread. Certain kinds of breads such as bulkie rolls have very little nutritional benefit.

Go green: Ask for twice the usual amount of lettuce and to-mato or sprouts.

Say cheese—maybe: Low-fat cheese, if they have it. If not, skip it.

Spread yourself thin: Choose mustard or reduced-fat mayo, but tell them to go easy on the spread.

Putting it all together, ordering a healthy turkey sandwich might sound like this: "Smoked turkey sandwich. Please just put half the amount of turkey you usually use—two or three slices is fine. I'd like that on whole-wheat bread. If you've got low-fat cheese, that's great; otherwise, no cheese, thanks. Extra lettuce and tomato [or sprouts]. Do you have 'lite' mayo? If not, I'll have a small amount of mustard."

Let's see what you save with just a few alterations:

Regular Deli Sandwich			DASH Deli Sandwich		
Ingredients	Calories	DASH Servings	Ingredients	Calories	DASH Servings
Roast beef, 6 oz.	324	2 meat	Turkey, 3 oz.	90	1 meat
Bulkie roll	250	3 grain	Bread, whole-wheat, 2 slices (1 oz. each)	200	2 grain
Lettuce and tomato	20	½ vegetable	Lettuce and tomato (double)	40	1 vegetable

Regular Deli Sandwich			DASH Deli Sandwich		
Mayo, 3 tbsp.	300	3 added fat	Mustard, 1 tbsp.	10	Mustard is not included in a DASH food group
Cheddar cheese, 3 slices (1 oz. each)	320	2 dairy			
Total	**1,214**		**Total**	**340**	

It's usual to have a beverage and a side order of something along with a sandwich. A bag of baby carrots will give you the crunch you might want from a bag of potato chips. If you must eat the chips, make it a 100-calorie bag. Nonfat milk will provide you with important DASH servings. If it's soda you want because your DASH dairy servings are covered, make it a no-calorie or low-calorie choice.

Using my approach to Hi-Lo-Slo sandwich building, not only are you cutting back on calories, fat, and sodium that in large quantities can be unhealthy, but you are including as part of your lunch foods that are important for health such as vegetables and dairy.

FAQ 19:
I recently lost my job and am wondering—isn't eating low-calorie and healthy food more expensive?

Lower-calorie living can sometimes feel like it's more expensive than the alternative. There's the cost of health club memberships, fresh produce and other healthy foods, and fitness equipment such as walking shoes and bicycles.

My opinion? It will save you money in the long term! Keeping your weight at a healthy level will help prevent the kinds of chronic diseases that can cost you big money. That's because people who are less healthy make less money, have higher insurance costs, and greater out-of-pocket expenses.

A University of Michigan health and retirement study on more than 7,000 men and women between the ages of 57 and 67 found that overweight women had a significantly smaller individual net worth, even after allowing for differences in health, marital status, and other factors. Overweight people earn less than their lean counterparts due to job discrimination (heavier people are less likely to be hired or promoted) and the inability to get or hold down jobs because of diseases and disabilities caused by obesity.

Sometimes it is cheaper to eat in a healthier way. For example, "plain" cereals like cornflakes and oatmeal are much less expensive than sugary processed ones and instant oatmeal with added sugar. Similarly, you can make a delicious spaghetti sauce almost as quickly as heating up a bottle of processed sauce for less money—the key is to have the ingredients on hand. Foods like brown rice and beans can be purchased in bulk for low cost compared to the high calorie and nutrient values they offer.

Here are some other ways to stick to your weight-loss goals and save money:

Eat less meat: To keep calories and saturated fat intake down, the DASH diet is relatively low in meats (especially red meat) compared to the average American diet. Since meat is one of the more expensive items on your shopping list, reducing your meat intake makes DASH more economical than the average American diet. You can cut costs further by replacing the meat in your diet with other protein sources such as legumes—beans and tofu, for example.

Grow your own: Yes, growing your own vegetables is a great way to save money. It's also good exercise. Bringing in tomatoes, lettuce, and herbs from your garden sure beats paying for them at the grocery store!

Brew your own coffee and tea: We all know how expensive it is to buy coffee and tea from upmarket coffee shops. You can save yourself a lot of money by making coffee or tea at home or at work and bringing it with you in a refillable mug. Best of all, this way you can experiment with your own coffee blends and teas, and not need to overload them with high-calorie dairy and sugar.

Eat local: Shopping at farmers' markets during the local growing season can be a great way to save on fresh fruits and vegetables, my top-rated Hi-Lo-Slo foods. Not just that, but you're supporting your local farmers and doing your bit for the environment, since these products don't have to be shipped from far away using fossil fuels. It's always a good idea to compare the cost of the products you're buying there with those found at your local supermarket. Not all farmers' markets save you money, but most do.

Quit cold cereals and cook oatmeal: Typical breakfast cereals are incredibly expensive. The good news is that there is a very inexpensive (and healthier) alternative to expensive cereals—oatmeal! You can make oatmeal with skim milk and add all sorts of fruits and nuts for a breakfast far healthier than any that comes in a box.

Eat in: Preparing your meals at home is always more economical than ordering in or going to a restaurant. Plus you can be sure you'll be eating Hi-Lo-Slo foods if you prepare them yourself. If you need some ideas for DASH-friendly meals, check out our meal plans—complete with recipes.

Skip bottled water—and *soda!* Most communities have healthy water and yet many of us continue to purchase bottled water thinking it is healthier. Buy a refillable container and fill it with water from your kitchen faucet and you'll be saving money—and saving the environment. If your local water isn't good, look into installing a filter. That still might be a cheaper solution than buying bottled water.

As for soda, Americans guzzle gallons of it a week, according to statistics. Some say the amount of it we drink accounts for the rise in obesity. Diet soda may be better for your waistline than regular soda, but it still hits you in the wallet. Drink tap water instead of soda, and your pocketbook—and waistline—will thank you.

As you can see, the down economy is no reason to cut back on your weight-loss efforts. You can eat healthy foods and also be frugal in these tough economic times, all the while sticking to your weight-loss goals.

FAQ 20:
Is it really true there's a connection between sleeping poorly and being overweight?
Regular sleep benefits many aspects of health, and that includes keeping weight down. This information comes from the ongoing National Health and Nutrition Examination Survey, which has lasted over thirty years. The study revealed that those participants who got less than seven hours of sleep a night were more likely to be obese. Even if they weren't already obese, people who slept less were more likely to become obese later on. Participants who slept just five hours per night were 73 percent more likely to become obese than those who got seven to nine nightly hours of sleep. Just one hour of sleep can make a significant difference—those who got six hours of sleep were 27 percent more likely to become obese than those who slept seven to nine hours per night. Those who slept the least were most likely to become obese—two to four hours of sleep resulted in a 67 percent increased chance of obesity compared to those who slept seven to nine hours.

A study at Britain's University of Warwick found comparable results. By studying 28,000 children and 15,000 adults, researchers found that sleeping less than five hours a night almost doubled the risk of obesity, greater increase in body mass index, and waist circumference over time.

So there you have it—getting a good night's sleep is vital for many aspects of our health. Here are some tips for how to achieve that nightly rest:

- Establish a regular pattern. Try to go to bed and get up at the same time every day.
- Avoid caffeine after lunchtime and avoid alcohol near bedtime. The famous nightcap might help you get to sleep but often causes awakening in the middle of the night.
- Don't exercise within four hours of retiring. Daytime exercise is great, but exercising before bedtime can be a source of stimulation and make it difficult to get to sleep.
- Avoid naps during the day and especially in the evening. Concentrate your sleep into the nighttime period.
- Begin to wind down an hour before bedtime. Avoid activities that might tend to wake you up.
- Don't stay up late to watch TV. Record it to watch later, or catch the details in the morning.

FAQ 21:

My weight-loss goals go out the window when I'm on the road. How can I stick to my goals when I'm on vacation?

We all love our vacation getaways, but we can feel we've let ourselves down if we return knowing we haven't been meeting our weight-management goals while traveling. What's more dispiriting than getting on the scale at home after you set your bags down to find you've gained 5 pounds in just a week away? Bottom line: You don't have to choose between a fun and enjoyable vacation on the one hand and meeting your weight goals on the other. These are not mutually exclusive!

How to enjoy a vacation that's enjoyable and also in line with your health goals? First of all, it's important not to overeat, and to stick to your customized DASH Diet for Weight Loss eating plan as much as possible.

Perhaps even more important is to be physically active while you're on vacation. After all, when we're in our usual routines it can be difficult to find time to exercise, but during our vacations all those hours in the day cry out to be filled with fun physical activity.

Exercise burns calories and makes us feel better, too. Adding ex-

ercise to your vacation can also enhance your vacation experience because it usually involves activities that get you off the beach towel or
chaise longue and involved in some activities that you don't get to do
at home, whether it's snorkeling, kayaking, or hiking.

Here are some tips for enjoying a fun- and activity-filled vacation
that will enable you to stick to your weight-management goals:

- Choose a vacation that offers fun physical activity options (kayaking, skiing, snorkeling, etc.). Research them ahead of time and
  come prepared.
- Take your walking shoes and other exercise clothing, and a pedometer if you own one.
- Enjoy a brisk morning walk before or after breakfast. Not a morning person? Do it after dinner.
- In addition to your morning walk, find one physically active
  thing to do every day, whether it's hiking or a walking tour of local sights or kayaking. Dancing counts!
- Choose a restaurant a good distance away for dinner, and walk
  there and back.

If you find you really enjoy the feeling of being active on vacation, consider taking an exercise-focused vacation the next time you
go away.

Part 3

Meal Plans

MEAL PLANS are a great way to get started quickly on a new dietary pattern. They leave out all of the guesswork! By following meal plans, you know you are eating the right number of calories each day, as well as getting the right number of servings from each DASH food group. Meal plans are also great teaching tools. Following a meal plan helps you learn about how to estimate a DASH serving of pasta or meat or just about any other food.

Here is where we will let you in on a little secret. We know from experience that people starting on a new diet *want* meal plans. When we start a new eating pattern, knowing what and how much to choose can be overwhelming. Meal plans spell it all out. Easy, right? Well, not quite.

In some ways, meal plans can be difficult to follow. Our seven-day meal plans lay out all your meals for a week. And breakfast is different every day, and so is lunch, and so is dinner. Most of us don't eat a different breakfast on each of the seven days of the week, and then a different lunch as well. It's a lot of work to eat that way. Not to mention, it can be expensive. If you are going to eat only ½ cup of grapes twice each week, how much do you buy? If you run into this same issue with all of the fruits and vegetables in your meal plan, you have to be a pretty savvy shopper so you aren't left with a refrigerator full of uneaten produce at the end of the week. In addition, maybe you won't like what we lay out for lunch on Day 2 or dinner on Day 6. So the best way to use our meal plans is to use swapping and substitution.

"Swapping" is the term we use for taking an entire meal, say lunch on Day 1, and using it on multiple days of the week. That's easy to do and easy to understand. "Substitution" is a little bit more difficult. Here you omit one item in a meal plan and substitute with another item that's equivalent. A good substitution is a food that has a similar calorie content and has the same number of DASH servings. So, for example, let's say your lunch meal plan calls for blueberries, but you don't have blueberries in your house. Substituting ½ cup of fresh pineapple chunks at 40 calories and 1 DASH serving of fruit for ½ cup of blueberries at 45 calories and 1 DASH serving of fruit is near perfect. A less perfect substitution would be ½ cup of sliced banana (at 70 calories) or ¾ cup of orange juice (at 80 calories). Both the banana and orange juice are 1 DASH serving of fruit, but are higher in calories than the blueberries would have been. Consistently making substitutions that are higher in calories (more calorically dense) are going to put you over your calorie target and slow your weight loss.

But don't get stressed about this. Even if you don't follow every meal plan to the letter every day, if you use them as a guide and try to pick Hi-Lo-Slo foods to meet your DASH goals, when you deviate from the meal plans you will be doing just fine.

Meat-Eater Meal Plans

||||||||||||||||||||||||||||||||||||||||||||||||||||||||||||||||||||||||||||||||||||||||||||||||||||||||||||

1,200 CALORIES: DAY 1
Target: 5 grain, 3 fruit, 4 vegetable, 2 dairy, 1½ meat, ¼ nuts/seeds/legumes,
*   ½ added fat, ½ sweets*

Breakfast *(160 calories)*
1 ounce bran flakes (about ¾ cup), *1 grain (90 calories)*
½ cup fresh strawberries, *1 fruit (25 calories)*
½ cup nonfat milk, *½ dairy (45 calories)*

Morning Snack *(150 calories)*
1 small low-fat granola bar, *1 grain (100 calories)*
1 medium apple, *1 fruit (50 calories)*

Lunch *(375 calories)*
2½ cups mixed raw leafy greens and vegetables (bell peppers, carrots, etc.),
   2½ vegetable (50 calories)
3 ounces grilled skinless chicken breast, *1 meat (150 calories)*
1 tablespoon unsalted, roasted sunflower seeds, *½ nuts/seeds/legumes*
   (50 calories)
1 tablespoon low-fat creamy Italian dressing, *½ added fat (40 calories)*
Half a 7-inch whole-wheat pita pocket, *1 grain (85 calories)*

Afternoon Snack *(160 calories)*
1 cup nonfat vanilla yogurt, *1 dairy (160 calories)*

Dinner *(310 calories)*
Piled-High Veggie Pizza (⅙ of a 14-inch pizza) (see recipe), *2 grain, 2 vegetable, ½ dairy (250 calories)*
1 medium orange, *1 fruit (60 calories)*

Evening Snack/Dessert *(40 calories)*
2 dark chocolate kisses, *½ sweets (40 calories)*

Nutrition analysis for the day: 1,995 calories, 5 grain, 3 fruit, 4½ vegetable, 2 dairy, 1 meat, ½ nuts/seeds/legumes, ½ added fat, ½ sweets

|||||||||||||||||||||||||||||||||||||||||||||||||||||||||||||||||||||||||||||||||||||||||||||||||||||||||||

1,200 CALORIES: DAY 2

Target: 5 grain, 3 fruit, 4 vegetable, 2 dairy, 1½ meat, ¼ nuts/seeds/legumes, ½ added fat, ½ sweets

Breakfast *(215 calories)*
1 ounce uncooked oatmeal, cooked with water (cooks to about ¾ cup), *1 grain (100 calories)*
½ cup cubed cantaloupe, *1 fruit (25 calories)*
1 cup nonfat milk, *1 dairy (90 calories)*

Morning Snack *(180 calories)*
1 ounce honey whole-wheat pretzels, *1 grain (110 calories)*
2 tablespoons hummus, *¼ nuts/seeds/legumes (70 calories)*

Lunch *(225 calories)*
Veggie Melt Panini made with just one slice of bread (see recipe), *1 grain, 2 vegetable, 1 dairy (225 calories)*

Afternoon Snack *(35 calories)*
½ cup mixed fresh berries, *1 fruit (35 calories)*

Dinner *(500 calories)*
4½ ounces grilled chicken, *1½ meat (200 calories)*
1 cup Roasted Cauliflower (see recipe), *2 vegetable (100 calories)*
1 cup cooked brown rice, *2 grain (200 calories)*

Evening Snack/Dessert *(60 calories)*
½ Baked Banana (see recipe), *1 fruit, ½ sweets (60 calories)*

Nutrition analysis for the day: 1,215 calories, 5 grain, 3 fruit, 4 vegetable, 2 dairy, 1½ meat, ¼ nuts/seeds/legumes, 0 added fat, ½ sweets

||||||||||||||||||||||||||||||||||||||||||||||||||||||||||||||||||||||||||||||||||||||||||||||||||||||||||||||||||||

1,200 CALORIES: DAY 3

Target: 5 grain, 3 fruit, 4 vegetable, 2 dairy, 1½ meat, ¼ nuts/seeds/legumes, ½ added fat, ½ sweets

Breakfast *(195 calories)*
6 egg whites, scrambled (cooked with cooking spray), *1 meat (100 calories)*
One 1-ounce slice whole-wheat bread, toasted, *1 grain (80 calories)*
½ teaspoon trans-fat-free margarine, *½ added fat (15 calories)*

Morning Snack *(115 calories)*
1 cup nonfat milk, *1 dairy (90 calories)*
½ cup fresh strawberries, *1 fruit (25 calories)*

Lunch *(255 calories)*
2½ cups mixed raw leafy greens and vegetables (peppers, carrots, etc.), *2½ vegetables (50 calories)*
¾ ounce shredded low-fat cheddar cheese (about 3 tablespoons), *½ dairy (40 calories)*
1½ ounces skinless grilled chicken breast, *½ meat (75 calories)*
2 tablespoons fat-free Italian dressing *(15 calories)*
One 4-inch whole-wheat pita pocket, *1 grain (75 calories)*

Afternoon Snack *(160 calories)*
½ cup fresh raspberries, *1 fruit (30 calories)*
2 teaspoons chocolate syrup, *½ sweets (30 calories)*
1 small low-fat granola bar, *1 grain (100 calories)*

Dinner *(530 calories)*
1 cup Fruity Chicken Stir-Fry (see recipe), *1 fruit, 1 vegetable, ½ meat (330 calories)*
1 cup cooked brown rice, *2 grain (200 calories)*

Nutrition analysis for the day: 1,255 calories, 5 grain, 3 fruit, 3½ vegetable, 1½ dairy, 2 meat, 0 nuts/seeds/legumes, ½ added fat, ½ sweets

||||||||||||||||||||||||||||||||||||||||||||||||||||||||||||||||||||||||||||||||||||||||||||||||||||||||||||||||||||||||||||

1,200 CALORIES: DAY 4
Target: 5 grain, 3 fruit, 4 vegetable, 2 dairy, 1½ meat, ¼ nuts/seeds/legumes,
½ added fat, ½ sweets

Breakfast *(225 calories)*
1 ounce toasted oat cereal, *1 grain (100 calories)*
½ cup mixed fresh berries, *1 fruit (35 calories)*
1 cup nonfat milk, *1 dairy (90 calories)*

Morning Snack *(25 calories)*
½ cup sliced melon, *1 fruit (25 calories)*

Lunch *(345 calories)*
3 ounces sliced roasted turkey breast, *1 meat (115 calories)*
One 4-inch whole-wheat pita pocket, *1 grain (75 calories)*
4 slices tomato, *1 vegetable (20 calories)*
4 leaves romaine lettuce, *1 vegetable (20 calories)*
1 teaspoon deli mustard *(5 calories)*
One 1-ounce snack bag pretzels, *1 grain (110 calories)*

Afternoon Snack *(110 calories)*
1 medium apple, *1 fruit (60 calories)*
1½ teaspoons peanut butter, *¼ nuts/seeds/legumes (50 calories)*

Dinner *(395 calories)*
1 Chicken Caesar Wrap (see recipe), *2 vegetable, ½ meat, 2 grain, ½ dairy, 1 added fat*
    (395 calories)

Evening Snack/Dessert *(60 calories)*
1 snack-size peppermint patty, *½ sweets (60 calories)*

Nutrition analysis for the day: 1,160 calories, 5 grain, 3 fruit, 4 vegetable, 1½ dairy,
1½ meat, ¼ nuts/seeds/legumes, 1 added fat, ½ sweets

|||||||||||||||||||||||||||||||||||||||||||||||||||||||||||||||||||||||||||||||||||||||||||||||||||||||||||||||||

1,200 CALORIES: DAY 5
Target: 5 grain, 3 fruit, 4 vegetable, 2 dairy, 1½ meat, ¼ nuts/seeds/legumes,
    ½ added fat, ½ sweets

Breakfast *(250 calories)*
1 Low-Fat Blueberry Muffin (see recipe), *2 grain (200 calories)*
1 medium apple, *1 fruit (50 calories)*

Morning Snack *(75 calories)*
¼ cup sliced nectarine, *1 fruit (35 calories)*
¾ ounce (1 small slice) low-fat cheddar cheese, *½ dairy (40 calories)*

Lunch *(310 calories)*
1 Cobb Salad (see recipe), *4 vegetable, ½ dairy, ½ meat, 1 added fat (225 calories)*
Half a 7-inch whole-wheat pita pocket, *1 grain (85 calories)*

Afternoon Snack *(105 calories)*
4 celery sticks (5 inches each), *1 vegetable (5 calories)*
1 tablespoon peanut butter, *½ nuts/seeds/legumes (100 calories)*

Dinner *(345 calories)*
Shrimp Scampi, 3 ounces shrimp with sauce (see recipe), *1 meat (145 calories)*
1 cup cooked whole-wheat linguine, *2 grain (200 calories)*

Evening Snack/Dessert *(165 calories)*
½ cup low-fat frozen yogurt, *1 dairy (140 calories)*
½ cup fresh strawberries, *1 fruit (25 calories)*

Nutrition analysis for the day: 1,250 calories, 5 grain, 3 fruit, 5 vegetable, 2 dairy,
1½ meat, ½ nuts/seeds/legumes, 1 added fat, 0 sweets

|||||||||||||||||||||||||||||||||||||||||||||||||||||||||||||||||||||||||||||||||||||||||||||||||||||||||||||||||

1,200 CALORIES: DAY 6
Target: 5 grain, 3 fruit, 4 vegetable, 2 dairy, 1½ meat, ¼ nuts/seeds/legumes,
    ½ added fat, ½ sweets

Breakfast *(170 calories)*
1 medium low-fat granola bar, *2 grain (140 calories)*
1 medium peach, *1 fruit (30 calories)*

Morning Snack *(130 calories)*
1 cup nonfat plain Greek-style yogurt, *1 dairy (130 calories)*

Lunch *(340 calories)*
Hummus sandwich with fresh tomatoes:
    Half a 7-inch whole-wheat pita pocket, *1 grain (85 calories)*
    ¾ ounce (1 thin slice) low-fat swiss cheese, *½ dairy (40 calories)*
    2 tablespoons hummus, *¼ nuts/seeds/legumes (70 calories)*
    3 thick slices tomato, *1 vegetable (15 calories)*
    ½ cup bean sprouts, *½ vegetable (15 calories)*
2 cups Simple Spinach Salad (see recipe), *2 vegetable, ¼ dairy, 1 added fat (115 calories)*

Afternoon Snack *(110 calories)*
1 ounce unsalted mini pretzels (about ½ cup), *1 grain (110 calories)*

Dinner *(370 calories)*
4 ounces Poached Salmon (see recipe), *1⅓ meat (195 calories)*
½ cup Roasted Brussels Sprouts (see recipe), *1 vegetable (50 calories)*
⅔ cup Quinoa, Corn, and Black Bean Salad (see recipe), *1 grain, ¼ vegetable, ¼ nuts/
    seeds/legumes (125 calories)*

Evening Snack/Dessert *(75 calories)*
1 cup fresh strawberries, *2 fruit (50 calories)*
1½ teaspoons sugar, *½ sweets (25 calories)*

*Nutrition analysis for the day: 1,195 calories, 5 grain, 3 fruit, 4¾ vegetable,
1¾ dairy, 1⅓ meat, ½ nuts/seeds/legumes, 1 added fat, ½ sweets*

1,200 CALORIES: DAY 7
*Target: 5 grain, 3 fruit, 4 vegetable, 2 dairy, 1½ meat, ¼ nuts/seeds/legumes,
    ½ added fat, ½ sweets*

Breakfast *(280 calories)*
1½ ounces shredded wheat squares, *1½ grain (150 calories)*
1 cup nonfat milk, *1 dairy (90 calories)*
½ cup blueberries, *1 fruit (40 calories)*

Morning Snack *(160 calories)*
1 ounce unsalted pretzels, *1 grain (110 calories)*
½ cup grapes, *1 fruit (50 calories)*

Lunch *(240 calories)*
Toasted cheese sandwich:
> Half a 7-inch whole-wheat pita pocket, *1 grain (85 calories)*
> 1½ ounces low-fat cheddar cheese (2 slices), *1 dairy (75 calories)*
1 cup baby carrots, *2 vegetable (50 calories)*
2 tablespoons fat-free ranch dressing *(30 calories)*

Afternoon Snack *(80 calories)*
2 dark-chocolate-covered strawberries, *1 fruit, ½ sweets (80 calories)*

Dinner *(310 calories)*
4 ounces baked cod,* *1⅓ meat (120 calories)*

*Place fish on a baking sheet sprayed with cooking spray. Bake at 425°F for 15 minutes or until fish flakes with a fork.

½ cup (5–6 small spears) Roasted Asparagus (see recipe), *1 vegetable (40 calories)*
½ small (2-ounce) whole-wheat dinner roll, *1 grain (75 calories)*
1 cup mixed raw leafy greens, *1 vegetable (15 calories)*
1 tablespoon Lemon Caper Vinaigrette (see recipe), *1 added fat (60 calories)*

Evening Snack/Dessert *(100 calories)*
1 small low-fat granola bar, *1 grain (100 calories)*

Nutrition analysis for the day: 1,170 calories, 5½ grain, 3 fruit, 4 vegetable, 2 dairy, 1⅓ meat, 0 nuts/seeds/legumes, 1 added fat, ½ sweets

||||||||||||||||||||||||||||||||||||||||||||||||||||||||||||||||||||||||||||||||||||||||||||||||||||||

1,400 CALORIES: DAY 1
Target: 5 grain, 4 fruit, 4 vegetable, 2 dairy, 1½ meat, ¼ nuts/seeds/legumes, ½ added fat, ½ sweets

Breakfast *(205 calories)*
1 ounce bran flakes (about ¾ cup), *1 grain (90 calories)*
½ cup sliced banana, *1 fruit (70 calories)*
½ cup nonfat milk, *½ dairy (45 calories)*

Morning Snack *(150 calories)*
1 small low-fat granola bar, *1 grain (100 calories)*
1 medium apple, *1 fruit (50 calories)*

Lunch *(465 calories)*
2½ cups mixed raw leafy greens and vegetables (bell peppers, carrots, etc.),
    2½ vegetable (50 calories)
4 ounces grilled skinless chicken breast, *1⅓ meat (160 calories)*
1 hard-boiled egg, *⅓ meat (80 calories)*
1 tablespoon unsalted roasted sunflower seeds, *½ nuts/seeds/legumes (50 calories)*
1 tablespoon low-fat creamy Italian dressing, *½ added fat (40 calories)*
Half a 7-inch whole-wheat pita pocket, *1 grain (85 calories)*

Afternoon Snack *(220 calories)*
1 cup nonfat vanilla yogurt, *1 dairy (160 calories)*
1 medium orange, *1 fruit (60 calories)*

Dinner *(305 calories)*
Piled-High Veggie Pizza (⅙ of a 14-inch pizza) (see recipe), *2 grain, 2 vegetable, ½ dairy*
    (250 calories)
½ cup sliced mango, *1 fruit (55 calories)*

Evening Snack/Dessert *(40 calories)*
2 dark chocolate kisses, *½ sweets (40 calories)*

Nutrition analysis for the day: 1,385 calories, 5 grain, 4 fruit, 4½ vegetable,
2 dairy, 1⅔ meat, ½ nuts/seeds/legumes, ½ added fat, ½ sweets

||||||||||||||||||||||||||||||||||||||||||||||||||||||||||||||||||||||||||||||||||||||||||||||||||

1,400 CALORIES: DAY 2
Target: 5 grain, 4 fruit, 4 vegetable, 2 dairy, 1½ meat, ¼ nuts/seeds/legumes,
    ½ added fat, ½ sweets

Breakfast *(250 calories)*
1 ounce uncooked oatmeal cooked with water (cooks to about ¾ cup), *1 grain*
    (100 calories)
1 medium orange, *1 fruit (60 calories)*
1 cup nonfat milk, *1 dairy (90 calories)*

Morning Snack *(230 calories)*
1 ounce whole-wheat snack crackers, *1 grain (130 calories)*
1 tablespoon peanut butter, *½ nuts/seeds/legumes (100 calories)*

Lunch *(335 calories)*
1 Veggie Melt Panini (see recipe), *2 grain, 2 vegetable, 1 dairy (335 calories)*

Afternoon Snack *(115 calories)*

½ cup nonfat vanilla yogurt, *½ dairy (80 calories)*
½ cup fresh berries, *1 fruit (35 calories)*

Dinner *(365 calories)*

4½ ounces grilled skinless chicken breast, *1½ meat (165 calories)*
1 cup Roasted Cauliflower (see recipe), *2 vegetable (100 calories)*
½ cup cooked brown rice, *1 grain (100 calories)*

Evening Snack/Dessert *(120 calories)*

1 Baked Banana (see recipe), *2 fruit, 1 sweets (120 calories)*

*Nutrition analysis for the day: 1,415 calories, 5 grain, 4 fruit, 4 vegetable,
2 ½ dairy, 1 ½ meat, ½ nuts/seeds/legumes, 0 added fat, 1 sweets*

IIIIIIIIIIIIIIIIIIIIIIIIIIIIIIIIIIIIIIIIIIIIIIIIIIIIIIIIIIIIIIIIIIIIIIIIIIIIIIIIIIIIIIIIIIIIIIIIIIIIIIIIIIIIIIIIIIIIIII

1,400 CALORIES: DAY 3

*Target: 5 grain, 4 fruit, 4 vegetable, 2 dairy, 1½ meat, ¼ nuts/seeds/legumes,
     ½ added fat, ½ sweets*

Breakfast *(180 calories)*

6 egg whites or ¾ cup egg substitute, scrambled (cooked with cooking spray), *1 meat
     (100 calories)*
One 1-ounce slice whole-wheat bread, toasted, *1 grain (80 calories)*

Morning Snack *(130 calories)*

1 medium peach, *1 fruit (30 calories)*
1 small low-fat granola bar, *1 grain (100 calories)*

Lunch *(350 calories)*

3 cups mixed raw leafy greens and vegetables, *3 vegetables (60 calories)*
1½ ounces reduced-fat cheddar cheese (about ⅓ cup shredded), *1 dairy (120 calories)*
1½ ounces skinless grilled chicken breast, *½ meat (55 calories)*
1 tablespoon reduced-fat ranch dressing, *½ added fat (40 calories)*
One 4-inch pita pocket, *1 grain (75 calories)*

Afternoon Snack *(270 calories)*

1 ounce unsalted mini pretzels (about ½ cup), *1 grain (110 calories)*
½ cup low-fat cottage cheese, *1 dairy (80 calories)*
1 cup pineapple chunks, *2 fruit (80 calories)*

Dinner *(430 calories)*

1 cup Fruity Chicken Stir-Fry (see recipe), *1 fruit, 1 vegetable, ½ meat (330 calories)*
½ cup cooked brown rice, *1 grain (100 calories)*

Evening Snack/Dessert *(60 calories)*
5 Tootsie Rolls, *½ sweets (60 calories)*

Nutrition analysis for the day: 1,420 calories, 5 grain, 4 fruit, 4 vegetable, 2 dairy, 2 meat, 0 nuts/seeds/legumes, ½ added fat, ½ sweets

‖‖‖

1,400 CALORIES: DAY 4
Target: 5 grain, 4 fruit, 4 vegetable, 2 dairy, 1½ meat, ¼ nuts/seeds/legumes, ½ added fat, ½ sweets

Breakfast *(260 calories)*
1 ounce toasted oat cereal, *1 grain (100 calories)*
½ cup sliced banana, *1 fruit (70 calories)*
1 cup nonfat milk, *1 dairy (90 calories)*

Morning Snack *(105 calories)*
1 cup unsweetened applesauce, *2 fruit (105 calories)*

Lunch *(345 calories)*
3 ounces sliced roasted turkey breast, *1 meat (115 calories)*
One 4-inch whole-wheat pita pocket, *1 grain (75 calories)*
4 slices tomato, *1 vegetable (20 calories)*
4 leaves romaine lettuce, *1 vegetable (20 calories)*
1 teaspoon deli mustard *(5 calories)*
One 1-ounce snack bag unsalted pretzels, *1 grain (110 calories)*

Afternoon Snack *(110 calories)*
1 medium apple, *1 fruit (60 calories)*
1½ teaspoons peanut butter, *¼ nuts/seeds/legumes (50 calories)*

Dinner *(395 calories)*
1 Chicken Caesar Wrap (see recipe), *2 vegetable, ½ meat, 2 grain, ½ dairy, 1 added fat (395 calories)*

Evening Snack/Dessert *(130 calories)*
¼ cup low-fat frozen yogurt, *½ dairy (70 calories)*
1 snack-size peppermint patty, *½ sweets (60 calories)*

Nutrition analysis for the day: 1,345 calories, 5 grain, 4 fruit, 4 vegetable, 2 dairy, 1½ meat, ¼ nuts/seeds/legumes, 1 added fat, ½ sweets

1,400 CALORIES: DAY 5
Target: 5 grain, 4 fruit, 4 vegetable, 2 dairy, 1½ meat, ¼ nuts/seeds/legumes, ½ added fat, ½ sweets

Breakfast *(290 calories)*
1 Low-Fat Blueberry Muffins (see recipe), *2 grain (200 calories)*
1 cup nonfat milk, *1 dairy (90 calories)*

Morning Snack *(110 calories)*
1 cup sliced mango, *2 fruit (110 calories)*

Lunch *(365 calories)*
1 Cobb Salad (see recipe), *4 vegetable, ½ dairy, ½ meat, 1 added fat (225 calories)*
½ cup low-fat vanilla yogurt, *½ dairy (80 calories)*
1 medium orange, *1 fruit (60 calories)*

Afternoon Snack *(180 calories)*
One 1-ounce slice whole-wheat bread, toasted, *1 grain (80 calories)*
1 tablespoon peanut butter, *½ nuts/seeds/legumes (100 calories)*

Dinner *(345 calories)*
Shrimp Scampi (see recipe), 3 ounces shrimp with sauce (see recipe), *1 meat (145 calories)*
1 cup whole-wheat linguine, *2 grain (200 calories)*

Evening Snack/Dessert *(105 calories)*
1 medium apple, *1 fruit (50 calories)*
2 tablespoons low-fat caramel sauce, *½ sweets (55 calories)*

Nutrition analysis for the day: 1,395 calories, 5 grain, 4 fruit, 4 vegetable, 2 dairy, 1½ meat, ½ nuts/seeds/legumes, 1 added fat, ½ sweets

1,400 CALORIES: DAY 6
Target: 5 grain, 4 fruit, 4 vegetable, 2 dairy, 1½ meat, ¼ nuts/seeds/legumes, ½ added fat, ½ sweets

Breakfast *(255 calories)*
1 small low-fat granola bar, *1 grain (100 calories)*
1 cup sliced peaches, *2 fruit (65 calories)*
1 cup nonfat milk, *1 dairy (90 calories)*

Morning Snack *(110 calories)*
3 cups air-popped popcorn, *1 grain (110 calories)*
Sparkling water with a squeeze of orange *(0 calories)*

Lunch *(290 calories)*
Hummus sandwich with fresh tomatoes:
    Half a 7-inch whole-wheat pita pocket, *1 grain (85 calories)*
    2 tablespoons hummus, *¼ nuts/seeds/legumes (50 calories)*
    3 thick slices tomato, *1 vegetable (15 calories)*
    ½ cup bean sprouts, *½ vegetable (15 calories)*
    ½ cup mixed raw leafy greens, *½ vegetable (10 calories)*
2 cups Simple Spinach Salad (see recipe), *2 vegetable, ¼ dairy, 1 added fat (115 calories)*

Afternoon Snack *(270 calories)*
1 ounce unsalted mini pretzels (about ½ cup), *1 grain (110 calories)*
1 cup nonfat vanilla yogurt, *1 dairy (160 calories)*

Dinner *(340 calories)*
4½ ounces Poached Salmon (see recipe), *1½ meat (215 calories)*
⅔ cup Quinoa, Corn, and Black Bean Salad (see recipe), *1 grain, ¼ vegetable, ¼ nuts/
    seeds/legumes (125 calories)*

Evening Snack/Dessert *(75 calories)*
1 cup fresh strawberries, *2 fruit (50 calories)*
1½ teaspoon sugar, *½ sweets (25 calories)*

*Nutrition analysis for the day: 1,340 calories, 5 grain, 4 fruit, 4¼ vegetable,
2¼ dairy, 1½ meat, ½ nuts/seeds, 1 added fat, ½ sweets*

||||||||||||||||||||||||||||||||||||||||||||||||||||||||||||||||||||||||||||||||||||||||||||||||||||

1,400 CALORIES: DAY 7
*Target: 5 grain, 4 fruit, 4 vegetable, 2 dairy, 1½ meat, ¼ nuts/seeds/legumes,
    ½ added fat, ½ sweets*

Breakfast *(320 calories)*
1½ ounces shredded wheat squares, *1½ grain (150 calories)*
1 tablespoon flaxseeds, *½ nuts/seeds/legumes (40 calories)*
1 cup nonfat milk, *1 dairy (90 calories)*
½ cup blueberries, *1 fruit (40 calories)*

Morning Snack *(210 calories)*
1 ounce unsalted pretzels, *1 grain (110 calories)*
¼ cup dried cherries, *1 fruit (100 calories)*

Lunch *(240 calories)*
Toasted cheese sandwich:
>Half a 7-inch whole-wheat pita pocket, *1 grain (85 calories)*
>1½ ounces low-fat cheddar cheese (about 2 slices), *1 dairy (75 calories)*
1 cup sliced carrots, *2 vegetable (50 calories)*
2 tablespoons fat-free ranch dressing *(30 calories)*

Afternoon Snack *(50 calories)*
½ cup grapes, *1 fruit (50 calories)*

Dinner *(455 calories)*
5 ounces baked cod,* *1⅔ meat (150 calories)*
1 cup (10–12 small spears) Roasted Asparagus (see recipe), *2 vegetable (80 calories)*
1 small (2-ounce) whole-wheat dinner roll, *2 grain (150 calories)*
1 cup mixed raw leafy greens, *1 vegetable (15 calories)*
1 tablespoon Lemon Caper Vinaigrette (see recipe), *1 added fat (60 calories)*

*Place fish on a baking sheet sprayed with cooking spray. Bake at 425°F for 15 minutes or until fish flakes with a fork.

Evening Snack/Dessert *(80 calories)*
2 dark-chocolate-covered strawberries, *1 fruit, ½ sweets (80 calories)*

Nutrition analysis for the day: 1,355 calories, 5½ grain, 4 fruit, 5 vegetable, 2 dairy, 1⅔ meat, ½ nuts/seeds, 1 added fat, ½ sweets

||||||||||||||||||||||||||||||||||||||||||||||||||||||||||||||||||||||||||||||||||||||||||||||||||||||||

1,600 CALORIES: DAY 1
Target: 6 grain, 4 fruit, 4 vegetable, 2 dairy, 1½ meat, ¼ nuts/seeds/legumes,
*   1 added fat, ½ sweets*

Breakfast *(350 calories)*
1 cup low-fat fruited yogurt, *1 dairy (200 calories)*
1 ounce low-fat granola (about ¼ cup), *1 grain (110 calories)*
½ cup blueberries, *1 fruit (40 calories)*

Morning Snack *(150 calories)*
1 small low-fat granola bar, *1 grain (100 calories)*
1 medium apple, *1 fruit (50 calories)*

Lunch *(525 calories)*
2½ cups mixed raw leafy greens and vegetables (bell peppers, carrots, etc.),
>2½ vegetable (50 calories)*

4 ounces grilled skinless chicken breast, *1⅓ meat (200 calories)*
1 hard-boiled egg, *⅓ meat (80 calories)*
1 tablespoon unsalted, roasted sunflower seeds, *½ nuts/seeds/legumes (50 calories)*
2 tablespoons low-fat balsamic vinaigrette, *1 added fat (60 calories)*
Half a 7-inch whole-wheat pita pocket, *1 grain (85 calories)*

Afternoon Snack *(185 calories)*
½ cup low-fat cottage cheese, *1 dairy (80 calories)*
1 medium (7-inch) banana, *2 fruit (105 calories)*

Dinner *(250 calories)*
Piled-High Veggie Pizza (⅙ of a 14-inch pizza) (see recipe), *2 grain, 2 vegetable, ½ dairy*
    (250 calories)

Evening Snack/Dessert *(170 calories)*
2 dark chocolate kisses, *½ sweets (50 calories)*
2 graham cracker rectangles, *1 grain (120 calories)*

Nutrition analysis for the day: 1,630 calories, 6 grain, 4 fruit, 4 ½ vegetable,
2 ½ dairy, 1⅔ meat, ½ nuts/seeds/legumes, 1 added fat, ½ sweets

||||||||||||||||||||||||||||||||||||||||||||||||||||||||||||||||||||||||||||||||||||||||||||||||||||||||

1,600 CALORIES: DAY 2
Target: 6 grain, 4 fruit, 4 vegetable, 2 dairy, 1½ meat, ¼ nuts/seeds/legumes,
    1 added fat, ½ sweets

Breakfast *(315 calories)*
1 ounce uncooked oatmeal cooked with water (cooks to about ¾ cup), *1 grain*
    (100 calories)
¼ cup raisins, *1 fruit (110 calories)*
1 cup low-fat milk, *1 dairy (110 calories)*

Morning Snack *(200 calories)*
1 ounce unsalted whole-wheat mini pretzels (about ½ cup), *1 grain (100 calories)*
1 tablespoon peanut butter, *½ nuts/seeds/legumes (100 calories)*

Lunch *(335 calories)*
1 Veggie Melt Panini (see recipe), *2 grain, 2 vegetable, 1 dairy (335 calories)*

Afternoon Snack *(25 calories)*
½ cup cubed melon, *1 fruit (25 calories)*

Dinner *(555 calories)*
4½ ounces grilled chicken, *1½ meat (165 calories)*
1 small (3-inch) baked potato, *1 vegetable (150 calories)*
½ cup grilled zucchini, *1 vegetable (15 calories)*
1 teaspoon trans-fat-free margarine, *1 added fat (25 calories)*
1 cup cooked brown rice, *2 grain (200 calories)*

Evening Snack/Dessert *(120 calories)*
1 Baked Banana (see recipe), *2 fruit, 1 sweets (120 calories)*

Nutrition analysis for the day: 1,550 calories, 6 grain, 4 fruit, 4 vegetable, 2 dairy, 1½ meat, ½ nuts/seeds/legumes, 1 added fat, 1 sweets

||||||||||||||||||||||||||||||||||||||||||||||||||||||||||||||||||||||||||||||||||||||||||||||||||||||||||||

1,600 CALORIES: DAY 3
Target: 6 grain, 4 fruit, 4 vegetable, 2 dairy, 1½ meat, ¼ nuts/seeds/legumes, 1 added fat, ½ sweets

Breakfast *(280 calories)*
6 egg whites or ¾ cup egg substitute, scrambled (cooked with cooking spray), *1 meat (100 calories)*
1½ ounces shredded low-fat cheddar cheese (about ⅓ cup), *1 dairy (75 calories)*
One 1-ounce slice whole-wheat bread, toasted, *1 grain (80 calories)*
½ cup fresh strawberries, *1 fruit (25 calories)*

Morning Snack *(130 calories)*
1 medium peach, *1 fruit (30 calories)*
1 small low-fat granola bar, *1 grain (100 calories)*

Lunch *(330 calories)*
3 cups mixed raw leafy greens and vegetables, *3 vegetables (60 calories)*
¾ ounce shredded low-fat cheddar cheese (about 3 tablespoons), *½ dairy (40 calories)*
1½ ounces skinless grilled chicken breast, *½ meat (75 calories)*
2 tablespoons reduced-fat ranch dressing, *1 added fat (80 calories)*
One 4-inch whole-wheat pita pocket, *1 grain (75 calories)*

Afternoon Snack *(240 calories)*
1 medium apple, *1 fruit (50 calories)*
1 ounce unsalted mini pretzels (about ½ cup), *1 grain (110 calories)*
½ cup nonfat vanilla yogurt, *1 dairy (80 calories)*

Dinner *(530 calories)*
1 cup Fruity Chicken Stir-Fry (see recipe), *1 fruit, 1 vegetable, ½ meat (330 calories)*
1 cup cooked brown rice, *2 grain (200 calories)*

Evening Snack/Dessert *(75 calories)*
Half a ¾-inch slice Gingerbread (see recipe), *½ sweets (75 calories)*

Nutrition analysis for the day: 1,585 calories, 6 grain, 4 fruit, 4 vegetable, 2½ dairy, 2 meat, 0 nuts/seed/legumes, 1 added fat, ½ sweets

||||||||||||||||||||||||||||||||||||||||||||||||||||||||||||||||||||||||||||||||||||||||||||||||||||||||

1,600 CALORIES: DAY 4

Target: 6 grain, 4 fruit, 4 vegetable, 2 dairy, 1½ meat, ¼ nuts/seeds/legumes,
*   1 added fat, ½ sweets*

Breakfast *(280 calories)*
1 ounce toasted oat cereal, *1 grain (100 calories)*
½ cup sliced banana, *1 fruit (70 calories)*
1 cup low-fat milk, *1 dairy (110 calories)*

Morning Snack *(105 calories)*
1 cup red grapes, *2 fruit (105 calories)*

Lunch *(465 calories)*
3 ounces sliced roasted beef tenderloin, *1 meat (150 calories)*
Two 1-ounce slices whole-wheat bread, *2 grain (160 calories)*
1 cup shredded lettuce, *1 vegetable (20 calories)*
4 slices tomato, *1 vegetable (20 calories)*
1 teaspoon deli mustard *(5 calories)*
One 1-ounce snack bag pretzels, *1 grain (110 calories)*

Afternoon Snack *(250 calories)*
1 ounce whole-wheat snack crackers, *1 grain (130 calories)*
¾ ounce (1 small slice) low-fat cheddar cheese, *½ dairy (40 calories)*
¼ cup dried apricots, *1 fruit (80 calories)*
Cranberry sparkling water with a squeeze of lime *(0 calories)*

Dinner *(395 calories)*
1 Chicken Caesar Wrap (see recipe), *2 vegetable, ½ meat, 2 grain, ½ dairy, 1 added fat (395 calories)*

Evening Snack/Dessert *(60 calories)*
1 snack-size peppermint patty, *½ sweets (60 calories)*

Nutrition analysis for the day: 1,555 calories, 7 grain, 4 fruit, 4 vegetables, 2 dairy, 1½ meat, 0 nuts/seeds/legumes, 1 added fat, ½ sweets

||||||||||||||||||||||||||||||||||||||||||||||||||||||||||||||||||||||||||||||||||||||||||||||||||||||

1,600 CALORIES: DAY 5
*Target: 6 grain, 4 fruit, 4 vegetable, 2 dairy, 1½ meat, ¼ nuts/seeds/legumes,
        1 added fat, ½ sweets*

Breakfast *(340 calories)*
1 Low-Fat Blueberry Muffin (see recipe), *2 grain (200 calories)*
½ cup raspberries, *1 fruit (30 calories)*
1 cup low-fat milk, *1 dairy (110 calories)*

Morning Snack *(160 calories)*
1 cup sliced mango, *2 fruit (110 calories)*
¾ ounce (1 small slice) low-fat cheddar cheese, *½ dairy (50 calories)*

Lunch *(325 calories)*
1 Cobb Salad (see recipe), *4 vegetable, ½ dairy, ½ meat, 1 added fat (225 calories)*
1 small chocolate chip granola bar, *1 grain (100 calories)*

Afternoon Snack *(160 calories)*
"Ants on a log":
        4 celery sticks (5 inches each), *1 vegetable (5 calories)*
        1 tablespoon peanut butter, *½ nuts/seeds/legumes (100 calories)*
        2 tablespoons raisins, *½ fruit (55 calories)*

Dinner *(445 calories)*
Shrimp Scampi, 3 ounces shrimp with sauce (see recipe), *1 meat (145 calories)*
1½ cups whole-wheat linguine, *3 grain (300 calories)*

Evening Snack/Dessert *(105 calories)*
1 medium apple, *1 fruit (50 calories)*
2 tablespoons low-fat caramel sauce, *½ sweets (55 calories)*

Nutrition analysis for the day: 1,535 calories, 6 grain, 4½ fruit, 5 vegetable, 2 dairy, 1½ meat, ½ nuts/seeds/legumes, 1 added fat, ½ sweets

||||||||||||||||||||||||||||||||||||||||||||||||||||||||||||||||||||||||||||||||||||||||||||||||||||||||||||||||||||||||||||||||||||

1,600 CALORIES: DAY 6

Target: 6 grain, 4 fruit, 4 vegetable, 2 dairy, 1½ meat, ¼ nuts/seeds/legumes,
*   1 added fat, ½ sweets*

Breakfast *(190 calories)*
1 small low-fat granola bar, *1 grain (100 calories)*
¾ cup 100% apple juice, *1 fruit (90 calories)*

Morning Snack *(110 calories)*
3 cups air-popped popcorn, *1 grain (110 calories)*
Sparkling water with a squeeze of orange *(0 calories)*

Lunch *(440 calories)*
Hummus sandwich with fresh tomatoes:
       One 7-inch whole-wheat pita pocket, *2 grain (170 calories)*
       2 tablespoons hummus, *¼ nuts/seeds/legumes (70 calories)*
       1 ounce slice low-fat swiss cheese, *⅔ dairy (55 calories)*
       3 thick slices tomato, *1 vegetable (15 calories)*
       Bean sprouts, ½ cup, *½ vegetable (15 calories)*
2 cups Simple Spinach Salad (see recipe), *2 vegetable, ¼ dairy, 1 added fat (115 calories)*

Afternoon Snack *(370 calories)*
1 ounce unsalted mini pretzels (about ½ cup), *1 grain (110 calories)*
1 cup nonfat vanilla yogurt, *1 dairy (160 calories)*
¼ cup dried cherries, *1 fruit (100 calories)*

Dinner *(390 calories)*
4½ ounces Poached Salmon (see recipe), *1½ meat (215 calories)*
½ cup Roasted Brussels Sprouts (see recipe), *1 vegetable (50 calories)*
⅔ cup Quinoa, Corn, and Black Bean Salad (see recipe), *1 grain, ¼ vegetable, ¼ nuts/*
    seeds/legumes (125 calories)

Evening Snack/Dessert *(90 calories)*
1 cup fresh strawberries, *2 fruit (50 calories)*
2 teaspoons chocolate syrup, *½ sweets (40 calories)*

Nutrition analysis for the day: 1,590 calories, 6 grain, 4 fruit, 4¾ vegetable,
1¾ dairy, 1½ meat, ½ nuts/seeds/legumes, 1 added fat, ½ sweets

III

1,600 CALORIES: DAY 7
Target: 6 grain, 4 fruit, 4 vegetable, 2 dairy, 1½ meat, ¼ nuts/seeds/legumes, 1 added fat, ½ sweets

Breakfast *(370 calories)*
1½ ounces shredded wheat squares, *1½ grain (150 calories)*
1 tablespoon flaxseeds, *½ nuts/seeds/legumes (40 calories)*
1 cup low-fat milk, *1 dairy (110 calories)*
½ cup sliced banana, *1 fruit (70 calories)*

Morning Snack *(210 calories)*
1 ounce unsalted pretzels, *1 grain (110 calories)*
1 cup grapes, *2 fruit (100 calories)*

Lunch *(375 calories)*
Toasted cheese sandwich:
     One 7-inch whole-wheat pita pocket, *2 grain (220 calories)*
     1½ ounces low-fat cheddar cheese (about 2 slices), *1 dairy (75 calories)*
1 cup sliced carrots, *2 vegetable (50 calories)*
2 tablespoons fat-free ranch dressing *(30 calories)*

Afternoon Snack *(160 calories)*
1 medium orange, *1 fruit (60 calories)*
1 ounce unsalted whole-wheat mini pretzels (about ½ cup), *1 grain (100 calories)*

Dinner *(305 calories)*
5 ounces baked cod,* *1⅔ meat (150 calories)*
1 cup (10–12 small spears) Roasted Asparagus (see recipe), *2 vegetable (80 calories)*
1 cup mixed raw leafy greens, *1 vegetable (15 calories)*
1 tablespoon Lemon Caper Vinaigrette (see recipe), *1 added fat (60 calories)*

* Place fish on a baking sheet sprayed with cooking spray. Bake at 425°F for 15 minutes or until fish flakes with a fork.

Evening Snack/Dessert *(190 calories)*
2 graham cracker rectangles, *1 grain (120 calories)*
10 mini marshmallows and 2 dark chocolate kisses, *½ sweets (70 calories)*

Nutrition analysis for the day: 1,610 calories, 6½ grain, 4 fruit, 5 vegetable, 2 dairy, 1⅔ meat, ½ nuts/seeds/legumes, 1 added fat, ½ sweets

1,800 CALORIES: DAY 1

*Target: 6½ grain, 4 fruit, 4 vegetable, 2½ dairy, 1½ meat, ½ nuts/seeds/legumes,
1½ added fat, ½ sweets*

Breakfast *(330 calories)*
Two 1-ounce slices whole-wheat bread, *2 grain (160 calories)*
1 tablespoon peanut butter, *½ nuts/seeds/legumes (100 calories)*
1 cup mixed fresh berries, *2 fruit (70 calories)*

Morning Snack *(170 calories)*
1 medium orange, *1 fruit (60 calories)*
1 ounce unsalted pretzels, *1 grain (110 calories)*

Lunch *(420 calories)*
Two 1-ounce slices whole-wheat bread, *2 grain (160 calories)*
3 ounces sliced roast beef, *1 meat (150 calories)*
¾ ounce shredded low-fat cheddar cheese (about 3 tablespoons), *½ dairy
(40 calories)*
2 tablespoons low-fat mayonnaise, *1 added fat (30 calories)*
4 slices tomato, *1 vegetable (20 calories)*
4 leaves lettuce, *1 vegetable (20 calories)*

Afternoon Snack *(240 calories)*
1 cup low-fat fruited yogurt, *1 dairy (200 calories)*
½ cup pineapple, *1 fruit (40 calories)*

Dinner *(350 calories)*
1 cup Beef and Vegetable Stir-Fry (see recipe), *½ meat, 2 vegetable (200 calories)*
¾ cup cooked brown rice, *1½ grain (150 calories)*

Evening Snack/Dessert *(230 calories)*
½ cup low-fat frozen yogurt, *1 dairy (140 calories)*
2 teaspoons chocolate syrup, *½ sweets (40 calories)*
1 tablespoon whipped cream, *½ added fat (50 calories)*

*Nutrition analysis for the day: 1,740 calories, 6½ grain, 4 fruit, 4 vegetable,
2½ dairy, 1½ meat, ½ nuts/seeds/legumes, 1½ added fat, ½ sweets*

|||||||||||||||||||||||||||||||||||||||||||||||||||||||||||||||||||||||||||||||||||||||||||||||||||||||||||||||

1,800 CALORIES: DAY 2
*Target: 6½ grain, 4 fruit, 4 vegetable, 2½ dairy, 1½ meat, ½ nuts/seeds/legumes,
1½ added fat, ½ sweets*

Breakfast *(325 calories)*
1 ounce uncooked oatmeal cooked with water (cooks to about ¾ cup), *1 grain
(100 calories)*
1 packet sugar substitute (optional) *(0 calories)*
¼ cup raisins, *1 fruit (110 calories)*
½ cup cubed cantaloupe, *1 fruit (25 calories)*
1 cup nonfat milk, *1 dairy (90 calories)*

Morning Snack *(235 calories)*
1 cup unsweetened applesauce, *2 fruit (105 calories)*
One 1-ounce snack bag pita chips, *1 grain (130 calories)*

Lunch *(330 calories)*
Two 1-ounce slices whole-wheat bread, *2 grain (160 calories)*
3 ounces sliced roasted turkey breast, *1 meat (115 calories)*
1 tablespoon low-fat mayonnaise, *¼ added fat (15 calories)*
4 slices tomato, *1 vegetable (20 calories)*
4 leaves lettuce, *1 vegetable (20 calories)*

Afternoon Snack *(250 calories)*
¼ cup canned black beans, drained and rinsed, *½ nuts/seeds/legumes (60 calories)*
½ cup cooked brown rice, *1 grain (100 calories)*
¼ cup tomato salsa, *½ vegetable (15 calories)*
1½ ounces shredded low-fat cheddar cheese (about ⅓ cup), *1 dairy (75 calories)*

Dinner *(395 calories)*
1 Chicken Caesar Wrap (see recipe), *2 vegetable, ½ meat, 2 grain, ½ dairy, 1 added fat
(395 calories)*

Evening Snack/Dessert *(265 calories)*
Strawberry Shortcake (see recipe), *1 sweets, 1 fruit (265 calories)*

*Nutrition analysis for the day: 1,800 calories, 7 grain, 5 fruit, 4½ vegetable,
2½ dairy, 1½ meat, ½ nuts/seeds/legumes, 1½ added fat, 1 sweets*

|||||||||||||||||||||||||||||||||||||||||||||||||||||||||||||||||||||||||||||||||||||||||||||||||||||||||||||||||||

1,800 CALORIES: DAY 3
Target: 6½ grain, 4 fruit, 4 vegetable, 2½ dairy, 1½ meat, ½ nuts/seeds/legumes,
*   1½ added fat, ½ sweets*

Breakfast *(460 calories)*
2 whole eggs plus 2 egg whites, scrambled (cooked with cooking spray), *1 meat*
*   (190 calories)*
1½ ounces shredded low-fat cheddar cheese (about ⅓ cup), *1 dairy (75 calories)*
Two 1-ounce slices whole-wheat bread, *2 grain (160 calories)*
½ teaspoon trans-fat-free margarine, *½ added fat (10 calories)*
1 tablespoon low-sodium ketchup (optional) *(25 calories)*

Morning Snack *(140 calories)*
1 Mango Smoothie (see recipe), *1 fruit, 1 dairy, ½ sweets (140 calories)*

Lunch *(375 calories)*
1 Cobb Salad (see recipe), *4 vegetable, ½ dairy, ½ meat, 1 added fat (225 calories)*
1 small (2-ounce) whole-wheat dinner roll, *2 grain (150 calories)*

Afternoon Snack *(105 calories)*
1 medium (7-inch) banana, *2 fruit (105 calories)*

Dinner *(480 calories)*
1 cup Fruity Chicken Stir-Fry (see recipe), *1 fruit, 1 vegetable, ½ meat (330 calories)*
¾ cup cooked brown rice, *1½ grain (150 calories)*

Evening Snack/Dessert *(220 calories)*
1 ounce unsalted mini pretzels (about ½ cup), *1 grain (110 calories)*
2 tablespoons peanuts, *¼ nuts/seeds/legumes (110 calories)*

Nutrition analysis for the day: 1,780 calories, 6½ grain, 4 fruit, 5 vegetable,
2½ dairy, 2 meat, ¼ nuts/seeds/legumes, 1½ added fat, ½ sweets

||||||||||||||||||||||||||||||||||||||||||||||||||||||||||||||||||||||||||||||||||||||||||||||||||||||||||||

1,800 CALORIES: DAY 4

Target: 6½ grain, 4 fruit, 4 vegetable, 2½ dairy, 1½ meat, ½ nuts/seeds/legumes, 1½ added fat, ½ sweets

Breakfast *(360 calories)*
2 ounces shredded wheat squares (about 1¼ cups), *2 grain (200 calories)*
½ cup sliced banana, *1 fruit (70 calories)*
1 cup nonfat milk, *1 dairy (90 calories)*

Morning Snack *(310 calories)*
1 cup low-fat fruited yogurt, *1 dairy (200 calories)*
1 ounce unsalted mini pretzels (about ½ cup), *1 grain (110 calories)*

Lunch *(390 calories)*
Hummus sandwich with fresh tomatoes:
      One 7-inch whole-wheat pita pocket, *2 grain (170 calories)*
      ¼ cup hummus, *½ nuts/seeds/legumes (140 calories)*
      3 thick slices tomato, *1 vegetable (15 calories)*
      ½ cup bean sprouts, *½ vegetable (15 calories)*
1 cup sliced melon, *2 fruit (50 calories)*

Afternoon Snack *(105 calories)*
½ cup baby carrots, *1 vegetable (25 calories)*
2 tablespoons low-fat creamy Italian dressing, *1 added fat (80 calories)*

Dinner *(555 calories)*
4½ ounces Poached Salmon (see recipe), *1½ meat (215 calories)*
1 medium (5-inch) baked sweet potato, *2 vegetable (180 calories)*
½ teaspoon trans-fat-free margarine, *½ added fat (10 calories)*
¾ cup brown rice, *1½ grain (150 calories)*

Evening Snack/Dessert *(60 calories)*
½ Baked Banana (see recipe), *1 fruit, ½ sweets (60 calories)*

Nutrition analysis for the day: 1,780 calories, 6½ grain, 4 fruit, 4½ vegetable, 2 dairy, 1½ meat, ½ nuts/seeds/legumes, 1½ added fat, ½ sweets

1,800 CALORIES: DAY 5

Target: 6½ grain, 4 fruit, 4 vegetable, 2½ dairy, 1½ meat, ½ nuts/seeds/legumes, 1½ added fat, ½ sweets

Breakfast *(425 calories)*
1 Low-Fat Blueberry Muffin (see recipe), *2 grain (200 calories)*
1 teaspoon trans-fat-free margarine, *1 added fat (25 calories)*
1 cup low-fat fruited yogurt, *1 dairy (200 calories)*

Morning Snack *(200 calories)*
¼ cup dried cherries, *1 fruit (100 calories)*
1 small low-fat granola bar, *1 grain (100 calories)*

Lunch *(405 calories)*
Toasted cheese sandwich:
        One 7-inch whole-wheat pita pocket, *2 grain (170 calories)*
        1½ ounces low-fat cheddar cheese (2 slices), *1 dairy (75 calories)*
1 medium apple, *1 fruit (60 calories)*
½ cup sliced bell peppers, *1 vegetable (20 calories)*
2 tablespoons low-fat raspberry walnut vinaigrette dressing, *1 added fat (80 calories)*

Afternoon Snack *(205 calories)*
"Ants on a log":
        4 celery sticks (5 inches each), *1 vegetable (5 calories)*
        1 tablespoon peanut butter, *½ nuts/seeds/legumes (90 calories)*
        ¼ cup raisins, *1 fruit (110 calories)*

Dinner *(490 calories)*
¾ cup cooked whole-wheat pasta, *1½ grain (150 calories)*
1 cup low-sodium marinara sauce, *2 vegetable (80 calories)*
4½ ounces ground turkey breast meat (cooked with cooking spray), *1½ meat (180 calories)*
¼ cup shredded parmesan cheese, *½ dairy (80 calories)*

Evening Snack/Dessert *(50 calories)*
½ cup fresh strawberries, *1 fruit (25 calories)*
1½ teaspoons sugar, *½ sweets (25 calories)*

Nutrition analysis for the day: 1,775 calories, 6½ grain, 4 fruit, 4 vegetable, 2½ dairy, 1½ meat, ½ nuts/seeds/legumes, 2 added fat, ½ sweets

|||||||||||||||||||||||||||||||||||||||||||||||||||||||||||||||||||||||||||||||||||||||||||||||||||||||||||||||||||||||||

1,800 CALORIES: DAY 6

Target: 6½ grain, 4 fruit, 4 vegetable, 2½ dairy, 1½ meat, ½ nuts/seeds/legumes, 1½ added fat, ½ sweets

Breakfast *(310 calories)*
1 ounce toasted oat cereal (about 1 cup), *1 grain (100 calories)*
½ cup blueberries, *1 fruit (40 calories)*
1 cup nonfat milk, *1 dairy (90 calories)*
¾ cup 100% orange juice, *1 fruit (80 calories)*

Morning Snack *(150 calories)*
3 cups air-popped popcorn, *1 grain (110 calories)*
½ cup sliced pineapple, *1 fruit (40 calories)*

Lunch *(370 calories)*
Two 1-ounce slices whole-wheat bread, *2 grain (160 calories)*
½ cup tuna fish (canned in water), *1 meat (120 calories)*
2 tablespoons low-fat mayonnaise, *1 added fat (30 calories)*
1 medium orange, *1 fruit (60 calories)*

Afternoon Snack *(215 calories)*
1 small (3-inch) baked potato, *1 vegetable (110 calories)*
½ cup salsa, *1 vegetable (30 calories)*
1½ ounces shredded low-fat cheddar cheese (about ⅓ cup), *1 dairy (75 calories)*

Dinner *(540 calories)*
2 Turkey Soft Tacos (see recipe), *2 grain, 2 vegetable, 1 added fat, 1 meat (500 calories)*
¾ ounce shredded low-fat cheddar cheese (about 3 tablespoons), *½ dairy (40 calories)*

Evening Snack/Dessert *(150 calories)*
7 dark-chocolate-covered almonds, *½ nuts/seeds/legumes, ½ sweets (150 calories)*

Nutrition analysis for the day: 1,735 calories, 6 grain, 4 fruit, 4 vegetable, 2½ dairy, 2 meat, ½ nuts/seeds/legumes, 2 added fat, ½ sweets

1,800 CALORIES: DAY 7
Target: 6½ grain, 4 fruit, 4 vegetable, 2½ dairy, 1½ meat, ½ nuts/seeds/legumes,
   1½ added fat, ½ sweets

Breakfast *(380 calories)*
1 cup low-fat fruited yogurt, *1 dairy (200 calories)*
1 ounce low-fat granola (about ¼ cup), *1 grain (110 calories)*
½ cup sliced banana, *1 fruit (70 calories)*

Morning Snack *(170 calories)*
1 cup mixed fresh berries, *2 fruit (70 calories)*
1 small low-fat granola bar, *1 grain (100 calories)*

Lunch *(460 calories)*
Black bean burrito:
   One 10-inch whole-wheat tortilla, *2 grain (180 calories)*
   ½ cup canned black beans, drained and rinsed, *1 nuts/seeds/legumes*
      (115 calories)
   1½ ounces shredded low-fat cheddar cheese (about ⅓ cup), *1 dairy (75 calories)*
   ¼ cup tomato salsa, *½ vegetable (15 calories)*
   2 tablespoons reduced-fat sour cream, *1 added fat (40 calories)*
½ cup chopped fresh tomato, *1 vegetable (15 calories)*
1 cup shredded lettuce, *1 vegetable (20 calories)*

Afternoon Snack *(140 calories)*
½ cup nonfat vanilla frozen yogurt, *1 dairy (140 calories)*

Dinner *(535 calories)*
Shrimp Scampi, 4½ ounces shrimp with sauce (see recipe), *1½ meat (185 calories)*
1¼ cups whole-wheat linguine, *2½ grain (250 calories)*
¾ cup green peas, *1½ vegetable (100 calories)*

Evening Snack/Dessert *(80 calories)*
2 dark-chocolate-covered strawberries, *1 fruit, ½ sweets (80 calories)*

Nutrition analysis for the day: 1,765 calories, 6½ grain, 4 fruit, 4 vegetable, 3 dairy,
1½ meat, 1 nuts/seeds/legumes, 1 added fat, ½ sweets

||||||||||||||||||||||||||||||||||||||||||||||||||||||||||||||||||||||||||||||||||||||||||||||||||||||||||||||||||||||||||||||||||||||||||||

2,000 CALORIES: DAY 1
Target: 7 grain, 4 fruit, 4 vegetable, 2½ dairy, 1½ meat, ½ nuts/seeds/legumes,
   2 added fat, ½ sweets

Breakfast *(330 calories)*
Two 1-ounce slices whole-wheat bread, *2 grain (160 calories)*
1 tablespoon peanut butter, *½ nuts/seeds/legumes (100 calories)*
½ cup sliced banana, *1 fruit (70 calories)*

Morning Snack *(170 calories)*
1 medium orange, *1 fruit (60 calories)*
1 ounce unsalted pretzels, *1 grain (110 calories)*

Lunch *(685 calories)*
Two 1-ounce slices whole-wheat bread, *2 grain (160 calories)*
3 ounces sliced roast beef, *1 meat (150 calories)*
¾ ounce (1 thin slice) reduced-fat swiss cheese, *½ dairy (55 calories)*
2 tablespoons low-fat mayonnaise, *1 added fat (30 calories)*
2 slices tomato, *½ vegetable (10 calories)*
¼ ripe avocado, *⅓ vegetable (60 calories)*
4 leaves lettuce, *1 vegetable (20 calories)*
½ cup reduced-fat cottage cheese, *1 dairy (100 calories)*
¼ cup dried cherries, *1 fruit (100 calories)*

Afternoon Snack *(220 calories)*
1 cup low-fat vanilla yogurt, *1 dairy (180 calories)*
½ cup pineapple, *1 fruit (40 calories)*

Dinner *(400 calories)*
1 cup Beef and Vegetable Stir-Fry (see recipe), *½ meat, 2 vegetable (200 calories)*
1 cup cooked brown rice, *2 grain (200 calories)*

Evening Snack/Dessert *(175 calories)*
Half a ¾-inch slice Gingerbread (see recipe), *½ sweets (75 calories)*
2 tablespoons whipped cream, *1 added fat (100 calories)*

Nutrition analysis for the day: 1,980 calories, 7 grain, 4 fruit, 4 vegetable, 2½ dairy,
1½ meat, ½ nuts/seeds/legumes, 2 added fat, ½ sweets

||||||||||||||||||||||||||||||||||||||||||||||||||||||||||||||||||||||||||||||||||||||||||||||||||||||||

2,000 CALORIES: DAY 2

Target: 7 grain, 4 fruit, 4 vegetable, 2½ dairy, 1½ meat, ½ nuts/seeds/legumes, 2 added fat, ½ sweets

Breakfast *(325 calories)*
1 ounce uncooked oatmeal cooked with water (cooks to about ¾ cup), *1 grain (100 calories)*
1 packet sugar substitute (optional) *(0 calories)*
¼ cup raisins, *1 fruit (110 calories)*
½ cup cantaloupe, *1 fruit (25 calories)*
1 cup nonfat milk, *1 dairy (90 calories)*

Morning Snack *(235 calories)*
1 cup unsweetened applesauce, *2 fruit (105 calories)*
One 1-ounce snack bag pita chips, *1 grain (130 calories)*

Lunch *(345 calories)*
Two 1-ounce slices whole-wheat bread, toasted, *2 grain (160 calories)*
3 ounces sliced roasted turkey breast, *1 meat (115 calories)*
2 tablespoons low-fat mayonnaise, *1 added fat (30 calories)*
4 slices tomato, *1 vegetable (20 calories)*
4 leaves lettuce, *1 vegetable (20 calories)*

Afternoon Snack *(440 calories)*
1 cup low-fat fruited yogurt, *1 dairy (200 calories)*
1 ounce low-fat granola (about ¼ cup), *1 grain (110 calories)*
3 tablespoons slivered almonds, *½ nuts/seeds/legumes (130 calories)*

Dinner *(395 calories)*
1 Chicken Caesar Wrap (see recipe), *2 vegetable, ½ meat, 2 grain, ½ dairy, 1 added fat (395 calories)*

Evening Snack/Dessert *(265 calories)*
Strawberry Shortcake (see recipe), *1 sweets, 1 fruit (265 calories)*

Nutrition analysis for the day: 2,005 calories, 7 grain, 5 fruit, 4 vegetable, 2½ dairy, 1½ meat, ½ nuts/seeds/legumes, 2 added fat, 1 sweets

‖‖

2,000 CALORIES: DAY 3

Target: 7 grain, 4 fruit, 4 vegetable, 2½ dairy, 1½ meat, ½ nuts/seeds/legumes,
*   2 added fat, ½ sweets*

Breakfast *(500 calories)*
3 whole eggs, scrambled (cooked with cooking spray), *1 meat (240 calories)*
1½ ounces shredded low-fat cheddar cheese (about ⅓ cup), *1 dairy (75 calories)*
Two 1-ounce slices whole-wheat bread, toasted, *2 grain (160 calories)*
1 teaspoon trans-fat-free margarine, *1 added fat (25 calories)*

Morning Snack *(260 calories)*
1 cup low-fat vanilla yogurt, *1 dairy (180 calories)*
1 cup blueberries, *2 fruit (80 calories)*

Lunch *(375 calories)*
1 Cobb Salad (see recipe), *4 vegetable, ½ dairy, ½ meat, 1 added fat (225 calories)*
1 small (2-ounce) whole-wheat dinner roll, *2 grain (150 calories)*

Afternoon Snack *(100 calories)*
1 medium pear, *1 fruit (100 calories)*

Dinner *(530 calories)*
1 cup Fruity Chicken Stir-Fry (see recipe), *1 fruit, 1 vegetable, ½ meat (330 calories)*
1 cup cooked brown rice, *2 grain (200 calories)*

Evening Snack/Dessert *(290 calories)*
1 ounce unsalted mini pretzels (about ½ cup), *1 grain (110 calories)*
2 tablespoons peanuts, *¼ nuts/seeds/legumes (110 calories)*
1 tablespoon chocolate chips, *½ sweets (70 calories)*

Nutrition analysis for the day: 2,055 calories, 7 grain, 4 fruit, 5 vegetable, 2½ dairy,
2 meat, ¼ nuts/seeds/legumes, 2 added fat, ½ sweets

|||||||||||||||||||||||||||||||||||||||||||||||||||||||||||||||||||||||||||||||||||||||||||||||||||||||||||||||

2,000 CALORIES: DAY 4

Target: 7 grain, 4 fruit, 4 vegetable, 2½ dairy, 1½ meat, ½ nuts/seeds/legumes, 2 added fat, ½ sweets

Breakfast *(345 calories)*
2 ounces shredded wheat squares (about 1¼ cup), *2 grain (200 calories)*
½ cup mixed fresh berries, *1 fruit (35 calories)*
1 cup low-fat milk, *1 dairy (110 calories)*

Morning Snack *(310 calories)*
1 cup low-fat fruited yogurt, *1 dairy (200 calories)*
1 ounce unsalted mini pretzels (about ½ cup), *1 grain (110 calories)*

Lunch *(390 calories)*
Hummus sandwich with fresh tomatoes:
    One 7-inch whole-wheat pita pocket, *2 grain (170 calories)*
    ¼ cup hummus, *½ nuts/seeds/legumes (140 calories)*
    3 thick slices tomato, *1 vegetable (15 calories)*
    ½ cup bean sprouts, *½ vegetable (15 calories)*
1 cup sliced melon, *2 fruit (50 calories)*

Afternoon Snack *(200 calories)*
½ ripe avocado, *1 vegetable (120 calories)*
2 tablespoons low-fat creamy Italian dressing, *1 added fat (80 calories)*

Dinner *(620 calories)*
4½ ounces Poached Salmon (see recipe), *1½ meat (215 calories)*
1 medium (5-inch) baked sweet potato, *2 vegetable (180 calories)*
1 teaspoon trans-fat-free margarine, *1 added fat (25 calories)*
1 cup brown rice, *2 grain (200 calories)*

Evening Snack/Dessert *(60 calories)*
½ Baked Banana (see recipe), *1 fruit, ½ sweets (60 calories)*

Nutrition analysis for the day: 1,925 calories, 7 grain, 4 fruit, 4½ vegetable, 2 dairy, 1½ meat, ½ nuts/seeds/legumes, 2 added fat, ½ sweets

|||||||||||||||||||||||||||||||||||||||||||||||||||||||||||||||||||||||||||||||||||||||||||||||||||||||||||||||||||||

2,000 CALORIES: DAY 5
Target: 7 grain, 4 fruit, 4 vegetable, 2½ dairy, 1½ meat, ½ nuts/seeds/legumes,
*   2 added fat, ½ sweets*

Breakfast *(395 calories)*
1 Low-Fat Blueberry Muffin (see recipe), *2 grain (200 calories)*
1 teaspoon trans-fat-free margarine, *1 added fat (25 calories)*
1 medium orange, *1 fruit (60 calories)*
1 cup low-fat milk, *1 dairy (110 calories)*

Morning Snack *(150 calories)*
1 medium apple, *1 fruit (50 calories)*
1 small low-fat granola bar, *1 grain (100 calories)*

Lunch *(495 calories)*
½ large (about 4-inch) whole-wheat bagel, *2 grain (200 calories)*
1 tablespoon low-fat cream cheese, *½ added fat (35 calories)*
1 cup low-fat fruited yogurt, *1 dairy (200 calories)*
½ cup sliced peppers, *1 vegetable (20 calories)*
1 tablespoon low-fat raspberry walnut vinaigrette, *½ fat (40 calories)*

Afternoon Snack *(215 calories)*
"Ants on a log":
    4 celery sticks (5 inches each), *1 vegetable (5 calories)*
    1 tablespoon peanut butter, *½ nuts/seeds/legumes (100 calories)*
    ¼ cup raisins, *1 fruit (110 calories)*

Dinner *(520 calories)*
1 cup cooked whole-wheat pasta, *2 grain (200 calories)*
1 cup low-sodium marinara sauce, *2 vegetable (80 calories)*
4½ ounces ground turkey breast meat (cooked with cooking spray), *1½ meat*
    (160 calories)
¼ cup shredded parmesan cheese, *½ dairy (80 calories)*

Evening Snack/Dessert *(165 calories)*
½ cup low-fat frozen yogurt, *1 dairy (140 calories)*
½ cup fresh strawberries, *1 fruit (25 calories)*

Nutrition analysis for the day: 1,940 calories, 7 grain, 4 fruit, 4 vegetable, 3½ dairy,
1½ meat, ½ nuts/seeds/legumes, 2 added fat, 0 sweets

III

2,000 CALORIES: DAY 6
Target: 7 grain, 4 fruit, 4 vegetable, 2½ dairy, 1½ meat, ½ nuts/seeds/legumes,
*   2 added fat, ½ sweets*

Breakfast *(345 calories)*
1 cup low-fat fruited yogurt, *1 dairy (200 calories)*
½ cup mixed fresh berries, *1 fruit (35 calories)*
1 ounce low-fat granola (about ¼ cup), *1 grain (110 calories)*

Morning Snack *(215 calories)*
3 cups air-popped popcorn, *1 grain (110 calories)*
1 teaspoon trans-fat-free margarine, *1 added fat (25 calories)*
1 cup sliced pineapple, *1 fruit (80 calories)*

Lunch *(480 calories)*
Two 1-ounce slices whole-wheat bread, *2 grain (160 calories)*
½ cup tuna fish (canned in water), *1 meat (120 calories)*
2 tablespoons low-fat mayonnaise, *1 added fat (30 calories)*
1 medium orange, *1 fruit (60 calories)*
One 1-ounce snack bag pretzels, *1 grain (110 calories)*

Afternoon Snack *(215 calories)*
1 small (3-inch) baked potato, *1 vegetable (110 calories)*
½ cup salsa, *1 vegetable (30 calories)*
1½ ounces shredded low-fat cheddar cheese (about ⅓ cup), *1 dairy (75 calories)*

Dinner *(540 calories)*
2 Turkey Soft Tacos (see recipe), *2 grain, 2 vegetable, 1 meat (500 calories)*
¾ ounce shredded low-fat cheddar cheese (about 3 tablespoons), *½ dairy (40 calories)*

Evening Snack/Dessert *(150 calories)*
7 dark-chocolate-covered almonds, *½ nuts/seeds/legumes, ½ sweets (150 calories)*

Nutrition analysis for the day: 1,945 calories, 7 grain, 4 fruit, 4 vegetable,
2½ dairy, 2 meat, ½ nuts/seeds/legumes, 2 added fat, ½ sweets

||||||||||||||||||||||||||||||||||||||||||||||||||||||||||||||||||||||||||||||||||||||||||||||||||||||||||||||||||||||

2,000 CALORIES: DAY 7

Target: 7 grain, 4 fruit, 4 vegetable, 2½ dairy, 1½ meat, ½ nuts/seeds/legumes, 2 added fat, ½ sweets

Breakfast *(445 calories)*

1 cup low-fat fruited yogurt, *1 dairy (200 calories)*
1 slice cinnamon raisin toast, *1 grain (80 calories)*
1 teaspoon trans-fat-free margarine, *1 added fat (25 calories)*
1 cup sliced banana, *2 fruit (140 calories)*

Morning Snack *(170 calories)*

1 cup mixed fresh berries, *2 fruit (70 calories)*
1 small low-fat granola bar, *1 grain (100 calories)*

Lunch *(530 calories)*

Black bean burrito:

> One 10-inch whole-wheat tortilla, *2 grain (180 calories)*
> ½ cup canned black beans, drained and rinsed, *1 nuts/seeds/legumes (115 calories)*
> ¼ ripe avocado, *½ vegetable (80 calories)*
> 1½ ounces shredded low-fat cheddar cheese (about ⅓ cup), *1 dairy (75 calories)*
> ¼ cup tomato salsa, *½ vegetable (25 calories)*
> 2 tablespoons reduced-fat sour cream, *1 added fat (40 calories)*

½ cup chopped fresh tomato, *1 vegetable (15 calories)*
1 cup shredded lettuce, *1 vegetable (20 calories)*

Afternoon Snack *(235 calories)*

1 small (3-inch) baked potato, *1 vegetable (110 calories)*
½ cup salsa, *1 vegetable (50 calories)*
¾ ounce shredded Monterey Jack cheese (about 3 tablespoons), *½ dairy (75 calories)*

Dinner *(485 calories)*

Shrimp Scampi (see recipe), 4½ ounces shrimp with sauce (see recipe), *1½ meat (185 calories)*
1½ cups whole-wheat linguine, *3 grain (300 calories)*

Evening Snack/Dessert *(80 calories)*

2 dark-chocolate-covered strawberries, *1 fruit, ½ sweets (80 calories)*

Nutrition analysis for the day: 1,945 calories, 7 grain, 5 fruit, 5 vegetable, 2½ dairy, 1½ meat, 1 nuts/seeds/legumes, 2 added fat, ½ sweets

2,200 CALORIES: DAY 1

Target: 8 grain, 4 fruit, 5 vegetable, 3 dairy, 2 meat, ½ nuts/seeds/legumes,
*   2½ added fat, 1 sweets*

Breakfast *(480 calories)*
Two 1-ounce slices whole-wheat bread, toasted, *2 grain (160 calories)*
1 tablespoon peanut butter, *½ nuts/seeds/legumes (90 calories)*
1 cup sliced banana, *2 fruit (140 calories)*
1 cup nonfat milk, *1 dairy (90 calories)*

Morning Snack *(120 calories)*
½ cup low-fat cottage cheese, *1 dairy (80 calories)*
½ cup fresh pineapple chunks, *1 fruit (40 calories)*

Lunch *(610 calories)*
Two 1-ounce slices whole-wheat bread, *2 grain (160 calories)*
4 ounces sliced grilled skinless chicken breast, *1⅓ meat (200 calories)*
2 tablespoons low-fat mayonnaise, *1 added fat (30 calories)*
4 slices tomato, *1 vegetable (20 calories)*
4 leaves romaine lettuce, *1 vegetable (20 calories)*
1 ounce honey whole-wheat pretzels, *1 grain (110 calories)*
1 medium apple, *1 fruit (50 calories)*

Afternoon Snack *(205 calories)*
1 ounce whole-wheat snack crackers, *1 grain (130 calories)*
1½ ounces low-fat cheddar cheese, *1 dairy (75 calories)*

Dinner *(550 calories)*
1½ cups Beef and Vegetable Stir-Fry (see recipe), *¾ meat, 3 vegetable (300 calories)*
1½ cups cooked brown rice, *2½ grain (250 calories)*

Evening Snack/Dessert *(180 calories)*
One ¾-inch slice Gingerbread (see recipe), *1 sweets (150 calories)*
3 tablespoons low-fat whipped topping, *1½ added fat (30 calories)*

Nutrition analysis for the day: 2,145 calories, 8½ grain, 4 fruit, 5 vegetable, 3 dairy,
2 meat, ½ nuts/seeds/legumes, 2½ added fat, 1 sweets

||||||||||||||||||||||||||||||||||||||||||||||||||||||||||||||||||||||||||||||||||||||||||||||||||||||||||||||||||||||||||

2,200 CALORIES: DAY 2
Target: 8 grain, 4 fruit, 5 vegetable, 3 dairy, 2 meat, ½ nuts/seeds/legumes,
2½ added fat, 1 sweets

Breakfast *(315 calories)*
2 ounces uncooked oatmeal cooked with water (cooks to about 1½ cup), *2 grain*
    (200 calories)
1 packet sugar substitute (optional) *(0 calories)*
½ cup cantaloupe, *1 fruit (25 calories)*
1 cup nonfat milk, *1 dairy (90 calories)*

Morning Snack *(235 calories)*
1 cup unsweetened applesauce, *2 fruit (105 calories)*
One 1-ounce snack bag baked pita chips, *1 grain (130 calories)*

Lunch *(600 calories)*
Two 1-ounce slices whole-wheat bread, *2 grain (160 calories)*
1½ ounces reduced-fat swiss cheese (1 big slice), *1 dairy (110 calories)*
1½ ounces sliced roast beef, *½ meat (75 calories)*
1 tablespoon low-fat mayonnaise, *½ added fat (15 calories)*
4 slices tomato, *1 vegetable (20 calories)*
4 leaves lettuce, *1 vegetable (20 calories)*
1 cup low-fat fruited yogurt, *1 dairy (200 calories)*

Afternoon Snack *(205 calories)*
"Ants on a Log":
        4 celery sticks (5 inches each), *1 vegetable (5 calories)*
        1 tablespoon peanut butter, *½ nuts/seeds/legumes (90 calories)*
        ¼ cup raisins, *1 fruit (110 calories)*

Dinner *(560 calories)*
4½ ounces Poached Salmon (see recipe), *1½ meat (220 calories)*
2 cups mixed raw leafy greens and vegetables, *2 vegetable (35 calories)*
2 tablespoons balsamic vinaigrette dressing, *2 added fat (100 calories)*
⅔ cup Quinoa, Corn, and Black Bean Salad (see recipe), *1 grain, ¼ vegetable, ¼ nuts/*
    seeds/legumes (125 calories)
One 1-ounce slice whole-wheat bread, toasted, *1 grain (80 calories)*

Evening Snack/Dessert *(210 calories)*
2 dark chocolate kisses, *½ sweets (40 calories)*
2 graham cracker rectangles, *1 grain (120 calories)*
2 marshmallows, *½ sweets (50 calories)*

Nutrition analysis for the day: 2,125 calories, 8 grain, 4 fruit, 5¼ vegetable, 3 dairy, 2 meat, ¾ nuts/seeds/legumes, 2½ added fat, 1 sweets

||||||||||||||||||||||||||||||||||||||||||||||||||||||||||||||||||||||||||||||||||||||||||||||||||||||||||||||||

2,200 CALORIES: DAY 3

Target: 8 grain, 4 fruit, 5 vegetable, 3 dairy, 2 meat, ½ nuts/seeds/legumes,
   2½ added fat, 1 sweets

Breakfast *(550 calories)*
2 whole eggs plus 2 egg whites, scrambled (cooked with cooking spray), *1 meat (195 calories)*
1½ ounces shredded low-fat cheddar cheese (about ⅓ cup), *1 dairy (75 calories)*
1 cup mixed fresh berries, *2 fruit (70 calories)*
Two 1-ounce slices whole-wheat bread, toasted, *2 grain (160 calories)*
1 teaspoon trans-fat-free margarine, *1 added fat (25 calories)*
1½ teaspoons fruit preserves, *½ sweets (25 calories)*

Morning Snack *(250 calories)*
1 cup low-fat vanilla yogurt, *1 dairy (180 calories)*
½ cup sliced banana, *1 fruit (70 calories)*

Lunch *(420 calories)*
1 Cobb Salad (see recipe), *4 vegetable, ½ dairy, ½ meat, 1 added fat (225 calories)*
One 1-ounce slice whole-wheat bread, *1 grain (80 calories)*
1½ ounces sliced roasted turkey breast, *½ meat (60 calories)*
¾ ounce low-fat American cheese (1 slice), *½ dairy (40 calories)*
1 tablespoon low-fat mayonnaise, *½ added fat (15 calories)*

Afternoon Snack *(190 calories)*
½ cup sliced pears, *1 fruit (50 calories)*
1 medium low-fat granola bar, *2 grain (140 calories)*

Dinner *(530 calories)*
1 cup Fruity Chicken Stir-Fry (see recipe), *1 fruit, 1 vegetable, ½ meat (330 calories)*
1 cup cooked brown rice, *2 grain (200 calories)*

Evening Snack/Dessert *(290 calories)*
1 ounce unsalted mini pretzels (about ½ cup), *1 grain (110 calories)*
2 tablespoons peanuts, *¼ nuts/seeds/legumes (110 calories)*
1 tablespoon chocolate chips, *½ sweets (70 calories)*

Nutrition analysis for the day: 2,230 calories, 8 grain, 5 fruit, 5 vegetable, 3 dairy, 2½ meat, ¼ nuts/seeds/legumes, 2½ added fat, 1 sweets

III

2,200 CALORIES: DAY 4

Target: 8 grain, 4 fruit, 5 vegetable, 3 dairy, 2 meat, ½ nuts/seeds/legumes,
*   2½ added fat, 1 sweets*

Breakfast *(380 calories)*
2 ounces shredded wheat squares (about 1¼ cup), *2 grain (200 calories)*
1 cup mixed fresh berries, *2 fruit (70 calories)*
1 cup low-fat milk, *1 dairy (110 calories)*

Morning Snack *(270 calories)*
1 cup nonfat vanilla yogurt, *1 dairy (160 calories)*
1 ounce unsalted mini pretzels (about ½ cup), *1 grain (110 calories)*

Lunch *(640 calories)*
1 Chicken Caesar Wrap (see recipe), *2 vegetable, ½ meat, 2 grain, ½ dairy, 1 added fat*
*   (395 calories)*
1 cup red and yellow bell pepper slices, *2 vegetable (25 calories)*
2 tablespoons low-fat creamy Italian dressing, *1 added fat (80 calories)*
½ cup nonfat vanilla frozen yogurt, *1 dairy (140 calories)*

Afternoon Snack *(220 calories)*
1 ounce whole-wheat snack crackers, *1 grain (130 calories)*
1 tablespoon peanut butter, *½ nuts/seeds/legumes (90 calories)*

Dinner *(605 calories)*
4½ ounces grilled chicken breast without skin, *1½ meat (210 calories)*
1 medium (5-inch) baked sweet potato, *2 vegetable (180 calories)*
½ teaspoon trans-fat-free margarine, *½ added fat (15 calories)*
1 cup cooked brown rice, *2 grain (200 calories)*

Evening Snack/Dessert *(120 calories)*
1 Baked Banana (see recipe), *2 fruit, 1 sweets (120 calories)*

Nutrition analysis for the day: 2,235 calories, 8 grain, 4 fruit, 6 vegetable, 3½ dairy,
2 meat, ½ nuts/seeds/legumes, 2½ added fat, 1 sweets

2,200 CALORIES: DAY 5
Target: 8 grain, 4 fruit, 5 vegetable, 3 dairy, 2 meat, ½ nuts/seeds/legumes,
   2½ added fat, 1 sweets

Breakfast *(540 calories)*
½ large (about 4-inch) whole-wheat bagel, *2 grain (200 calories)*
1½ teaspoons trans-fat-free margarine, *1½ added fat (40 calories)*
1 cup grapes, *2 fruit (100 calories)*
1 cup low-fat fruited yogurt, *1 dairy (200 calories)*

Morning Snack *(150 calories)*
1 medium apple, *1 fruit (50 calories)*
1 small low-fat granola bar, *1 grain (100 calories)*

Lunch *(515 calories)*
Two 1-ounce slices whole-wheat bread, *2 grain (160 calories)*
3 ounces sliced roast beef, *1 meat (150 calories)*
1 tablespoon low-fat mayonnaise, *½ added fat (15 calories)*
4 slices tomato, *1 vegetable (20 calories)*
4 leaves romaine lettuce, *1 vegetable (20 calories)*
2 ounces low-fat swiss cheese (about 2 thick slices), *1½ dairy (150 calories)*

Afternoon Snack *(380 calories)*
Trail mix:
        3 tablespoons peanuts, *½ nuts/seeds/legumes (160 calories)*
        1 ounce unsalted mini pretzels (about ½ cup), *1 grain (110 calories)*
        ¼ cup raisins, *1 fruit (110 calories)*

Dinner *(535 calories)*
1 cup cooked whole-wheat pasta, *2 grain (200 calories)*
1 cup low-sodium marinara sauce, *2 vegetable (80 calories)*
½ cup sweet green peas, *1 vegetable (65 calories)*
3 ounces ground turkey breast (cooked with cooking spray), *1 meat (110 calories)*
¾ ounce shredded parmesan cheese (about ¼ cup), *½ dairy (80 calories)*

Evening Snack/Dessert *(80 calories)*
½ cup fresh strawberries, *1 fruit (25 calories)*
1 tablespoon sugar, *1 sweets (45 calories)*
1 tablespoon low-fat whipped topping, *½ added fat (10 calories)*

Nutrition analysis for the day: 2,200 calories, 8 grain, 5 fruit, 5 vegetable, 3 dairy,
2 meat, ½ nuts/seeds/legumes, 2½ added fat, 1 sweets

|||||||||||||||||||||||||||||||||||||||||||||||||||||||||||||||||||||||||||||||||||||||||||||||||||||||||||||||||||||||||||||||

2,200 CALORIES: DAY 6
*Target: 8 grain, 4 fruit, 5 vegetable, 3 dairy, 2 meat, ½ nuts/seeds/legumes,
    2½ added fat, 1 sweets*

Breakfast *(395 calories)*
2 ounces toasted oat cereal (about 2 cups), *2 grain (200 calories)*
1 medium (7-inch) banana, *2 fruit (105 calories)*
1 cup nonfat milk, *1 dairy (90 calories)*

Morning Snack *(335 calories)*
1 cup low-fat fruited yogurt, *1 dairy (200 calories)*
1 ounce low-fat granola (about ¼ cup), *1 grain (110 calories)*
½ cup sliced fresh strawberries, *1 fruit (25 calories)*

Lunch *(590 calories)*
Two 1-ounce slices whole-wheat bread, *2 grain (160 calories)*
½ cup tuna fish (canned in water), *1 meat (120 calories)*
1½ ounces low-fat swiss cheese, *1 dairy (150 calories)*
2 leaves lettuce, *½ vegetable (10 calories)*
2 slices tomato, *½ vegetable (10 calories)*
2 tablespoons low-fat mayonnaise, *1 added fat (30 calories)*
1 medium orange, *1 fruit (60 calories)*
1 small chocolate chip cookie, *½ sweets (50 calories)*

Afternoon Snack *(175 calories)*
1 small (3-inch) baked potato, *1 vegetable (110 calories)*
½ cup salsa, *1 vegetable (30 calories)*
2 tablespoons low-fat sour cream, *1 added fat (35 calories)*

Dinner *(520 calories)*
Shrimp Scampi, 3 ounces shrimp with sauce (see recipe), *1 meat (145 calories)*
1½ cup whole-wheat linguine, *3 grain (300 calories)*
2 cups mixed raw leafy greens and vegetables, *2 vegetable (35 calories)*
1 tablespoon low-fat Italian dressing, *½ added fat (40 calories)*

Evening Snack/Dessert *(150 calories)*
7 dark-chocolate-covered almonds, *½ nuts/seeds/legumes, ½ sweets (150 calories)*

*Nutrition analysis for the day: 2,165 calories, 8 grain, 4 fruit, 5 vegetable, 3 dairy,
2 meat, ½ nuts/seeds/legumes, 2½ added fat, 1 sweets*

2,200 CALORIES: DAY 7
Target: 8 grain, 4 fruit, 5 vegetable, 3 dairy, 2 meat, ½ nuts/seeds/legumes,
2½ added fat, 1 sweets

Breakfast *(420 calories)*
1 Low-Fat Blueberry Muffin (see recipe), *2 grain (200 calories)*
1 teaspoon trans-fat-free margarine, *1 added fat (25 calories)*
1 cup nonfat milk, *1 dairy (90 calories)*
1 cup grapes, *2 fruit (105 calories)*

Morning Snack *(275 calories)*
One 4-ounce snack cup applesauce, *1 fruit (55 calories)*
2 ounces honey whole-wheat pretzels, *2 grain (220 calories)*

Lunch *(520 calories)*
Black bean burrito:
      One 10-inch whole-wheat tortilla, *2 grain (180 calories)*
      ½ cup canned black beans, drained and rinsed, *1 nuts/seeds/legumes*
        (115 calories)
      ¼ ripe avocado, *½ vegetable (60 calories)*
      1½ ounces shredded low-fat cheddar cheese (about ⅓ cup), *1 dairy (75 calories)*
      ¼ cup tomato salsa, *½ vegetable (15 calories)*
      2 tablespoons reduced-fat sour cream, *1 added fat (40 calories)*
½ cup chopped fresh tomato, *1 vegetable (15 calories)*
1 cup shredded lettuce, *1 vegetable (20 calories)*

Afternoon Snack *(380 calories)*
1 ounce whole-wheat snack crackers, *1 grain (130 calories)*
1 cup low-fat fruited yogurt, *1 dairy (200 calories)*
1 medium apple, *1 fruit (50 calories)*

Dinner *(480 calories)*
6 ounces baked cod,* *2 meat (180 calories)*
1 cup brown rice pilaf, *2 grain (200 calories)*
1 cup Roasted Brussels Sprouts (see recipe), *2 vegetable (100 calories)*

* Place fish on a baking sheet sprayed with cooking spray. Bake at 425°F for 15 minutes or until fish flakes with a fork.

Evening Snack/Dessert *(140 calories)*
1 ounce dark chocolate, *1 sweets (140 calories)*

*Nutrition analysis for the day: 2,215 calories, 9 grain, 4 fruit, 5 vegetable, 3 dairy,
2 meat, 1 nuts/seeds/legumes, 2 added fat, 1 sweets*

||||||||||||||||||||||||||||||||||||||||||||||||||||||||||||||||||||||||||||||||||||||||||||||||||||||||||||

2,400 CALORIES: DAY 1
*Target: 9 grain, 5 fruit, 5 vegetable, 3 dairy, 2 meat, ½ nuts/seeds/legumes,
    3 added fat, 1 sweets*

Breakfast *(565 calories)*
Two 1-ounce slices whole-wheat bread, toasted, *2 grain (160 calories)*
1 tablespoon peanut butter, *½ nuts/seeds/legumes (100 calories)*
1 medium (7-inch) banana, *2 fruit (105 calories)*
1 cup low-fat fruited yogurt, *1 dairy (200 calories)*

Morning Snack *(120 calories)*
½ cup low-fat cottage cheese, *1 dairy (80 calories)*
½ cup fresh pineapple, *1 fruit (40 calories)*

Lunch *(640 calories)*
Two 1-ounce slices whole-wheat bread, *2 grain (160 calories)*
4 ounces sliced grilled chicken breast, *1½ meat (200 calories)*
2 tablespoons low-fat mayonnaise, *1 added fat (30 calories)*
4 slices tomato, *1 vegetable (20 calories)*
4 leaves romaine lettuce, *1 vegetable (20 calories)*
1 ounce honey whole-wheat pretzels, *1 grain (110 calories)*
1 medium pear, *1 fruit (100 calories)*

Afternoon Snack *(255 calories)*
1 ounce whole-wheat snack crackers, *1 grain (130 calories)*
1½ ounces low-fat cheddar cheese, *1 dairy (75 calories)*
1 medium apple, *1 fruit (50 calories)*

Dinner *(600 calories)*
1½ cups Beef and Vegetable Stir-Fry (see recipe), *¾ meat, 3 vegetable (300 calories)*
1½ cups cooked brown rice, *3 grain (300 calories)*

Evening Snack/Dessert *(190 calories)*
One ¾-inch slice Gingerbread (see recipe), *1 sweets (150 calories)*
¼ cup low-fat whipped topping, *2 added fat (40 calories)*

*Nutrition analysis for the day: 2,370 calories, 9 grain, 5 fruit, 5 vegetable, 3 dairy,
2 meat, ½ nuts/seeds/legumes, 3 added fat, 1 sweets*

|||||||||||||||||||||||||||||||||||||||||||||||||||||||||||||||||||||||||||||||||||||||||||||||||||||||||||||

2,400 CALORIES: DAY 2
Target: 9 grain, 5 fruit, 5 vegetable, 3 dairy, 2 meat, ½ nuts/seeds/legumes, 3 added fat, 1 sweets

Breakfast *(520 calories)*
2 ounce uncooked oatmeal cooked with water (cooks to about 1½ cups), *2 grain (200 calories)*
1 packet sugar substitute (optional) *(0 calories)*
½ cup pear slices, *1 fruit (50 calories)*
¾ cup 100% apple juice, *1 fruit (90 calories)*
1 cup low-fat vanilla yogurt, *1 dairy (180 calories)*

Morning Snack *(235 calories)*
1 cup unsweetened applesauce, *2 fruit (105 calories)*
One 1-ounce snack bag pita chips, *1 grain (130 calories)*

Lunch *(540 calories)*
Two 1-ounce slices whole-wheat bread, toasted, *2 grain (160 calories)*
3 ounces reduced-fat swiss cheese (2 big slices), *2 dairy (220 calories)*
2 ounces roast beef, *⅔ meat (90 calories)*
2 tablespoons low-fat mayonnaise, *1 added fat (30 calories)*
4 slices tomato, *1 vegetable (20 calories)*
4 leaves lettuce, *1 vegetable (20 calories)*

Afternoon Snack *(215 calories)*
"Ants on a Log":
    4 celery sticks (5 inches each), *1 vegetable (5 calories)*
    1 tablespoon peanut butter, *½ nuts/seeds/legumes (100 calories)*
    ¼ cup raisins, *1 fruit (110 calories)*

Dinner *(655 calories)*
4 ounces Poached Salmon (see recipe), *1⅓ meat (195 calories)*
1 cup boiled yellow corn, *2 vegetable (135 calories)*
2 teaspoons trans-fat-free margarine, *2 added fat (50 calories)*
⅔ cup Quinoa, Corn, and Black Bean Salad (see recipe), *1 grain, ¼ vegetable, ¼ nuts/seeds/legumes (125 calories)*
1 small (2-ounce) whole-wheat dinner roll, *2 grain (150 calories)*

Evening Snack/Dessert *(210 calories)*
2 dark chocolate kisses, *½ sweets (40 calories)*
2 graham cracker rectangles, *1 grain (120 calories)*
2 marshmallows, *½ sweets (50 calories)*

Nutrition analysis for the day: 2,375 calories, 9 grain, 5 fruit, 5¼ vegetable, 3 dairy, 2 meat, ¾ nuts/seeds/legumes, 3 added fat, 1 sweets

||||||||||||||||||||||||||||||||||||||||||||||||||||||||||||||||||||||||||||||||||||||||||||||||||||||||||||||||||

2,400 CALORIES: DAY 3

Target: 9 grain, 5 fruit, 5 vegetable, 3 dairy, 2 meat, ½ nuts/seeds/legumes, 3 added fat, 1 sweets

Breakfast *(605 calories)*
2 whole eggs plus 2 egg whites, scrambled (cooked with cooking spray), *1 meat (195 calories)*
1½ ounces shredded low-fat cheddar cheese (about ⅓ cup), *1 dairy (75 calories)*
1 cup pitted sweet cherries, *2 fruit (100 calories)*
Two 1-ounce slices whole-wheat bread, toasted, *2 grain (160 calories)*
2 teaspoons trans-fat-free margarine, *2 added fat (50 calories)*
1½ teaspoons fruit preserves, *½ sweets (25 calories)*

Morning Snack *(250 calories)*
1 cup low-fat vanilla yogurt, *1 dairy (180 calories)*
½ cup sliced banana, *1 fruit (70 calories)*

Lunch *(450 calories)*
1 Cobb Salad (see recipe), *4 vegetable, ½ dairy, ½ meat, 1 added fat (225 calories)*
Two 1-ounce slices whole-wheat bread, *2 grain (160 calories)*
1½ ounces sliced roasted turkey breast, *½ meat (60 calories)*
1 teaspoon deli mustard *(5 calories)*

Afternoon Snack *(270 calories)*
1 medium apple, *1 fruit (50 calories)*
2 ounces honey whole-wheat pretzels, *2 grain (220 calories)*

Dinner *(530 calories)*
1 cup Fruity Chicken Stir-Fry (see recipe), *1 fruit, 1 vegetable, ½ meat (330 calories)*
1 cup cooked brown rice, *2 grain (200 calories)*

Evening Snack/Dessert *(290 calories)*
1 ounce unsalted mini pretzels (about ½ cup), *1 grain (110 calories)*
2 tablespoons peanuts, *¼ nuts/seeds/legumes (110 calories)*
1 tablespoon chocolate chips, *½ sweets (70 calories)*

Nutrition analysis for the day: 2,395 calories, 9 grain, 5 fruit, 5 vegetable, 2½ dairy, 2½ meat, ¼ nuts/seeds/legumes, 3 added fat, 1 sweets

|||||||||||||||||||||||||||||||||||||||||||||||||||||||||||||||||||||||||||||||||||||||||||||||||||||||||||||||||||||||||

2,400 CALORIES: DAY 4

Target: 9 grain, 5 fruit, 5 vegetable, 3 dairy, 2 meat, ½ nuts/seeds/legumes, 3 added fat, 1 sweets

Breakfast *(530 calories)*
2 ounces shredded wheat squares (about 1 cup), *2 grain (200 calories)*
1 cup sliced banana, *2 fruit (140 calories)*
¾ cup 100% orange juice, *1 fruit (80 calories)*
1 cup low-fat milk, *1 dairy (110 calories)*

Morning Snack *(420 calories)*
1 cup low-fat fruited yogurt, *1 dairy (200 calories)*
2 ounces unsalted mini pretzels (about 1 cup), *2 grain (220 calories)*

Lunch *(500 calories)*
1 Chicken Caesar Wrap (see recipe), *2 vegetable, ½ meat, 2 grain, ½ dairy, 1 added fat (395 calories)*
1 cup red and yellow bell pepper slices, *2 vegetable (25 calories)*
2 tablespoons "lite" creamy Italian dressing, *1 added fat (80 calories)*

Afternoon Snack *(230 calories)*
1 ounce whole-wheat snack crackers, *1 grain (130 calories)*
1 tablespoon peanut butter, *½ nuts/seeds/legumes (100 calories)*

Dinner *(630 calories)*
4½ ounces grilled chicken breast, *1½ meat (225 calories)*
1 medium (5-inch) baked sweet potato, *2 vegetable (180 calories)*
1 teaspoon trans-fat-free margarine, *1 added fat (25 calories)*
1 cup cooked brown rice, *2 grain (200 calories)*

Evening Snack/Dessert *(120 calories)*
1 Baked Banana (see recipe), *2 fruit, 1 sweets (120 calories)*

Nutrition analysis for the day: 2,430 calories, 9 grain, 5 fruit, 6 vegetable, 2½ dairy, 2 meat, ½ nuts/seeds/legumes, 3 added fat, 1 sweets

||||||||||||||||||||||||||||||||||||||||||||||||||||||||||||||||||||||||||||||||||||||||||||||||||||||||||||||||

2,400 CALORIES: DAY 5
Target: 9 grain, 5 fruit, 5 vegetable, 3 dairy, 2 meat, ½ nuts/seeds/legumes,
3 added fat, 1 sweets

Breakfast *(525 calories)*
½ large (about 4-inch) whole-wheat bagel, *2 grain (200 calories)*
1 teaspoon trans-fat-free margarine, *1 added fat (25 calories)*
1 cup grapes, *2 fruit (100 calories)*
1 cup low-fat fruited yogurt, *1 dairy (200 calories)*

Morning Snack *(190 calories)*
1 medium apple, *1 fruit (50 calories)*
1 medium low-fat granola bar, *2 grain (140 calories)*

Lunch *(420 calories)*
Two 1-ounce slices whole-wheat bread, *2 grain (160 calories)*
3 ounces sliced roast beef, *1 meat (150 calories)*
1 tablespoon low-fat mayonnaise, *½ added fat (15 calories)*
4 slices tomato, *1 vegetable (20 calories)*
4 leaves romaine lettuce, *1 vegetable (20 calories)*
¾ ounce low-fat swiss cheese (1 thin slice), *½ dairy (55 calories)*

Afternoon Snack *(410 calories)*
Trail mix:
      3 tablespoons peanuts, *½ nuts/seeds/legumes (160 calories)*
      1 ounce chocolate candies, *1 sweets (140 calories)*
      ¼ cup raisins, *1 fruit (110 calories)*

Dinner *(645 calories)*
1 cup cooked whole-wheat pasta, *2 grain (200 calories)*
1 cup low-sodium marinara sauce, *2 vegetable (80 calories)*
3 ounces ground turkey breast meat (cooked with cooking spray), *1 meat*
    (120 calories)
¾ ounce shredded parmesan cheese (about ¼ cup), *½ dairy (80 calories)*
½ small (2-ounce) whole-wheat dinner roll, *1 grain (75 calories)*
1 teaspoon trans-fat-free margarine, *1 added fat (25 calories)*
1 cup chopped romaine lettuce, *1 vegetable (20 calories)*
1 tablespoon reduced-fat caesar dressing, *1 added fat (45 calories)*

Evening Snack/Dessert *(190 calories)*
1 cup fresh strawberries, *2 fruit (50 calories)*
½ cup low-fat frozen yogurt, *1 dairy (140 calories)*

Nutrition analysis for the day: 2,380 calories, 9 grain, 6 fruit, 5 vegetable, 3 dairy, 2 meat, ½ nuts/seeds/legumes, 3½ added fat, 1 sweets

||||||||||||||||||||||||||||||||||||||||||||||||||||||||||||||||||||||||||||||||||||||||||||||||||||||||

2,400 CALORIES: DAY 6

Target: 9 grain, 5 fruit, 5 vegetable, 3 dairy, 2 meat, ½ nuts/seeds/legumes, 3 added fat, 1 sweets

Breakfast *(545 calories)*
2 ounces toasted oat cereal (about 2 cups), *2 grain (200 calories)*
One 1-ounce slice whole-wheat bread, toasted, *1 grain (80 calories)*
1½ teaspoons fruit preserves, *½ sweets (25 calories)*
½ cup sliced banana, *1 fruit (70 calories)*
¾ cup 100% orange juice, *1 fruit (80 calories)*
1 cup nonfat milk, *1 dairy (90 calories)*

Morning Snack *(470 calories)*
1 cup low-fat fruited yogurt, *1 dairy (200 calories)*
1 ounce low-fat granola (about ¼ cup), *1 grain (110 calories)*
½ cup dried apricots, *2 fruit (160 calories)*

Lunch *(540 calories)*
Two 1-ounce slices whole-wheat bread, *2 grain (160 calories)*
½ cup tuna fish (canned in water), *1 meat (120 calories)*
1½ ounces low-fat swiss cheese, *1 dairy (150 calories)*
2 leaves lettuce, *½ vegetable (10 calories)*
2 slices tomato, *½ vegetable (10 calories)*
2 tablespoons low-fat mayonnaise, *1 added fat (30 calories)*
1 medium orange, *1 fruit (60 calories)*

Afternoon Snack *(175 calories)*
1 small (3-inch) baked potato, *1 vegetable (110 calories)*
½ cup salsa, *1 vegetable (30 calories)*
2 tablespoons low-fat sour cream, *1 added fat (35 calories)*

Dinner *(500 calories)*
Shrimp Scampi, 3 ounces shrimp with sauce (see recipe), *1 meat (145 calories)*
1½ cups cooked whole-wheat linguine, *3 grain (300 calories)*
2 cups mixed raw leafy greens and vegetables (shredded carrots, sliced bell peppers)
    2 vegetable (35 calories)
2 tablespoons fat-free Italian dressing *(20 calories)*

Evening Snack/Dessert *(150 calories)*
7 dark-chocolate-covered almonds, *½ nuts/seeds/legumes, ½ sweets (150 calories)*

Nutrition analysis for the day: 2,380 calories, 9 grain, 5 fruit, 5 vegetable, 3 dairy, 2 meat, ½ nuts/seeds/legumes, 2 added fat, 1 sweets

----

2,400 CALORIES: DAY 7
Target: 9 grain, 5 fruit, 5 vegetable, 3 dairy, 2 meat, ½ nuts/seeds/legumes, 3 added fat, 1 sweets

Breakfast *(415 calories)*
1 Low-Fat Blueberry Muffin (see recipe), *2 grain (200 calories)*
1 teaspoon trans-fat-free margarine, *1 added fat (25 calories)*
1 cup nonfat milk, *1 dairy (90 calories)*
1 cup grapes, *2 fruit (100 calories)*

Morning Snack *(290 calories)*
One 4-ounce snack cup peaches in juice, *1 fruit (70 calories)*
2 ounces honey whole-wheat pretzels, *2 grain (220 calories)*

Lunch *(580 calories)*
Black bean burrito:
      One 10-inch whole-wheat tortilla, *2 grain (180 calories)*
      ½ cup canned black beans, drained and rinsed, *1 nuts/seeds/legumes (115 calories)*
      ½ ripe avocado, *1 vegetable (120 calories)*
      1½ ounces shredded low-fat cheddar cheese (about ⅓ cup), *1 dairy (75 calories)*
      ¼ cup tomato salsa, *½ vegetable (15 calories)*
      2 tablespoons reduced-fat sour cream, *1 added fat (40 calories)*
½ cup chopped fresh tomato, *1 vegetable (15 calories)*
1 cup shredded lettuce, *1 vegetable (20 calories)*

Afternoon Snack *(380 calories)*
1 ounce whole-wheat snack crackers, *1 grain (130 calories)*
1 cup low-fat fruited yogurt, *1 dairy (200 calories)*
1 medium apple, *1 fruit (50 calories)*

Dinner *(585 calories)*
6 ounces baked cod,* *2 meat (180 calories)*
1 cup brown rice pilaf, *2 grain (200 calories)*
1 cup Roasted Brussels Sprouts (see recipe), *2 vegetable (100 calories)*

One 1-ounce slice whole-wheat bread, toasted, *1 grain (80 calories)*
1 teaspoon trans-fat-free margarine, *1 added fat (25 calories)*

*Place fish on a baking sheet sprayed with cooking spray. Bake at 425°F for 15 minutes or until fish flakes with a fork.

Evening Snack/Dessert *(170 calories)*
1 ounce dark chocolate, *1 sweets (140 calories)*
½ cup fresh raspberries, *1 fruit (30 calories)*

Nutrition analysis for the day: 2,420 calories, 10 grain, 5 fruit, 5½ vegetable, 3 dairy, 2 meat, 1 nuts/seeds/legumes, 3 added fat, 1 sweets

||||||||||||||||||||||||||||||||||||||||||||||||||||||||||||||||||||||||||||||||||||||||||||||||||||||||||||

2,600 CALORIES: DAY 1
Target: 10 grain, 5 fruit, 5 vegetable, 3 dairy, 2½ meat, 1 nuts/seeds/legumes, 3 added fat, 1½ sweets

Breakfast *(680 calories)*
Two 1-ounce slices whole-wheat bread, toasted, *2 grain (160 calories)*
2 whole eggs plus 2 egg whites, scrambled (cooked with cooking spray), *1 meat (195 calories)*
1 teaspoon trans-fat-free margarine, *1 added fat (25 calories)*
1 medium (7-inch) banana, *2 fruit (140 calories)*
1 cup nonfat vanilla yogurt, *1 dairy (160 calories)*

Morning Snack *(300 calories)*
½ cup low-fat cottage cheese, *1 dairy (80 calories)*
½ cup fresh pineapple, *1 fruit (40 calories)*
One 1-ounce slice whole-wheat bread, *1 grain (80 calories)*
1 tablespoon peanut butter, *½ nuts/seeds/legumes (100 calories)*

Lunch *(610 calories)*
Two 1-ounce slices whole-wheat bread, *2 grain (160 calories)*
3 ounces sliced grilled chicken breast, *1 meat (150 calories)*
2 tablespoons low-fat mayonnaise, *1 added fat (30 calories)*
4 slices tomato, *1 vegetable (20 calories)*
4 leaves romaine lettuce, *1 vegetable (20 calories)*
1 ounce honey whole-wheat pretzels, *1 grain (110 calories)*
1 cup sliced apple, *2 fruit (60 calories)*
1 tablespoon low-fat caramel dipping sauce, *½ sweets (60 calories)*

Afternoon Snack *(205 calories)*
1 ounce whole-wheat snack crackers, *1 grain (130 calories)*
1½ ounces low-fat cheddar cheese, *1 dairy (75 calories)*

Dinner *(600 calories)*
1½ cups Beef and Vegetable Stir-Fry (see recipe), *¾ meat, 3 vegetable (300 calories)*
1½ cups cooked brown rice, *3 grain (300 calories)*

Evening Snack/Dessert *(170 calories)*
One ¾-inch slice Gingerbread (see recipe), *1 sweets (150 calories)*
2 tablespoons low-fat whipped topping, *1 added fat (20 calories)*

Nutrition analysis for the day: 2,565 calories, 10 grain, 5 fruit, 5 vegetable, 3 dairy, 2¾ meat, ½ nuts/seeds/legumes, 3 added fat, 1½ sweets

||||||||||||||||||||||||||||||||||||||||||||||||||||||||||||||||||||||||||||||||||||||||||||||||||||||||||

2,600 CALORIES: DAY 2
Target: 10 grain, 5 fruit, 5 vegetable, 3 dairy, 2½ meat, 1 nuts/seeds/legumes,
   3 added fat, 1½ sweets

Breakfast *(420 calories)*
1 ounce uncooked oatmeal cooked with water (cooks to about ¾ cup), *1 grain*
   (100 calories)
1 cup low-fat milk, *1 dairy (110 calories)*
1 packet sugar substitute (optional) *(0 calories)*
One 1-ounce slice whole-wheat bread, toasted, *1 grain (80 calories)*
1 teaspoon trans-fat-free margarine, *1 added fat (25 calories)*
1 medium (7-inch) banana, *2 fruit (105 calories)*

Morning Snack *(235 calories)*
1 cup unsweetened applesauce, *2 fruit (105 calories)*
One 1-ounce snack bag pita chips, *1 grain (130 calories)*

Lunch *(665 calories)*
Two 1-ounce slices whole-wheat bread, toasted, *2 grain (160 calories)*
1½ ounces reduced-fat swiss cheese (2 small slices), *1 dairy (110 calories)*
3 ounces sliced roast beef, *1 meat (150 calories)*
1 teaspoon deli mustard *(5 calories)*
4 slices tomato, *1 vegetable (20 calories)*
4 leaves lettuce, *1 vegetable (20 calories)*
1 cup low-fat fruited yogurt, *1 dairy (200 calories)*

Afternoon Snack *(205 calories)*
"Ants on a log":
>   4 celery sticks (5 inches each), *1 vegetable (5 calories)*
>   1 tablespoon peanut butter, *½ nuts/seeds/legumes (90 calories)*
>   ¼ cup raisins, *1 fruit (110 calories)*

Dinner *(850 calories)*
6 ounces Poached Salmon (see recipe), *2 meat (290 calories)*
1 cup steamed corn kernels, *2 vegetable (135 calories)*
1 teaspoon trans-fat-free margarine, *1 added fat (25 calories)*
1 tablespoon balsamic vinaigrette dressing, *1 added fat (50 calories)*
1 cup cooked brown rice, *2 grain (200 calories)*
1 small (2-ounce) whole-wheat dinner roll, *2 grain (150 calories)*

Evening Snack/Dessert *(250 calories)*
4 dark chocolate kisses, *1 sweets (80 calories)*
2 graham cracker rectangles, *1 grain (120 calories)*
2 marshmallows, *½ sweets (50 calories)*

Nutrition analysis for the day: 2,625 calories, 10 grain, 5 fruit, 5 vegetable, 3 dairy, 3 meat, ½ nuts/seeds/legumes, 3 added fat, 1½ sweets

||||||||||||||||||||||||||||||||||||||||||||||||||||||||||||||||||||||||||||||||||||||||

2,600 CALORIES: DAY 3
Target: 10 grain, 5 fruit, 5 vegetable, 3 dairy, 2½ meat, 1 nuts/seeds/legumes, 3 added fat, 1½ sweets

Breakfast *(625 calories)*
3 whole eggs, scrambled (cooked with cooking spray), *1 meat (240 calories)*
1½ ounces shredded low-fat cheddar cheese (about ⅓ cup), *1 dairy (75 calories)*
1 cup pitted sweet cherries, *2 fruit (100 calories)*
Two 1-ounce slices whole-wheat bread, toasted, *2 grain (160 calories)*
1 teaspoon trans-fat-free margarine, *1 added fat (25 calories)*
1½ teaspoons fruit preserves, *½ sweets (25 calories)*

Morning Snack *(250 calories)*
1 cup low-fat vanilla yogurt, *1 dairy (180 calories)*
½ cup sliced banana, *1 fruit (70 calories)*

Lunch *(525 calories)*
1 Cobb Salad (see recipe), *4 vegetable, ½ dairy, ½ meat, 1 added fat (225 calories)*
Two 1-ounce slices whole-wheat bread, *2 grain (160 calories)*

1½ ounces sliced roasted turkey breast, *½ meat (60 calories)*
¾ ounce (1 slice) reduced-fat American cheese, *½ dairy (50 calories)*
2 tablespoons low-fat mayonnaise, *1 added fat (30 calories)*

Afternoon Snack *(320 calories)*
1 medium pear, *1 fruit (100 calories)*
2 ounces honey whole-wheat pretzels, *2 grain (220 calories)*

Dinner *(530 calories)*
1 cup Fruity Chicken Stir-Fry (see recipe), *1 fruit, 1 vegetable, ½ meat (330 calories)*
1 cup cooked brown rice, *2 grain (200 calories)*

Evening Snack/Dessert *(360 calories)*
1 ounce unsalted mini pretzels (about ½ cup), *1 grain (110 calories)*
2 tablespoons peanuts, *¼ nuts/seeds/legumes (110 calories)*
2 tablespoons chocolate chips, *1 sweets (140 calories)*

Nutrition analysis for the day: 2,610 calories, 9 grain, 5 fruit, 5 vegetable, 3 dairy, 2½ meat, ¼ nuts/seeds/legumes, 3 added fat, 1½ sweets

||||||||||||||||||||||||||||||||||||||||||||||||||||||||||||||||||||||||||||||||||||||||||||||

2,600 CALORIES: DAY 4
Target: 10 grain, 5 fruit, 5 vegetable, 3 dairy, 2½ meat, 1 nuts/seeds/legumes, 3 added fat, 1½ sweets

Breakfast *(610 calories)*
2 ounces shredded wheat squares (about 1 cup), *2 grain (200 calories)*
½ cup raisins, *2 fruit (220 calories)*
¾ cup 100% orange juice, *1 fruit (80 calories)*
1 cup low-fat milk, *1 dairy (110 calories)*

Morning Snack *(420 calories)*
1 cup low-fat fruited yogurt, *1 dairy (200 calories)*
2 ounces unsalted mini pretzels (about 1 cup), *2 grain (220 calories)*

Lunch *(515 calories)*
1 Chicken Caesar Wrap (see recipe), *2 vegetable, ½ meat, 2 grain, ½ dairy, 1 added fat (395 calories)*
1 cup red and yellow bell pepper slices, *2 vegetable (40 calories)*
2 tablespoons "lite" creamy Italian dressing, *1 added fat (80 calories)*

Afternoon Snack *(220 calories)*
1 ounce whole-wheat snack crackers, *1 grain (130 calories)*
1 tablespoon peanut butter, *½ nuts/seeds/legumes (90 calories)*

Dinner *(590 calories)*
6 ounces grilled trimmed beef sirloin, *2 meat (335 calories)*
1 cup grilled sliced zucchini and summer squash, *2 vegetable (30 calories)*
1 teaspoon trans-fat-free margarine, *1 added fat (25 calories)*
1 cup cooked brown rice, *2 grain (200 calories)*

Evening Snack/Dessert *(190 calories)*
1 Baked Banana (see recipe), *2 fruit, 1 sweets (120 calories)*
½ ounce shaved milk chocolate (about 1 tablespoon), *½ sweets (70 calories)*

Nutrition analysis for the day: 2,545 calories, 9 grain, 5 fruit, 6 vegetable, 2½ dairy, 2½ meat, ½ nuts/seeds/legumes, 3 added fat, 1½ sweets

||||||||||||||||||||||||||||||||||||||||||||||||||||||||||||||||||||||||||||||||||||||||||||||||||||||||

2,600 CALORIES: DAY 5

Target: 10 grain, 5 fruit, 5 vegetable, 3 dairy, 2½ meat, 1 nuts/seeds/legumes, 3 added fat, 1½ sweets

Breakfast *(625 calories)*
½ large (about 4-inch) whole-wheat bagel, *2 grain (200 calories)*
1 tablespoon peanut butter, *½ nuts/seeds/legumes (100 calories)*

1½ teaspoons fruit preserves, *½ sweets (25 calories)*
1 cup grapes, *2 fruit (100 calories)*
1 cup low-fat fruited yogurt, *1 dairy (200 calories)*

Morning Snack *(190 calories)*
1 medium apple, *1 fruit (50 calories)*
1 medium low-fat granola bar, *2 grain (140 calories)*

Lunch *(530 calories)*
Two 1-ounce slices whole-wheat bread, *2 grain (160 calories)*
3 ounces sliced roast beef, *1 meat (150 calories)*
2 tablespoons low-fat mayonnaise, *1 added fat (30 calories)*
4 slices tomato, *1 vegetable (20 calories)*
4 leaves romaine lettuce, *1 vegetable (20 calories)*
¾ ounce low-fat swiss cheese (1 thin slice), *½ dairy (40 calories)*
One 1-ounce snack bag pretzels, *1 grain (110 calories)*

Afternoon Snack *(410 calories)*
Trail mix:
>3 tablespoons peanuts, *½ nuts/seeds/legumes (160 calories)*
>1 ounce chocolate candies, *1 sweets (140 calories)*
>¼ cup raisins, *1 fruit (110 calories)*

Dinner *(680 calories)*
1 cup cooked whole-wheat pasta, *2 grain (200 calories)*
1 cup low-sodium marinara sauce, *2 vegetable (80 calories)*
4 ounces ground turkey breast meat (cooked with cooking spray), *1⅓ meat (155 calories)*
¾ ounce shredded parmesan cheese (about ¼ cup), *½ dairy (80 calories)*
½ small (2-ounce) whole-wheat dinner roll, *1 grain (75 calories)*
1 teaspoon trans-fat-free margarine, *1 added fat (25 calories)*
1 cup chopped romaine lettuce, *1 vegetable (20 calories)*
1 tablespoon reduced-fat caesar dressing, *1 added fat (45 calories)*

Evening Snack/Dessert *(165 calories)*
½ cup fresh strawberries, *1 fruit (25 calories)*
½ cup low-fat frozen yogurt, *1 dairy (140 calories)*

Nutrition analysis for the day: 2,600 calories, 10 grain, 5 fruit, 5 vegetable, 3 dairy, 2⅓ meat, 1 nuts/seeds/legumes, 3 added fat, 1½ sweets

||||||||||||||||||||||||||||||||||||||||||||||||||||||||||||||||||||||||||||||||||||||||||||||||||||||

2,600 CALORIES: DAY 6
Target: 10 grain, 5 fruit, 5 vegetable, 3 dairy, 2½ meat, 1 nuts/seeds/legumes, 3 added fat, 1½ sweets

Breakfast *(545 calories)*
2 ounces toasted oat cereal (about 2 cups), *2 grain (200 calories)*
One 1-ounce slice whole-wheat bread, toasted, *1 grain (80 calories)*
1½ teaspoons fruit preserves, *½ sweets (25 calories)*
½ cup sliced banana, *1 fruit (70 calories)*
¾ cup 100% orange juice, *1 fruit (80 calories)*
1 cup nonfat milk, *1 dairy (90 calories)*

Morning Snack *(510 calories)*
1 cup low-fat fruited yogurt, *1 dairy (200 calories)*
1 ounce low-fat granola (about ¼ cup), *1 grain (110 calories)*
½ cup dried cherries, *2 fruit (200 calories)*

Lunch *(580 calories)*
Two 1-ounce slices whole-wheat bread, *2 grain (160 calories)*
½ cup tuna fish (canned in water, drained), *1 meat (120 calories)*
1½ ounces low-fat swiss cheese, *1 dairy (80 calories)*
2 leaves lettuce, *½ vegetable (10 calories)*
2 slices tomato, *½ vegetable (10 calories)*
2 tablespoons low-fat mayonnaise, *1 added fat (30 calories)*
1 medium orange, *1 fruit (60 calories)*
1 ounce unsalted pretzels, *1 grain (110 calories)*

Afternoon Snack *(175 calories)*
1 small (3-inch) baked potato, *1 vegetable (110 calories)*
½ cup salsa, *1 vegetable (30 calories)*
2 tablespoons low-fat sour cream, *1 added fat (35 calories)*

Dinner *(655 calories)*
Shrimp Scampi, 5 ounces shrimp with sauce (see recipe), *1⅔ meat (205 calories)*
1½ cup whole-wheat linguine, *3 grain (300 calories)*
1 cup cooked green peas, *2 vegetable (125 calories)*
1 teaspoon trans-fat-free margarine, *1 added fat (25 calories)*

Evening Snack/Dessert *(150 calories)*
7 dark-chocolate-covered almonds, *½ nuts/seeds/legumes, ½ sweets (150 calories)*

Nutrition analysis for the day: 2,615 calories, 10 grain, 5 fruit, 5 vegetable, 3 dairy, 2⅔ meat, ½ nuts/seeds/legumes, 3 added fat, 1 sweets

||||||||||||||||||||||||||||||||||||||||||||||||||||||||||||||||||||||||||||||||||||||||||||||

2,600 CALORIES: DAY 7
Target: 10 grain, 5 fruit, 5 vegetable, 3 dairy, 2½ meat, 1 nuts/seeds/legumes,
    3 added fat, 1½ sweets

Breakfast *(415 calories)*
1 Low-Fat Blueberry Muffin (see recipe), *2 grain (200 calories)*
1 teaspoon trans-fat-free margarine, *1 added fat (25 calories)*
1 cup nonfat milk, *1 dairy (90 calories)*
1 cup grapes, *2 fruit (100 calories)*

Morning Snack *(290 calories)*
One 4-ounce snack cup peaches in juice, *1 fruit (70 calories)*
2 ounces honey whole-wheat pretzels, *2 grain (220 calories)*

Lunch *(730 calories)*

Chicken and black bean burrito:

> One 10-inch whole-wheat tortilla, *2 grain (180 calories)*
>
> 3 ounces grilled chicken breast, cubed, *1 meat (150 calories)*
>
> ½ cup canned black beans, drained and rinsed, *1 nuts/seeds/legumes (115 calories)*
>
> ½ ripe avocado, *1 vegetable (120 calories)*
>
> 1½ ounces shredded low-fat cheddar cheese (about ⅓ cup), *1 dairy (75 calories)*
>
> ¼ cup tomato salsa, *½ vegetable (15 calories)*
>
> 2 tablespoons reduced-fat sour cream, *1 added fat (40 calories)*

½ cup chopped fresh tomato, *1 vegetable (15 calories)*

1 cup shredded lettuce, *1 vegetable (20 calories)*

Afternoon Snack *(380 calories)*

1 ounce whole-wheat snack crackers, *1 grain (130 calories)*

1 cup low-fat fruited yogurt, *1 dairy (200 calories)*

1 medium apple, *1 fruit (50 calories)*

Dinner *(550 calories)*

5 ounces baked cod,* *1⅔ meat (150 calories)*

1 cup brown rice pilaf, *2 grain (200 calories)*

1 cup Roasted Brussels Sprouts (see recipe), *2 vegetable (100 calories)*

½ small (2-ounce) whole-wheat dinner roll, *1 grain (75 calories)*

1 teaspoon trans-fat-free margarine, *1 added fat (25 calories)*

*Place fish on a baking sheet sprayed with cooking spray. Bake at 425°F for 15 minutes or until fish flakes with a fork.

Evening Snack/Dessert *(170 calories)*

1 ounce dark chocolate, *1 sweets (140 calories)*

½ cup fresh raspberries, *1 fruit (30 calories)*

Nutrition analysis for the day: 2,535 calories, 10 grain, 5 fruit, 5½ vegetable, 3 dairy, 2⅔ meat, 1 nuts/seeds/legumes, 3 added fat, 1 sweets

Vegetarian Meal Plans

As you have learned, the original design of the DASH Diet included meat, fish, and poultry. To revise the DASH Diet meal plans so that they would be acceptable to vegetarians, we replaced the meat/fish/poultry servings with other protein-rich foods, primarily legumes and meat alternatives. You will see that as you read through these meal plans. Because some of you may be pesco-vegetarians, we have included fish in some menus, but we also offer a non-fish alternative in those menus as well.

We encourage you to experiment with these meal plans. For example, if you don't like tofu, substitute a different meat alternative, like tempeh. In the table below, all the servings of foods that can be substituted for meat contain about the same amount of protein (roughly 20 grams), so they are interchangeable in that regard. This is true except for legumes—a serving of legumes (½ cup) provides about 6–8 grams of protein. So if you will be using legumes for most of your meat substitutions, try to select high-protein items from the other food groups such as high-protein grains (like quinoa and oats) and vegetables (broccoli and spinach). See Chapter 10 for more high-protein selections.

And because you are interested in losing weight, you need to keep the calorie content of these substitutes in mind. We repeat here the table from Chapter 10 that shows the calories per serving. If you are going to substitute, don't always use the highest calorie alternative.

Serving size and calories for meat alternatives		
	Size of 1 DASH serving	**Calories per serving**
Meat/fish	3 ounces	140–220
Tofu (firm)	9 ounces	180
Tempeh	4 ounces	215
TVP*	½ cup (dehydrated)	160
Whole eggs	3	210
Egg whites	6	100
Seitan	3 ounces	120
Legumes	½ cup (cooked)	110–120

*Texturized Vegetable Protein

|||||||||||||||||||||||||||||||||||||||||||||||||||||||||||||||||||||||||||||||||||||||||||||||||||||||||

1,200 CALORIES: DAY 1
Target: 5 grain, 3 fruit, 4 vegetable, 2 dairy, 1¾ nuts/legumes/protein, ½ added fat,
   ½ sweets

Breakfast *(260 calories)*
1 whole egg plus 4 egg whites, scrambled (cooked with cooking spray), *1 nuts/*
   legumes/protein (150 calories)
One 1-ounce slice whole-wheat bread, *1 grain (80 calories)*
½ cup sliced cantaloupe, *1 fruit (30 calories)*

Morning Snack *(160 calories)*
1 cup nonfat vanilla yogurt, *1 dairy (160 calories)*

Lunch *(245 calories)*
2½ cups mixed raw leafy greens and vegetables (bell peppers, carrots, etc.),
   2½ vegetable (50 calories)
1½ ounces low-fat shredded cheddar cheese (about ⅓ cup), *1 dairy (70 calories)*
Half a 7-inch whole-wheat pita pocket, *1 grain (85 calories)*
1 tablespoon low-fat creamy Italian dressing, *½ added fat (40 calories)*

Afternoon Snack *(170 calories)*
1 cup mixed fresh berries, *2 fruit (70 calories)*
1 small low-fat granola bar, *1 grain (100 calories)*

Dinner *(360 calories)*
1 Tempeh Burger (see recipe), *2 grains, 1 nuts/legumes/protein (330 calories)*
1 cup grilled zucchini and portabella mushroom slices, *2 vegetables (30 calories)*

Evening Snack/Dessert *(40 calories)*
2 dark chocolate kisses, *½ sweets (40 calories)*

Nutrition analysis for the day: 1,235 calories, 5 grain, 3 fruit, 4½ vegetable, 2 dairy, 2 nuts/legumes/protein, ½ added fat, ½ sweets

|||||||||||||||||||||||||||||||||||||||||||||||||||||||||||||||||||||||||||||||||||||||||||||||||||||||||

1,200 CALORIES: DAY 2
Target: 5 grain, 3 fruit, 4 vegetable, 2 dairy, 1¾ nuts/legumes/protein, ½ added fat,
*   ½ sweets*

Breakfast *(160 calories)*
1 cup nonfat sugar-free yogurt, *1 dairy (120 calories)*
½ cup blueberries, *1 fruit (40 calories)*

Morning Snack *(150 calories)*
1 medium apple, *1 fruit (50 calories)*
One 100-calorie snack pack (of choice), *1 grain (100 calories)*

Lunch *(320 calories)*
½ cup cooked chickpeas, *1 nuts/legumes/protein (110 calories)*
Dressing: 1 teaspoon olive oil, 1 teaspoon lemon juice, 1 teaspoon minced cilantro,
    1 teaspoon minced parsley, *1 added fat (40 calories)*
2 cup raw spinach with ¼ cup diced cucumber and ¼ cup diced onion, *2½ vegetable
    (30 calories)*
1 ounce low-fat feta cheese, crumbled, *⅔ dairy (60 calories)*
One 1-ounce slice whole-wheat bread, *1 grain (80 calories)*

Afternoon Snack *(125 calories)*
1 small low-fat granola bar, *1 grain (100 calories)*
½ cup baby carrots, *1 vegetable (25 calories)*

Dinner *(380 calories)*
3 ounces grilled seitan, *1 nuts/legumes/protein (90 calories)*
2 tablespoons low-sodium teriyaki sauce *(40 calories)*

½ cup Roasted Brussels Sprouts (see recipe), *1 vegetable (50 calories)*
1 cup cooked brown rice, *2 grains (200 calories)*

Evening Snack/Dessert *(40 calories)*
1 medium peach, *1 fruit (30 calories)*
½ teaspoon honey, *½ sweets (10 calories)*

Nutrition analysis for the day: 1,175 calories, 5 grain, 3 fruit, 4½ vegetable,
1⅔ dairy, 2 nuts/legumes/protein, 1 added fat, ½ sweets

||||||||||||||||||||||||||||||||||||||||||||||||||||||||||||||||||||||||||||||||||||||||||||||||||||||||||||

1,200 CALORIES: DAY 3

Target: 5 grain, 3 fruit, 4 vegetable, 2 dairy, 1¾ nuts/legumes/protein, ½ added fat,
   ½ sweets

Breakfast *(150 calories)*
1 cup nonfat plain yogurt, *1 dairy (120 calories)*
½ cup sliced peaches, *1 fruit (30 calories)*

Morning Snack *(105 calories)*
4 celery sticks (5 inches each), *1 vegetable (5 calories)*
1 tablespoon peanut butter, *½ nuts/legumes/protein (100 calories)*

Lunch *(375 calories)*
Two 1-ounce slices whole-wheat bread, *2 grain (160 calories)*
3 ounces grilled seitan, *1 nuts/legumes/protein (90 calories)*
1 cup lettuce, tomato, *1 vegetable (35 calories)*
1 cup alfalfa sprouts and diced cucumber, *1 vegetable (30 calories)*
1 teaspoon fat-free honey mustard *(10 calories)*
½ cup grapes, *1 fruit (50 calories)*

Afternoon Snack *(110 calories)*
1 ounce unsalted pretzels, *1 grain (110 calories)*

Dinner *(410 calories)*
1½ cups Pasta Primavera (see recipe), *2 grains, 2 vegetable, ½ dairy, 1 added fat*
   (410 calories)

Evening Snack/Dessert *(60 calories)*
1 medium orange, *1 fruit (60 calories)*

Nutrition analysis for the day: 1,210 calories, 5 grain, 3 fruit, 5 vegetable, 1½ dairy,
1½ nuts/legumes/protein, 1 added fat, 0 sweets

||||||||||||||||||||||||||||||||||||||||||||||||||||||||||||||||||||||||||||||||||||||||||||||||||

1,200 CALORIES: DAY 4

Target: 5 grain, 3 fruit, 4 vegetable, 2 dairy, 1¾ nuts/legumes/protein, ½ added fat,
   ½ sweets

Breakfast *(305 calories)*
2 ounces bran flakes (about 1½ cups), *2 grain (180 calories)*
½ cup mixed fresh berries, *1 fruit (35 calories)*
1 cup nonfat milk, *1 dairy (90 calories)*

Morning Snack *(210 calories)*
2 rye crackers, *1 grain (70 calories)*
¼ cup hummus, *½ nuts/legumes/protein (140 calories)*

Lunch *(225 calories)*
Half a 7-inch whole-wheat pita pocket, *1 grain (85 calories)*
3 ounces grilled seitan, *1 nuts/legumes/protein (90 calories)*
1 cup raw spinach, *1 vegetable (10 calories)*
1 tablespoon "lite" creamy Italian dressing, *½ added fat (40 calories)*

Afternoon Snack *(130 calories)*
½ cup low-fat cottage cheese, *1 dairy (80 calories)*
1 cup cantaloupe slices, *2 fruit (50 calories)*

Dinner *(310 calories)*
1 cup Tofu and Vegetable Stir-Fry (see recipe), *2 vegetable, ½ nuts/legumes/protein*
   (180 calories)
½ cup cooked brown rice, *1 grain (100 calories)*
½ cup steamed sugar snap peas, *1 vegetable (30 calories)*

Evening Snack/Dessert *(35 calories)*
10 pieces chocolate candies, *½ sweets (35 calories)*

Nutrition analysis for the day: 1,215 calories, 5 grain, 3 fruit, 4 vegetable, 2 dairy,
2 nuts/legumes/protein, ½ added fat, ½ sweets

II

1,200 CALORIES: DAY 5

Target: 5 grain, 3 fruit, 4 vegetable, 2 dairy, 1¾ nuts/legumes/protein, ½ added fat, ½ sweets

Breakfast *(190 calories)*
1 cup nonfat plain yogurt, *1 dairy (120 calories)*
1 cup mixed fresh berries, *2 fruit (70 calories)*

Morning Snack *(190 calories)*
1 ounce unsalted pretzels, *1 grain (110 calories)*
½ cup low-fat cottage cheese, *1 dairy (80 calories)*

Lunch *(315 calories)*
1 cup Butternut Squash and Apple Soup (see recipe), *1 vegetable, 1 fruit (180 calories)*
One 1-ounce slice whole-wheat bread, *1 grain (80 calories)*
1 cup mixed raw leafy greens and vegetables, *1 vegetable (25 calories)*
1 tablespoon low-fat balsamic vinaigrette, *½ added fat (30 calories)*

Afternoon Snack *(110 calories)*
2 rye crackers, *1 grain (70 calories)*
¼ cup Black Bean Dip (see recipe), *½ nuts/legumes/protein (40 calories)*

Dinner *(345 calories)*
3 ounces Poached Salmon (see recipe), *1 nuts/legumes/protein (145 calories)*
1 cup boiled carrots, *2 vegetable (50 calories)*
1 small (2-ounce) whole-wheat dinner roll, *2 grain (150 calories)*
OR **Dinner 2** *(345 calories)*
3 ounces sautéed seitan,* *1 nuts/legumes/protein (130 calories)*
1 cup sautéed string beans*, *2 vegetable (35 calories)*
1 cup cooked whole-wheat couscous, *2 grain (180 calories)*

*Sauté seitan and string beans in 1 teaspoon olive oil over medium heat until seitan is firm and string beans are crisp-tender. Finish with a squeeze of lemon and dried basil.

Evening Snack/Dessert *(50 calories)*
1 small chocolate chip cookie, *½ sweets (50 calories)*

Nutrition analysis for the day: 1,200 calories, 5 grain, 3 fruit, 4 vegetable, 2 dairy, 1½ nuts/legumes/protein, ½ added fat, ½ sweets

||||||||||||||||||||||||||||||||||||||||||||||||||||||||||||||||||||||||||||||||||||||||||||||||||||||||||

1,200 CALORIES: DAY 6
*Target: 5 grain, 3 fruit, 4 vegetable, 2 dairy, 1¾ nuts/legumes/protein, ½ added fat,
½ sweets*

Breakfast *(220 calories)*
½ cup low-fat cottage cheese, *1 dairy (80 calories)*
½ cup pineapple chunks, *1 fruit (40 calories)*
1 small low-fat granola bar, *1 grain (100 calories)*

Morning Snack *(100 calories)*
1 medium pear, *1 fruit (100 calories)*

Lunch *(345 calories)*
2 cups mixed raw leafy greens and vegetables (shredded carrots, sliced bell peppers)
    2 vegetable (35 calories)
3 ounces grilled seitan, *1 nuts/legumes/protein (90 calories)*
1 tablespoon unsalted roasted sunflower seeds, *½ nuts/legumes/protein (50 calories)*
1 tablespoon low-fat creamy Italian dressing, *½ added fat (20 calories)*
1 small (2-ounce) whole-wheat dinner roll, *2 grain (150 calories)*

Afternoon Snack *(150 calories)*
1 medium apple, *1 fruit (50 calories)*
1 tablespoon peanut butter, *½ nuts/legumes/protein (100 calories)*

Dinner *(320 calories)*
Piled-High Veggie Pizza (⅙ of a 14-inch pizza) (see recipe), *2 grain, 2 vegetable, ½ dairy
    (250 calories)*
One 4-ounce snack cup peaches in juice, *1 fruit (70 calories)*

Evening Snack/Dessert *(50 calories)*
1 chocolate sandwich cookie, *½ sweets (50 calories)*

*Nutrition analysis for the day: 1,185 calories, 5 grain, 4 fruit, 4 vegetable, 1½ dairy,
2 nuts/legumes/protein, ½ added fat, ½ sweets*

‖‖

1,200 CALORIES: DAY 7

Target: 5 grain, 3 fruit, 4 vegetable, 2 dairy, 1¾ nuts/legumes/protein, ½ added fat, ½ sweets

Breakfast *(230 calories)*

1 ounce uncooked oatmeal cooked with water (cooks to about ¾ cup), *1 grain (100 calories)*

½ cup blueberries, *1 fruit (40 calories)*

1 cup nonfat milk, *1 dairy (90 calories)*

Morning Snack *(50 calories)*

½ cup unsweetened applesauce, *1 fruit (50 calories)*

Lunch *(335 calories)*

1 Veggie Melt Panini (see recipe), *2 grains, 2 vegetable, 1 dairy (335 calories)*

Afternoon Snack *(160 calories)*

3 cups air-popped popcorn, *1 grain (110 calories)*

1 kiwi, *1 fruit (50 calories)*

Dinner *(340 calories)*

5 ounces Poached Cod (see recipe), *1⅔ nuts/legumes/protein (150 calories)*

½ cup brown rice pilaf, *1 grain (100 calories)*

1½ cups mixed raw leafy greens with ½ cup sliced roasted red peppers, *2 vegetable (60 calories)*

1 tablespoon low-fat balsamic vinaigrette, *½ added fat (30 calories)*

OR Dinner 2 *(340 calories)*

5 ounces sautéed seitan,* *1⅔ nuts/legumes/protein (190 calories)*

1 cup sautéed peppers and onion, *2 vegetable (20 calories)*

1 tablespoon low-fat balsamic vinaigrette, *½ added fat (30 calories)*

½ cup brown rice pilaf, *1 grain (100 calories)*

*Sauté peppers and onion in 1 teaspoon olive oil until soft. Add seitan and sauté until firm. Drizzle with vinaigrette.

Evening Snack/Dessert *(80 calories)*

2 dark-chocolate-covered strawberries, *½ fruit, ½ sweets (80 calories)*

Nutrition analysis for the day: 1,195 calories, 5 grain, 3½ fruit, 4 vegetable, 2 dairy, 1⅔ nuts/legumes/protein, ½ added fat, ½ sweets

|||||||||||||||||||||||||||||||||||||||||||||||||||||||||||||||||||||||||||||||||||||||||||||||||||||||||||||||||||||||

1,400 CALORIES: DAY 1

Target: 5 grain, 4 fruit, 4 vegetable, 2 dairy, 1¾ nuts/legumes/protein, ½ added fat,
½ sweets

Breakfast *(320 calories)*
2 whole eggs plus 2 egg whites, scrambled (cooked with cooking spray), *1 nuts/
legumes/protein (200 calories)*
One 1-ounce slice whole-grain bread, *1 grain (80 calories)*
½ teaspoon trans-fat-free margarine, *½ added fat (15 calories)*
½ cup sliced cantaloupe, *1 fruit (25 calories)*

Morning Snack *(225 calories)*
1 cup nonfat plain yogurt, *1 dairy (120 calories)*
1 medium (7-inch) banana, *2 fruit (105 calories)*

Lunch *(345 calories)*
2½ cups mixed raw leafy greens and vegetables, *2½ vegetable (50 calories)*
1½ ounces low-fat shredded cheddar cheese (about ⅓ cup), *1 dairy (70 calories)*
Half a 7-inch whole-wheat pita pocket, *1 grain (85 calories)*
1 tablespoon low-fat creamy Italian dressing, *½ added fat (40 calories)*
1 medium pear, *1 fruit (100 calories)*

Afternoon Snack *(135 calories)*
½ cup mixed fresh berries, *1 fruit (35 calories)*
1 small low-fat granola bar, *1 grain (100 calories)*

Dinner *(360 calories)*
1 Tempeh Burger (see recipe), *2 grains, 1 nuts/legumes/protein (330 calories)*
1 cup grilled zucchini and portabella mushrooms slices, *2 vegetable (30 calories)*

Evening Snack/Dessert *(40 calories)*
2 dark chocolate kisses, *½ sweets (40 calories)*

*Nutrition analysis for the day: 1,425 calories, 5 grain, 5 fruit, 4½ vegetable,
2 dairy, 2 nuts/legumes/protein, 1 added fat, ½ sweets*

|||||||||||||||||||||||||||||||||||||||||||||||||||||||||||||||||||||||||||||||||||||||||||||||||||||||||||||

1,400 CALORIES: DAY 2

Target: 5 grain, 4 fruit, 4 vegetable, 2 dairy, 1¾ nuts/legumes/protein, ½ added fat, ½ sweets

Breakfast *(360 calories)*

1 ounce uncooked oatmeal, cooked with water (cooks to about ¾ cup), *1 grain (100 calories)*
1 tablespoon low-fat peanut butter, *½ nuts/legumes/protein (100 calories)*
½ cup sliced banana, *1 fruit (70 calories)*
1 cup nonfat milk, *1 dairy (90 calories)*

Morning Snack *(150 calories)*

1 medium apple, *1 fruit (50 calories)*
One 100-calorie snack pack (of choice), *1 grain (100 calories)*

Lunch *(235 calories)*

Half a 7-inch whole-wheat pita pocket, *1 grain (85 calories)*
¼ cup hummus, *½ nuts/legumes/protein (140 calories)*
1 cup raw spinach, *1 vegetable (10 calories)*

Afternoon Snack *(130 calories)*

1 cup carrot sticks, *2 vegetable (50 calories)*
2 tablespoons low-fat ranch dressing, *1 added fat (80 calories)*

Dinner *(380 calories)*

1 cup Tofu and Vegetable Stir-Fry (see recipe), *2 vegetables, ½ nuts/legumes/protein (180 calories)*
1 cup cooked brown rice, *2 grain (200 calories)*

Evening Snack/Dessert *(210 calories)*

½ cup low-fat frozen yogurt, *1 dairy (140 calories)*
1 cup mixed fresh berries, *2 fruit (70 calories)*

Nutrition analysis for the day: 1,465 calories, 5 grain, 4 fruit, 5 vegetable, 2 dairy, 1½ nuts/legumes/protein, 1 added fat, 0 sweet

||||||||||||||||||||||||||||||||||||||||||||||||||||||||||||||||||||||||||||||||||||||||||||||||||||||||||||||

1,400 CALORIES: DAY 3
Target: 5 grain, 4 fruit, 4 vegetable, 2 dairy, 1¾ nuts/legumes/protein, ½ added fat,
*   ½ sweets*

Breakfast *(160 calories)*
1 ounce bran flakes (about ¾ cup), *1 grain (90 calories)*
½ cup sliced fresh strawberries, unsweetened, *1 fruit (25 calories)*
½ cup nonfat milk, *½ dairy (45 calories)*

Morning Snack *(280 calories)*
½ cup shelled edamame, *1 nuts/legumes/protein (180 calories)*
1 small low-fat granola bar, *1 grain (100 calories)*

Lunch *(390 calories)*
2 cups raw spinach, *2 vegetables (15 calories)*
½ medium tomato, chopped, and ½ cup sliced cucumber, *2 vegetables (25 calories)*
½ cup cooked chickpeas, *1 nuts/legumes/protein (145 calories)*
1 ounce honey whole-wheat pretzels, *1 grain (110 calories)*
Dressing: 2 teaspoons lemon juice, 1 teaspoon olive oil, 2 tablespoons white wine
    vinegar, *1 added fat (45 calories)*
1 medium apple, *1 fruit (50 calories)*

Afternoon Snack *(115 calories)*
½ cup low-fat cottage cheese, *1 dairy (80 calories)*
½ cup mixed fresh berries, *1 fruit (35 calories)*

Dinner *(410 calories)*
1½ cups Pasta Primavera (see recipe), *2 grains, 2 vegetable, ½ dairy (410 calories)*

Evening Snack/Dessert *(55 calories)*
1 fig bar, *½ sweets (55 calories)*

Nutrition analysis for the day: 1,410 calories, 5 grain, 3 fruit, 6 vegetable, 2 dairy,
2 nuts/legumes/protein, 1 added fat, ½ sweets

||||||||||||||||||||||||||||||||||||||||||||||||||||||||||||||||||||||||||||||||||||||||||||||||||||||||||||||||||

1,400 CALORIES: DAY 4

Target: 5 grain, 4 fruit, 4 vegetable, 2 dairy, 1¾ nuts/legumes/protein, ½ added fat, ½ sweets

Breakfast *(290 calories)*
½ grapefruit, *1 fruit (50 calories)*
1 cup nonfat plain Greek-style yogurt, *1 dairy (130 calories)*
1 ounce low-fat granola (about ¼ cup), *1 grain (110 calories)*

Morning Snack *(50 calories)*
1 cup carrot sticks, *1 vegetable (50 calories)*

Lunch *(340 calories)*
Sauté with 1 teaspoon olive oil:
    ½ cup canned black beans, drained and rinsed, *1 nuts/legumes/protein*
      (115 calories)
    ½ cup low-sodium canned diced tomatoes, *1 vegetable (30 calories)*
    ½ teaspoon ground cumin *(0 calories)*
Half a 7-inch whole-wheat pita pocket, *1 grain (85 calories)*
1 cup chopped lettuce with ½ cup sliced raw vegetables, *2 vegetable (40 calories)*
1 tablespoon "lite" vinaigrette, *½ fat (20 calories)*
1 medium apple, *1 fruit (50 calories)*

Afternoon Snack *(170 calories)*
½ cup nonfat milk, *½ dairy (45 calories)*
1 ounce shredded wheat squares (about ½ cup), *1 grain (100 calories)*
½ cup sliced fresh strawberries, unsweetened, *1 fruit (25 calories)*

Dinner *(380 calories)*
3 ounces grilled seitan, *1 nuts/legumes/protein (90 calories)*
2 tablespoons low-sodium teriyaki sauce *(40 calories)*
½ cup Roasted Brussels Sprouts (see recipe), *1 vegetable (50 calories)*
1 cup cooked brown rice, *2 grain (200 calories)*

Evening Snack/Dessert *(135 calories)*
¼ cup dried cherries, *1 fruit (100 calories)*
10 pieces chocolate candies, *½ sweets (35 calories)*

Nutrition analysis for the day: 1,365 calories, 5 grain, 4 fruit, 5 vegetable, 1½ dairy, 2 nuts/legumes/protein, ½ added fat, ½ sweets

||||||||||||||||||||||||||||||||||||||||||||||||||||||||||||||||||||||||||||||||||||||||||||||||||||||||||||||||||||||||||||||

1,400 CALORIES: DAY 5

Target: 5 grain, 4 fruit, 4 vegetable, 2 dairy, 1¾ nuts/legumes/protein, ½ added fat, ½ sweets

Breakfast *(155 calories)*
1 cup nonfat plain yogurt, *1 dairy (120 calories)*
½ cup mixed fresh berries, *1 fruit (35 calories)*

Morning Snack *(190 calories)*
1 cup sliced mango, *2 fruit (120 calories)*
2 rye crackers, *1 grain (70 calories)*

Lunch *(305 calories)*
⅔ cup Quinoa, Corn, and Black Bean Salad (see recipe), *¼ vegetable, 1 grain, ¼ nuts/legumes/protein (125 calories)*
3 ounces stir-fried firm tofu (about ⅓ block), *⅓ nuts/legumes/protein (115 calories)*
1 cup red bell pepper and celery slices, *2 vegetable (25 calories)*
1 tablespoon low-fat ranch dressing, *½ added fat (40 calories)*

Afternoon Snack *(200 calories)*
1 small low-fat granola bar, *1 grain (100 calories)*
1 medium pear, *1 fruit (100 calories)*

Dinner *(345 calories)*
3 ounces Poached Salmon (see recipe), *1 nuts/legumes/protein (145 calories)*
1 cup boiled carrots, *2 vegetable (50 calories)*
1 small (2-ounce) whole-wheat dinner roll, *2 grain (150 calories)*
OR **Dinner 2** *(345 calories)*
3 ounces sautéed seitan,* *1 nuts/legumes/protein (130 calories)*
1 cup sautéed string beans*, *2 vegetable (35 calories)*
1 cup cooked whole-wheat couscous, *2 grain (180 calories)*

*Sauté seitan and string beans in 1 teaspoon olive oil over medium heat until seitan is firm and string beans are crisp-tender. Finish with a squeeze of lemon and dried basil.

Evening Snack/Dessert *(170 calories)*
½ cup low-fat frozen yogurt, *1 dairy (140 calories)*
2 teaspoons chocolate syrup, *½ sweets (30 calories)*

Nutrition analysis for the day: 1,365 calories, 5 grain, 4 fruit, 4¼ vegetable, 2 dairy, 1¾ nuts/legumes/protein, ½ added fat, ½ sweets

III

1,400 CALORIES: DAY 6

Target: 5 grain, 4 fruit, 4 vegetable, 2 dairy, 1¾ nuts/legumes/protein, ½ added fat, ½ sweets

Breakfast *(240 calories)*
One 1-ounce slice cinnamon raisin bread, toasted, *1 grain (80 calories)*
1 tablespoon low-fat peanut butter, *½ nuts/seeds/legume (90 calories)*
½ cup sliced banana, *1 fruit (70 calories)*

Morning Snack *(140 calories)*
½ cup low-fat cottage cheese, *1 dairy (80 calories)*
1 cup fresh raspberries, *2 fruit (60 calories)*

Lunch *(350 calories)*
Piled-High Veggie Pizza (⅙ of a 14-inch pizza) (see recipe), *2 grain, 2 vegetable, ½ dairy (250 calories)*
1 medium pear, *1 fruit (100 calories)*

Afternoon Snack *(200 calories)*
1 ounce unsalted pretzels, *1 grain (110 calories)*
3 tablespoons hummus, *½ nuts/legumes/protein (90 calories)*

Dinner *(405 calories)*
1 cup cooked whole-wheat pasta, *2 grain (200 calories)*
1 cup low-sodium marinara sauce, *2 vegetable (80 calories)*
½ cup reconstituted TVP,* *½ nuts/legumes/protein (80 calories)*
1½ cups mixed raw leafy greens, *1½ vegetable (20 calories)*
1 tablespoon low-fat Thousand Island dressing, *½ added fat (25 calories)*

*See Chapter 10 for more on TVP (texturized vegetable protein).

Evening Snack/Dessert *(40 calories)*
1 low-fat chocolate sandwich cookie, *½ sweets (40 calories)*

Nutrition analysis for the day: 1,375 calories, 6 grain, 4 fruit, 5½ vegetable, 1½ dairy, 1½ nuts/legumes/protein, ½ added fat, ½ sweets

|||||||||||||||||||||||||||||||||||||||||||||||||||||||||||||||||||||||||||||||||||||||||||||||||||||||||||||||||||||||||||||||||||||||||

1,400 CALORIES: DAY 7
Target: 5 grain, 4 fruit, 4 vegetable, 2 dairy, 1¾ nuts/legumes/protein, ½ added fat, ½ sweets

Breakfast *(325 calories)*
1 ounce uncooked oatmeal cooked with water (cooks to about ¾ cup), *1 grain (100 calories)*
1 cup nonfat milk, *1 dairy (90 calories)*
2 tablespoons raisins, *½ fruit (50 calories)*
2 tablespoons chopped pecans, *¼ nuts/legumes/protein (85 calories)*

Morning Snack *(160 calories)*
2 graham cracker rectangles, *1 grain (110 calories)*
½ cup unsweetened applesauce, *1 fruit (50 calories)*

Lunch *(385 calories)*
1 Veggie Melt Panini (see recipe), *2 grains, 2 vegetable, 1 dairy (335 calories)*
1 medium apple, *1 fruit (50 calories)*

Afternoon Snack *(100 calories)*
1½ cups air-popped popcorn, *½ grain (50 calories)*
1 kiwi, *1 fruit (50 calories)*

Dinner *(340 calories)*
5 ounces Poached Cod (see recipe), *1⅔ nuts/legumes/protein (150 calories)*
½ cup brown rice pilaf, *1 grain (100 calories)*
1½ cups mixed raw leafy greens with ½ cup sliced roasted red bell peppers, *2 vegetable (60 calories)*
1 tablespoon low-fat balsamic vinaigrette, *½ added fat (30 calories)*
OR Dinner 2 *(340 calories)*
5 ounces sautéed seitan,* *1⅔ nuts/legumes/protein (190 calories)*
1 cup sautéed peppers and onion, *2 vegetable (20 calories)*
1 tablespoon low-fat balsamic vinaigrette, *½ added fat (30 calories)*
½ cup brown rice pilaf, *1 grain (100 calories)*

*Sauté peppers and onion in 1 teaspoon olive oil until soft. Add seitan and sauté until firm. Drizzle with vinaigrette.

Evening Snack/Dessert *(80 calories)*
2 dark-chocolate-covered strawberries, *½ fruit, ½ sweets (80 calories)*

Nutrition analysis for the day: 1,390 calories, 5½ grain, 4 fruit, 4 vegetable, 2 dairy, 2 nuts/legumes/protein, ½ added fat, ½ sweets

IIIIIIIIIIIIIIIIIIIIIIIIIIIIIIIIIIIIIIIIIIIIIIIIIIIIIIIIIIIIIIIIIIIIIIIIIIIIIIIIIIIIIIIIIIIIIIIIIIIIIIIIIIIIIIIIIIIIIII

1,600 CALORIES: DAY 1

Target: 6 grain, 4 fruit, 4 vegetable, 2 dairy, 1¾ nuts/legumes/protein, 1 added fat, ½ sweets

Breakfast *(335 calories)*
2 whole eggs, fried (cooked with cooking spray), *⅔ nuts/legumes/protein (160 calories)*
1½ ounces shredded low-fat cheddar cheese (about ⅓ cup), *1 dairy (70 calories)*
One 1-ounce slice whole-grain bread, *1 grain (80 calories)*
½ cup sliced cantaloupe, *1 fruit (25 calories)*

Morning Snack *(155 calories)*
1 cup nonfat plain yogurt, *1 dairy (120 calories)*
½ cup mixed fresh berries, *1 fruit (35 calories)*

Lunch *(525 calories)*
1½ cups Tortellini and Bean Soup (see recipe), *2 vegetable, ½ grain, ½ dairy (330 calories)*
2 cups baby arugula, *2 vegetable (15 calories)*
2 tablespoons "lite" balsamic vinaigrette, *1 added fat (60 calories)*
6 unsalted saltine crackers, *1 grain (120 calories)*

Afternoon Snack *(165 calories)*
1 ounce unsalted pretzels, *1 grain (110 calories)*
½ medium (7-inch) banana, *1 fruit (55 calories)*

Dinner *(360 calories)*
1 Tempeh Burger (see recipe), *2 grains, 1 nuts/legumes/protein (330 calories)*
1 cup grilled zucchini and portabella mushrooms slices, *1 vegetable (30 calories)*

Evening Snack/Dessert *(85 calories)*
½ cup fresh strawberries, *1 fruit (25 calories)*
3 dark chocolate kisses, *½ sweets (60 calories)*

Nutrition analysis for the day: 1,625 calories, 5½ grain, 4 fruit, 5 vegetable, 2½ dairy, 1⅔ nuts/legumes/protein, 1 added fat, ½ sweets

||||||||||||||||||||||||||||||||||||||||||||||||||||||||||||||||||||||||||||||||||||||||||||||||||||||||||||||||||||||||||

1,600 CALORIES: DAY 2
Target: 6 grain, 4 fruit, 4 vegetable, 2 dairy, 1¾ nuts/legumes/protein, 1 added fat, ½ sweets

Breakfast *(325 calories)*
1 ounce uncooked oatmeal cooked with water (cooks to about ¾ cup), *1 grain (100 calories)*
½ medium (7-inch) banana, sliced, *1 fruit (60 calories)*
3 tablespoons chopped walnuts, *½ nuts/legumes/protein (120 calories)*
½ cup nonfat milk, *½ dairy (45 calories)*

Morning Snack *(130 calories)*
1 reduced-fat string cheese stick, *⅔ dairy (80 calories)*
1 medium apple, *1 fruit (50 calories)*

Lunch *(490 calories)*
Middle Eastern lunch special:
     Half a 7-inch whole-wheat pita pocket, *1 grain (85 calories)*
     ¼ cup hummus, *½ nuts/legumes/protein (140 calories)*
     1½ cups grilled vegetables (red/green bell peppers, zucchini, onions, mushrooms), *3 vegetable (115 calories)*
½ cup cooked whole-wheat couscous, *1 grain (90 calories)*
1 medium orange, *1 fruit (60 calories)*

Afternoon Snack *(100 calories)*
1 small low-fat granola bar, *1 grain (100 calories)*

Dinner *(380 calories)*
1 cup Tofu and Vegetable Stir-Fry (see recipe), *2 vegetables, ½ nuts/legumes/protein (180 calories)*
1 cup cooked brown rice, *2 grain (200 calories)*

Evening Snack/Dessert *(220 calories)*
½ cup low-fat frozen yogurt, *1 dairy (140 calories)*
½ cup fresh raspberries, *1 fruit (30 calories)*
2 teaspoons chocolate syrup, *½ sweets (30 calories)*
2 tablespoons low-fat whipped topping, *1 added fat (20 calories)*

Nutrition analysis for the day: 1,645 calories, 6 grain, 4 fruit, 5 vegetable, 2 dairy, 1½ nuts/legumes/protein, 1 added fat, ½ sweets

|||||||||||||||||||||||||||||||||||||||||||||||||||||||||||||||||||||||||||||||||||||||||||||||||||||||

1,600 CALORIES: DAY 3
*Target: 6 grain, 4 fruit, 4 vegetable, 2 dairy, 1¾ nuts/legumes/protein, 1 added fat,
     ½ sweets*

Breakfast *(250 calories)*
1 ounce bran flakes (about ¾ cup), *1 grain (90 calories)*
½ cup sliced banana, *1 fruit (70 calories)*
1 cup nonfat milk, *1 dairy (90 calories)*

Morning Snack *(280 calories)*
½ cup shelled edamame, *1 nuts/legumes/protein (180 calories)*
1 small low-fat granola bar, *1 grain (100 calories)*

Lunch *(390 calories)*
2 cups raw spinach, *2 vegetable (15 calories)*
½ medium tomato, chopped, and ½ cup sliced cucumber, *2 vegetable (25 calories)*
½ cup cooked chickpeas, *1 nuts/legumes/protein (145 calories)*
Dressing: 2 teaspoons lemon juice, 1 teaspoon extra virgin olive oil, 2 tablespoons
     white wine vinegar, *1 added fat (45 calories)*
1 ounce honey whole-wheat pretzels, *1 grain (110 calories)*
1 medium apple, *1 fruit (50 calories)*

Afternoon Snack *(265 calories)*
1 cup nonfat plain Greek-style yogurt, *1 dairy (130 calories)*
1 ounce low-fat granola (about ¼ cup), *1 grain (110 calories)*
½ cup sliced fresh strawberries, *1 fruit (25 calories)*

Dinner *(410 calories)*
1½ cups Pasta Primavera (see recipe), *2 grains, 2 vegetable, ½ dairy (410 calories)*

Evening Snack/Dessert *(55 calories)*
1 fig bar, *½ sweets (55 calories)*

*Nutrition analysis for the day: 1,650 calories, 6 grain, 3 fruit, 6 vegetable, 2½ dairy,
2 nuts/legumes/protein, 1 added fat, ½ sweets*

||||||||||||||||||||||||||||||||||||||||||||||||||||||||||||||||||||||||||||||||||||||||||||||||||||||||||

1,600 CALORIES: DAY 4
Target: 6 grain, 4 fruit, 4 vegetable, 2 dairy, 1¾ nuts/legumes/protein, 1 added fat,
*   ½ sweets*

Breakfast *(380 calories)*
1 Low-Fat Blueberry Muffin (see recipe), *2 grain (200 calories)*
½ grapefruit, *1 fruit (50 calories)*
1 cup nonfat plain Greek-style yogurt, *1 dairy (130 calories)*

Morning Snack *(200 calories)*
1 ounce whole-wheat snack crackers, *1 grain (130 calories)*
2 tablespoons hummus, *¼ nuts/legumes/protein (70 calories)*

Lunch *(340 calories)*
Sauté with 1 teaspoon olive oil:
        ½ cup canned black beans, drained and rinsed, *1 nuts/legumes/protein*
            (115 calories)
        ½ cup low-sodium canned diced tomatoes, *1 vegetable (30 calories)*
        ½ teaspoon ground cumin *(0 calories)*
Half a 7-inch whole-wheat pita pocket, *1 grain (85 calories)*
1 cup chopped lettuce with ½ cup sliced raw vegetables, *2 vegetable (40 calories)*
1 tablespoon "lite" vinaigrette, *½ added fat (20 calories)*
1 medium apple, *1 fruit (50 calories)*

Afternoon Snack *(170 calories)*
½ cup nonfat milk, *1 dairy (45 calories)*
1 ounce toasted oat cereal, *1 grain (100 calories)*
½ cup sliced fresh strawberries, *1 fruit (25 calories)*

Dinner *(380 calories)*
3 ounces grilled seitan, *1 nuts/legumes/protein (90 calories)*
2 tablespoons low-sodium teriyaki sauce *(40 calories)*
½ cup Roasted Brussels Sprouts (see recipe), *1 vegetable (50 calories)*
1 cup cooked brown rice, *2 grains (200 calories)*

Evening Snack/Dessert *(100 calories)*
½ cup sliced peaches, *1 fruit (30 calories)*
2 small gingersnaps, *½ sweets (60 calories)*
1 tablespoon low-fat whipped topping, *½ added fat (10 calories)*

Nutrition analysis for the day: 1,570 calories, 7 grain, 4 fruit, 4 vegetable, 2 dairy,
2¼ nuts/legumes/protein, 1 added fat, ½ sweets

1,600 CALORIES: DAY 5
Target: 6 grain, 4 fruit, 4 vegetable, 2 dairy, 1¾ nuts/legumes/protein, 1 added fat,
   ½ sweets

Breakfast *(195 calories)*
1 cup nonfat vanilla yogurt, *1 dairy (160 calories)*
½ cup mixed fresh berries, *1 fruit (35 calories)*

Morning Snack *(230 calories)*
1 ounce honey whole-wheat pretzels, *1 grain (110 calories)*
1 cup sliced mango, *2 fruit (120 calories)*

Lunch *(355 calories)*
1⅓ cups Quinoa, Corn, and Black Bean Salad (see recipe), *½ vegetable, 2 grain, ½ nuts/*
   legumes/protein (250 calories)
1 ounce stir-fried seitan, *¼ nuts/legumes/protein (35 calories)*
½ cup sliced red bell pepper and ½ cup sliced carrots, *2 vegetable (30 calories)*
1 tablespoon low-fat ranch dressing, *½ added fat (40 calories)*

Afternoon Snack *(300 calories)*
1 medium pear, *1 fruit (100 calories)*
1½ ounces low-fat cheddar cheese, *1 dairy (70 calories)*
1 ounce whole-wheat snack crackers, *1 grain (130 calories)*

Dinner *(345 calories)*
3 ounces Poached Salmon (see recipe), *1 nuts/legumes/protein (145 calories)*
1 cup boiled carrots, *2 vegetable (50 calories)*
1 small (2-ounce) whole-wheat dinner roll, *2 grain (150 calories)*
OR **Dinner 2** *(345 calories)*
3 ounces sautéed seitan,* *1 nuts/legumes/protein (130 calories)*
1 cup sautéed string beans,* *2 vegetable (35 calories)*
1 cup cooked whole-wheat couscous, *2 grain (180 calories)*

*Sauté seitan and string beans in 1 teaspoon olive oil over medium heat until seitan is firm and
string beans are crisp tender. Finish with a squeeze of lemon and dried basil.

Evening Snack/Dessert *(140 calories)*
3 cups air-popped popcorn, *1 grain (100 calories)*
½ teaspoon trans-fat-free margarine, *½ added fat (15 calories)*
2 teaspoons cinnamon sugar, *½ sweets (25 calories)*

Nutrition analysis for the day: 1,565 calories, 7 grain, 4 fruit, 4½ vegetable,
2 dairy, 1¾ nuts/legumes/protein, 1 added fat, ½ sweets

||||||||||||||||||||||||||||||||||||||||||||||||||||||||||||||||||||||||||||||||||||||||||||||||||||||||||||||

1,600 CALORIES: DAY 6
Target: 6 grain, 4 fruit, 4 vegetable, 2 dairy, 1¾ nuts/legumes/protein, 1 added fat,
   ½ sweets

Breakfast *(295 calories)*
One 1-ounce slice cinnamon raisin bread, toasted, *1 grain (80 calories)*
1 tablespoon peanut butter, *½ nuts/legumes/protein (90 calories)*
½ cup sliced banana, *1 fruit (70 calories)*
½ cup unsweetened applesauce, *1 fruit (55 calories)*

Morning Snack *(185 calories)*
½ cup low-fat cottage cheese, *1 dairy (80 calories)*
½ cup cantaloupe, *1 fruit (30 calories)*
2 tablespoons sliced almonds, *¼ nuts/legumes/protein (75 calories)*

Lunch *(350 calories)*
Piled-High Veggie Pizza (⅙ of a 14-inch pizza) (see recipe), *2 grain, 2 vegetable, ½ dairy*
   (250 calories)
1 medium pear, *1 fruit (100 calories)*

Afternoon Snack *(200 calories)*
½ cup nonfat chocolate milk, *½ dairy (80 calories)*
2 graham cracker rectangles, *1 grain (120 calories)*

Dinner *(485 calories)*
1 cup cooked whole-wheat pasta, *2 grain (200 calories)*
1 cup low-sodium marinara sauce, *2 vegetable (80 calories)*
1 cup reconstituted TVP,* *1 nuts/legumes/protein (160 calories)*
1½ cups mixed raw leafy greens, *1½ vegetable (20 calories)*
1 tablespoon low-fat Thousand Island dressing, *½ added fat (25 calories)*

* See Chapter 10 for more on TVP (texturized vegetable protein).

Evening Snack/Dessert *(85 calories)*
Half a ¾-inch slice Gingerbread (see recipe), *½ sweets (75 calories)*
1 tablespoon low-fat whipped topping, *½ added fat (10 calories)*

Nutrition analysis for the day: 1,600 calories, 6 grain, 4 fruit, 5½ vegetable, 2 dairy, 1¾ nuts/legumes/protein, 1 added fat, ½ sweets

||||||||||||||||||||||||||||||||||||||||||||||||||||||||||||||||||||||||||||||||||||||||||||||||||||||||||||||||||||

1,600 CALORIES: DAY 7
Target: 6 grain, 4 fruit, 4 vegetable, 2 dairy, 1¾ nuts/legumes/protein, 1 added fat, ½ sweets

Breakfast *(375 calories)*
Apple, onion, and cheddar omelet (cooked with cooking spray):
    2 whole eggs, *⅔ nuts/legumes/protein (160 calories)*
    ½ cup diced apple, *1 fruit (30 calories)*
    ½ cup diced white onion (cooked until soft), *1 vegetable (50 calories)*
    1½ ounces shredded low-fat cheddar cheese (about ⅓ cup), *1 dairy (70 calories)*
½ whole-grain or whole-wheat English muffin, *1 grain (65 calories)*

Morning Snack *(170 calories)*
2 graham cracker rectangles, *1 grain (120 calories)*
½ cup unsweetened applesauce, *1 fruit (50 calories)*

Lunch *(435 calories)*
1 Veggie Melt Panini (see recipe), *2 grains, 2 vegetable, 1 dairy (335 calories)*
¼ cup dried cherries, *1 fruit (100 calories)*

Afternoon Snack *(105 calories)*
1½ cups air-popped popcorn, *½ grain (55 calories)*
1 kiwi, *1 fruit (50 calories)*

Dinner *(430 calories)*
5 ounces Poached Cod (see recipe), *1⅔ nuts/legumes/protein (150 calories)*
1 cup butternut squash, boiled and mashed *2 vegetable (80 calories)*
½ cup brown rice pilaf, *1 grain (100 calories)*
½ small (2-ounce) whole-wheat dinner roll, *1 grain (75 calories)*
1 teaspoon trans-fat-free margarine, *1 added fat (25 calories)*
OR **Dinner 2** *(440 calories)*
5 ounces sautéed seitan,* *1⅔ nuts/legumes/protein (190 calories)*
1 cup boiled carrots, *2 vegetable (50 calories)*
½ cup brown rice pilaf, *1 grain (100 calories)*
½ small (2-ounce) whole-wheat dinner roll, *1 grain (75 calories)*
1 teaspoon trans-fat-free margarine, *1 added fat (25 calories)*

*Sauté seitan in 1 teaspoon olive oil over medium heat until seitan is firm.

Evening Snack/Dessert *(60 calories)*
½ Baked Banana (see recipe), *1 fruit, ½ sweets (60 calories)*

Nutrition analysis for the day: 1,575 calories, 6½ grain, 5 fruit, 5 vegetable, 2 dairy, 2⅓ nuts/legumes/protein, 1 added fat, ½ sweets

||||||||||||||||||||||||||||||||||||||||||||||||||||||||||||||||||||||||||||||||||||||||||||||||||||||||||||||||||

1,800 CALORIES: DAY 1
Target: 6½ grain, 4 fruit, 4 vegetable, 2½ dairy, 2 nuts/legumes/protein, 1½ added fat, ½ sweets

Breakfast *(520 calories)*
3 whole eggs, fried (cooked with cooking spray), *1 nuts/legumes/protein (240 calories)*
1½ ounces shredded low-fat cheddar cheese (about ⅓ cup), *1 dairy (70 calories)*
Two 1-ounce slices whole-grain bread, *2 grain (160 calories)*
1 teaspoon trans-fat-free margarine, *1 added fat (25 calories)*
½ cup sliced cantaloupe, *1 fruit (25 calories)*

Morning Snack *(150 calories)*
½ cup low-fat cottage cheese, *1 dairy (80 calories)*
½ cup fruit salad (water-packed peach, pear, pineapple, apricot, cherry), *1 fruit (70 calories)*

Lunch *(525 calories)*
1½ cups Tortellini and Bean Soup (see recipe), *2 vegetable, ½ grain, ½ dairy (330 calories)*
2 cups baby arugula, *2 vegetable (15 calories)*
2 tablespoons "lite" balsamic vinaigrette, *1 added fat (60 calories)*
6 unsalted saltine crackers, *1 grain (120 calories)*

Afternoon Snack *(180 calories)*
½ cup sliced banana, *1 fruit (70 calories)*
1 ounce unsalted pretzels, *1 grain (110 calories)*

Dinner *(360 calories)*
1 Tempeh Burger (see recipe), *2 grains, 1 nuts/legumes/protein (330 calories)*
1 cup grilled zucchini and portabella mushrooms slices, *1 vegetable (30 calories)*

Evening Snack/Dessert *(140 calories)*
¼ cup dried apricots, *1 fruit (80 calories)*
3 dark chocolate kisses, *½ sweets (60 calories)*

Nutrition analysis for the day: 1,875 calories, 6½ grain, 4 fruit, 5 vegetable, 2½ dairy, 2 nuts/legumes/protein, 2 added fat, ½ sweets

||||||||||||||||||||||||||||||||||||||||||||||||||||||||||||||||||||||||||||||||||||||||||||||||||||||||||

1,800 CALORIES: DAY 2

*Target: 6½ grain, 4 fruit, 4 vegetable, 2½ dairy, 2 nuts/legumes/protein, 1½ added
    fat, ½ sweets*

Breakfast *(425 calories)*
2 ounces uncooked oatmeal, cooked with water (cooks to about 1½ cups), *2 grain
    (200 calories)*
½ medium (7-inch) banana sliced, *1 fruit (60 calories)*
3 tablespoons chopped walnuts, *½ nuts/legumes/protein (120 calories)*
½ cup nonfat milk, *½ dairy (45 calories)*

Morning Snack *(130 calories)*
1 reduced-fat string cheese stick, *⅔ dairy (80 calories)*
1 medium apple, *1 fruit (50 calories)*

Lunch *(460 calories)*
Middle Eastern lunch special:
      Half a 7-inch whole-wheat pita pocket, *1 grain (85 calories)*
      2 tablespoons hummus, *¼ nuts/legumes/protein (70 calories)*
      1½ cups grilled vegetables (red/green bell peppers, zucchini, onions,
          mushrooms), *3 vegetable (115 calories)*
½ cup cooked whole-wheat couscous, *1 grain (90 calories)*
1 medium pear, *1 fruit (100 calories)*

Afternoon Snack *(220 calories)*
1 ounce unsalted pretzels, *1 grain (110 calories)*
2 tablespoons peanuts, *¼ nuts/legumes/protein (110 calories)*

Dinner *(280 calories)*
1 cup Tofu and Vegetable Stir-Fry (see recipe), *2 vegetables, ½ nuts/legumes/protein
    (180 calories)*
½ cup cooked brown rice, *1 grain (100 calories)*

Evening Snack/Dessert *(220 calories)*
½ cup low-fat frozen yogurt, *1 dairy (140 calories)*
½ cup fresh raspberries, *1 fruit (30 calories)*
2 teaspoons chocolate syrup, *½ sweets (30 calories)*
2 tablespoons low-fat whipped topping, *1 added fat (20 calories)*

*Nutrition analysis for the day: 1,735 calories, 6 grain, 4 fruit, 5 vegetable, 2 dairy,
1½ nuts/legumes/protein, 1 added fat, ½ sweets*

|||||||||||||||||||||||||||||||||||||||||||||||||||||||||||||||||||||||||||||||||||||||||||||||||||||||||||||||||||

1,800 CALORIES: DAY 3
Target: 6½ grain, 4 fruit, 4 vegetable, 2½ dairy, 2 nuts/legumes/protein, 1½ added fat, ½ sweets

Breakfast *(350 calories)*
1 ounce bran flakes (about ¾ cup), *1 grain (90 calories)*
¼ cup golden raisins, *1 fruit (110 calories)*
½ cup sliced banana, *1 fruit (60 calories)*
1 cup nonfat milk, *1 dairy (90 calories)*

Morning Snack *(280 calories)*
½ cup shelled edamame, *1 nuts/legumes/protein (180 calories)*
1 small low-fat granola bar, *1 grain (100 calories)*

Lunch *(390 calories)*
2 cups raw spinach, *2 vegetable (15 calories)*
½ medium tomato, chopped, and ½ cup sliced cucumber, *2 vegetable (25 calories)*
½ cup cooked chickpeas, *1 nuts/legumes/protein (145 calories)*
Dressing: 2 teaspoons lemon juice, 1 teaspoon extra virgin olive oil, 2 tablespoons white wine vinegar, *1 added fat (45 calories)*
1 ounce honey whole-wheat pretzels, *1 grain (110 calories)*
1 medium apple, *1 fruit (50 calories)*

Afternoon Snack *(265 calories)*
1 cup nonfat plain Greek-style yogurt, *1 dairy (130 calories)*
1 ounce low-fat granola (about ¼ cup), *1 grain (110 calories)*
½ cup sliced fresh strawberries, *1 fruit (25 calories)*

Dinner *(485 calories)*
1½ cups Pasta Primavera (see recipe), *2 grains, 2 vegetable, ½ dairy (410 calories)*
½ small (2-ounce) whole-wheat dinner roll, *1 grain (75 calories)*

Evening Snack/Dessert *(55 calories)*
1 fig bar, *½ sweets (55 calories)*

Nutrition analysis for the day: 1,825 calories, 7 grain, 4 fruit, 6 vegetable, 2½ dairy, 2 nuts/legumes/protein, 1 added fat, ½ sweets

|||||||||||||||||||||||||||||||||||||||||||||||||||||||||||||||||||||||||||||||||||||||||||||||||||||||||||||||||||||||||||||

1,800 CALORIES: DAY 4

Target: 6½ grain, 4 fruit, 4 vegetable, 2½ dairy, 2 nuts/legumes/protein, 1½ added fat, ½ sweets

Breakfast *(405 calories)*
1 Low-Fat Blueberry Muffin (see recipe), *2 grain (200 calories)*
1 teaspoon trans-fat-free margarine, *1 added fat (25 calories)*
½ grapefruit, *1 fruit (50 calories)*
1 cup nonfat plain Greek-style yogurt, *1 dairy (130 calories)*

Morning Snack *(200 calories)*
1 ounce whole-wheat snack crackers, *1 grain (130 calories)*
2 tablespoons hummus, *¼ nuts/legumes/protein (70 calories)*

Lunch *(340 calories)*
Sauté with 1 teaspoon olive oil:
    ½ cup canned black beans, drained and rinsed, *1 nuts/legumes/protein*
      (115 calories)
    ½ cup low-sodium canned diced tomatoes, *1 vegetable (30 calories)*
    ½ teaspoon ground cumin *(0 calories)*
Half a 7-inch whole-wheat pita pocket, *1 grain (85 calories)*
1 cup shredded lettuce with ½ cup sliced raw vegetables, *2 vegetable (40 calories)*
1 tablespoon "lite" vinaigrette, *½ fat (20 calories)*
1 medium apple, *1 fruit (50 calories)*

Afternoon Snack *(325 calories)*
1 cup low-fat fruited yogurt, *1 dairy (200 calories)*
1 ounce toasted oat cereal, *1 grain (100 calories)*
½ cup sliced fresh strawberries, *1 fruit (25 calories)*

Dinner *(380 calories)*
3 ounces grilled seitan, *1 nuts/legumes/protein (90 calories)*
2 tablespoons low-sodium teriyaki sauce *(40 calories)*
½ cup Roasted Brussels Sprouts (see recipe), *1 vegetable (50 calories)*
1 cup cooked brown rice, *2 grains (200 calories)*

Evening Snack/Dessert *(100 calories)*
½ cup sliced peaches, *1 fruit (30 calories)*
2 small gingersnaps, *½ sweets (60 calories)*
1 tablespoon low-fat whipped topping, *½ added fat (10 calories)*

Nutrition analysis for the day: 1,750 calories, 7 grain, 4 fruit, 4 vegetable, 2 dairy, 2¼ nuts/legumes/protein, 2 added fat, ½ sweets

||||||||||||||||||||||||||||||||||||||||||||||||||||||||||||||||||||||||||||||||||||||||||||||||||||||||||||||||||||||||||||

1,800 CALORIES: DAY 5

Target: 6½ grain, 4 fruit, 4 vegetable, 2½ dairy, 2 nuts/legumes/protein, 1½ added fat, ½ sweets

Breakfast *(385 calories)*
1 cup nonfat vanilla yogurt, *1 dairy (160 calories)*
1 ounce low-fat granola (about ¼ cup), *1 grain (110 calories)*
2 tablespoons chopped walnuts, *¼ nuts/legumes/protein (80 calories)*
½ cup mixed fresh berries, *1 fruit (35 calories)*

Morning Snack *(155 calories)*
1 cup sliced mango, *2 fruit (120 calories)*
¾ ounce low-fat cheddar cheese (1 small slice), *½ dairy (35 calories)*

Lunch *(520 calories)*
1⅓ cups Quinoa, Corn, and Black Bean Salad (see recipe), *½ vegetable, 2 grain, ½ nuts/legumes/protein (250 calories)*
3 ounces crumbled tempeh, *¼ nuts/legumes/protein (160 calories)*
½ cup sliced red bell pepper and ½ cup sliced carrots, *2 vegetable (30 calories)*
2 tablespoons low-fat ranch dressing, *½ added fat (80 calories)*

Afternoon Snack *(300 calories)*
1 medium pear, *1 fruit (100 calories)*
1½ ounces low-fat cheddar cheese, *1 dairy (70 calories)*
1 ounce whole-wheat snack crackers, *1 grain (130 calories)*

Dinner *(345 calories)*
3 ounces Poached Salmon (see recipe), *1 nuts/legumes/protein (145 calories)*
1 cup boiled carrots, *2 vegetables (50 calories)*
1 small (2-ounce) whole-wheat dinner roll, *2 grain (150 calories)*
OR **Dinner 2** *(345 calories)*
3 ounces sautéed seitan,* *1 nuts/legumes/protein (130 calories)*
1 cup sautéed string beans,* *2 vegetable (35 calories)*
1 cup cooked whole-wheat couscous, *2 grain (180 calories)*

* Sauté seitan and string beans in 1 teaspoon olive oil over medium heat until seitan is firm and string beans are crisp-tender. Finish with a squeeze of lemon and dried basil.

Evening Snack/Dessert *(140 calories)*
3 cups air-popped popcorn, *1 grain (100 calories)*
½ teaspoon trans-fat-free margarine, *½ added fat (15 calories)*
2 teaspoons cinnamon sugar, *½ sweets (25 calories)*

Nutrition analysis for the day: 1,845 calories, 7 grain, 4 fruit, 4½ vegetable, 2½ dairy, 2 nuts/legumes/protein, 1 added fat, ½ sweets

1,800 CALORIES: DAY 6

Target: 6½ grain, 4 fruit, 4 vegetable, 2½ dairy, 2 nuts/legumes/protein, 1½ added fat, ½ sweets

Breakfast *(340 calories)*
One 1-ounce slice cinnamon raisin bread, toasted, *1 grain (80 calories)*
1 tablespoon peanut butter, *½ nuts/legumes/protein (90 calories)*
½ cup sliced banana, *1 fruit (70 calories)*
½ cup unsweetened applesauce, *1 fruit (55 calories)*
½ cup nonfat milk, *½ dairy (45 calories)*

Morning Snack *(145 calories)*
¼ cup low-fat cottage cheese, *½ dairy (40 calories)*
½ cup cubed cantaloupe, *1 fruit (30 calories)*
2 tablespoons sliced almonds, *¼ nuts/legumes/protein (75 calories)*

Lunch *(350 calories)*
Piled-High Veggie Pizza (⅙ of a 14-inch pizza) (see recipe), *2 grain, 2 vegetable, ½ dairy (250 calories)*
1 medium pear, *1 fruit (100 calories)*

Afternoon Snack *(280 calories)*
1 cup nonfat chocolate milk, *1 dairy (160 calories)*
2 graham cracker rectangles, *1 grain (120 calories)*

Dinner *(485 calories)*
1 cup cooked whole-wheat pasta, *2 grain (200 calories)*
1 cup low-sodium marinara sauce, *2 vegetable (80 calories)*
1 cup reconstituted TVP,* *1 nuts/legumes/protein (160 calories)*
1½ cups mixed raw leafy greens, *1½ vegetable (20 calories)*
1 tablespoon low-fat Thousand Island dressing, *½ added fat (25 calories)*

* See Chapter 10 for more on TVP (texturized vegetable protein).

Evening Snack/Dessert *(205 calories)*

Half a ¾-inch slice Gingerbread (see recipe), *½ sweets (75 calories)*

2 tablespoons chopped peanuts, *¼ nuts/legumes/protein (110 calories)*

2 tablespoons low-fat whipped topping, *1 added fat (20 calories)*

Nutrition analysis for the day: 1,805 calories, 6 grain, 4 fruit, 5½ vegetable, 2½ dairy, 2 nuts/legumes/protein, 1½ added fat, ½ sweets

||||||||||||||||||||||||||||||||||||||||||||||||||||||||||||||||||||||||||||||||||||||||||||||||||||||||||||||

1,800 CALORIES: DAY 7

Target: 6½ grain, 4 fruit, 4 vegetable, 2½ dairy, 2 nuts/legumes/protein, 1½ added fat, ½ sweets

Breakfast *(375 calories)*

Apple, onion, and cheddar omelet, cooked with cooking spray:

2 whole eggs, *⅔ nuts/legumes/protein (160 calories)*

½ cup diced apple, *1 fruit (30 calories)*

½ cup diced white onion (cooked until soft), *1 vegetable (50 calories)*

1½ ounces shredded low-fat cheddar cheese (about ⅓ cup), *1 dairy (70 calories)*

½ whole-grain or whole-wheat English muffin, *1 grain (65 calories)*

Morning Snack *(170 calories)*

2 graham cracker rectangles, *1 grain (120 calories)*

½ cup unsweetened applesauce, *1 fruit (50 calories)*

Lunch *(435 calories)*

1 Veggie Melt Panini (see recipe), *2 grains, 2 vegetable, 1 dairy (335 calories)*

¼ cup dried cherries, *1 fruit (100 calories)*

Afternoon Snack *(105 calories)*

1½ cups air-popped popcorn, *½ grain (55 calories)*

1 kiwi, *1 fruit (50 calories)*

Dinner *(470 calories)*

5 ounces Poached Cod (see recipe), *1⅔ nuts/legumes/protein (150 calories)*

½ cup brown rice pilaf, *1 grain (100 calories)*

1½ cups mixed raw leafy greens with ½ cup sliced roasted red peppers, *2 vegetable (60 calories)*

2 tablespoons low-fat balsamic vinaigrette, *1 added fat (60 calories)*

½ small (2-ounce) whole-wheat dinner roll, *1 grain (75 calories)*

1 teaspoon trans-fat–free margarine, *1 added fat (25 calories)*

OR Dinner 2 *(470 calories)*

5 ounces sautéed seitan,* *1⅔ nuts/legumes/protein (190 calories)*
1 cup sautéed peppers and onion,* *2 vegetable (20 calories)*
2 tablespoons low-fat balsamic vinaigrette, *1 added fat (60 calories)*
½ cup brown rice pilaf, *1 grain (100 calories)*
½ small (2-ounce) whole-wheat dinner roll, *1 grain (75 calories)*
1 teaspoon trans-fat-free margarine, *1 added fat (25 calories)*

*Sauté peppers and onion in 1 teaspoon olive oil until soft. Add seitan and sauté until firm. Drizzle with vinaigrette.

Evening Snack/Dessert *(200 calories)*

½ cup low-fat frozen yogurt, *1 dairy (140 calories)*
½ Baked Banana (see recipe), *1 fruit, ½ sweets (60 calories)*

Nutrition analysis for the day: 1,755 calories, 6½ grain, 5 fruit, 5 vegetable, 3 dairy, 2⅓ nuts/legumes/protein, 2 added fat, ½ sweets

‖‖‖

2,000 CALORIES: DAY 1

***Target: 7 grain, 4 fruit, 4 vegetable, 2½ dairy, 2 nuts/legumes/protein, 2 added fat,
½ sweets***

Breakfast *(520 calories)*

3 whole eggs, fried (cooked with cooking spray), *1 nuts/legumes/protein
      (240 calories)*
1½ ounces shredded low-fat cheddar cheese (about ⅓ cup), *1 dairy (70 calories)*
Two 1-ounce slices whole-wheat bread, *2 grain (160 calories)*
1 teaspoon trans-fat-free margarine, *1 added fat (25 calories)*
½ cup sliced cantaloupe, *1 fruit (25 calories)*

Morning Snack *(210 calories)*

1 cup nonfat plain yogurt, *1 dairy (120 calories)*
½ cup mixed fresh berries, *1 fruit (35 calories)*
½ ounce low-fat granola (about 2 tablespoons), *½ grain (55 calories)*

Lunch *(525 calories)*

1½ cups Tortellini and Bean Soup (see recipe), *2 vegetable, ½ grain, ½ dairy (330 calories)*
2 cups baby arugula, *2 vegetable (15 calories)*
2 tablespoons "lite" balsamic vinaigrette, *1 added fat (60 calories)*
6 unsalted saltine crackers, *1 grain (120 calories)*

Afternoon Snack *(200 calories)*
½ cup sliced banana, *1 fruit (70 calories)*
1 ounce whole-wheat snack crackers, *1 grain (130 calories)*

Dinner *(360 calories)*
1 Tempeh Burger (see recipe), *2 grains, 1 nuts/legumes/protein (330 calories)*
1 cup grilled zucchini and portabella mushroom slices, *1 vegetable (30 calories)*

Evening Snack/Dessert *(220 calories)*
½ cup dried apricots, *2 fruit (160 calories)*
3 dark chocolate kisses, *½ sweets (60 calories)*

*Nutrition analysis for the day: 2,035 calories, 7 grain, 5 fruit, 5 vegetable, 2½ dairy,
2 nuts/legumes/protein, 2 added fat, ½ sweets*

|||||||||||||||||||||||||||||||||||||||||||||||||||||||||||||||||||||||||||||||||||||||||

2,000 CALORIES: DAY 2

*Target: 7 grain, 4 fruit, 4 vegetable, 2½ dairy, 2 nuts/legumes/protein, 2 added fat,
½ sweets*

Breakfast *(385 calories)*
2 ounces uncooked oatmeal, cooked with water (cooks to about 1½ cups), *2 grain
(200 calories)*
½ medium (7-inch) banana, sliced, *1 fruit (60 calories)*
2 tablespoons chopped walnuts, *¼ nuts/legumes/protein (80 calories)*
½ cup nonfat milk, *½ dairy (45 calories)*

Morning Snack *(210 calories)*
2 reduced-fat string cheese sticks, *1⅓ dairy (160 calories)*
1 medium apple, *1 fruit (50 calories)*

Lunch *(530 calories)*
Middle Eastern lunch special:
 Half a 7-inch whole-wheat pita pocket, *1 grain (85 calories)*
 ¼ cup hummus, *½ nuts/legumes/protein (140 calories)*
 1½ cups grilled vegetables (red/green bell peppers, zucchini, onions,
  mushrooms), *3 vegetable (115 calories)*
½ cup cooked whole-wheat couscous, *1 grain (90 calories)*
1 medium pear, *1 fruit (100 calories)*

Afternoon Snack *(220 calories)*
1 ounce unsalted mini pretzels (about ½ cup), *1 grain (110 calories)*
2 tablespoons peanuts, *¼ nuts/legumes/protein (110 calories)*

Dinner *(470 calories)*

1 cup Tofu and Vegetable Stir-Fry (see recipe), *2 vegetables, ½ nuts/legumes/protein (180 calories)*

1 cup cooked brown rice, *2 grain (200 calories)*

½ cup steamed green peas, *1 vegetable (65 calories)*

1 teaspoon trans-fat-free margarine, *1 added fat (25 calories)*

Evening Snack/Dessert *(220 calories)*

½ cup low-fat frozen yogurt, *1 dairy (140 calories)*

½ cup fresh raspberries, *1 fruit (30 calories)*

2 teaspoons chocolate syrup, *½ sweets (30 calories)*

2 tablespoons low-fat whipped topping, *1 added fat (20 calories)*

Nutrition analysis for the day: 2,035 calories, 7 grain, 4 fruit, 6 vegetable, 2¾ dairy, 1½ nuts/legumes/protein, 2 added fat, ½ sweets

|||||||||||||||||||||||||||||||||||||||||||||||||||||||||||||||||||||||||||||||||||||||||||||||||||||||||||||||||

2,000 CALORIES: DAY 3
Target: 7 grain, 4 fruit, 4 vegetable, 2½ dairy, 2 nuts/legumes/protein, 2 added fat, ½ sweets

Breakfast *(350 calories)*

1 ounce bran flakes (about ¾ cup), *1 grain (90 calories)*

¼ cup golden raisins, *1 fruit (110 calories)*

½ medium (7-inch) banana, sliced, *1 fruit (60 calories)*

1 cup nonfat milk, *1 dairy (90 calories)*

Morning Snack *(280 calories)*

½ cup shelled edamame, *1 nuts/legumes/protein (180 calories)*

1 small low-fat granola bar, *1 grain (100 calories)*

Lunch *(390 calories)*

2 cups raw spinach, *2 vegetable (15 calories)*

½ medium tomato, chopped, and ½ cup sliced cucumber, *2 vegetable (25 calories)*

½ cup cooked chickpeas, *1 nuts/legumes/protein (145 calories)*

Dressing: 2 teaspoons lemon juice, 1 teaspoon extra virgin olive oil, 2 tablespoons white wine vinegar, *1 added fat (45 calories)*

1 ounce honey whole-wheat pretzels, *1 grain (110 calories)*

1 medium apple, *1 fruit (50 calories)*

Afternoon Snack *(335 calories)*
1 cup low-fat fruited yogurt, *1 dairy (200 calories)*
1 ounce low-fat granola (about ¼ cup), *1 grain (110 calories)*
½ cup sliced fresh strawberries, *1 fruit (25 calories)*

Dinner *(510 calories)*
1½ cups Pasta Primavera (see recipe), *2 grains, 2 vegetable, ½ dairy (410 calories)*
½ small (2-ounce) whole-wheat dinner roll, *1 grain (75 calories)*
1 teaspoon trans-fat-free margarine, *1 added fat (25 calories)*

Evening Snack/Dessert *(55 calories)*
1 fig bar, *½ sweets (55 calories)*

Nutrition analysis for the day: 1,920 calories, 7 grain, 4 fruit, 6 vegetable, 2½ dairy, 2 nuts/legumes/protein, 2 added fat, ½ sweets

‖‖‖

2,000 CALORIES: DAY 4
*Target: 7 grain, 4 fruit, 4 vegetable, 2½ dairy, 2 nuts/legumes/protein, 2 added fat,
   ½ sweets*

Breakfast *(405 calories)*
1 Low-Fat Blueberry Muffin (see recipe), *2 grain (200 calories)*
1 teaspoon trans-fat-free margarine, *1 added fat (25 calories)*
½ grapefruit, *1 fruit (50 calories)*
1 cup nonfat plain Greek-style yogurt, *1 dairy (130 calories)*

Morning Snack *(270 calories)*
1 ounce whole-wheat snack crackers, *1 grain (130 calories)*
¼ cup hummus, *½ nuts/legumes/protein (140 calories)*

Lunch *(390 calories)*
Sauté with 1 teaspoon olive oil:
½ cup canned black beans, drained and rinsed, *1 nuts/legumes/protein (115 calories)*
        ½ cup low-sodium canned diced tomatoes, *1 vegetable (30 calories)*
        ½ teaspoon ground cumin *(0 calories)*
Half a 7-inch whole-wheat pita pocket, *1 grain (85 calories)*
1 cup chopped lettuce with ½ cup sliced raw vegetables, *2 vegetable (40 calories)*
1 tablespoon "lite" vinaigrette, *½ fat (20 calories)*
1 medium pear, *1 fruit (100 calories)*

Afternoon Snack *(325 calories)*
1 cup low-fat fruited yogurt, *1 dairy (200 calories)*
1 ounce toasted oat cereal, *1 grain (100 calories)*
½ cup sliced fresh strawberries, *1 fruit (25 calories)*

Dinner *(445 calories)*
4½ ounces grilled firm tofu, *½ nuts/legumes/protein (105 calories)*
2 tablespoons low-sodium teriyaki sauce *(40 calories)*
1 cup Roasted Brussels Sprouts (see recipe), *2 vegetable (100 calories)*
1 cup cooked brown rice, *2 grain (200 calories)*

Evening Snack/Dessert *(100 calories)*
½ cup sliced peaches, *1 fruit (30 calories)*
2 small gingersnaps, *½ sweets (60 calories)*
1 tablespoon low-fat whipped topping, *½ added fat (10 calories)*

Nutrition analysis for the day: 1,935 calories, 7 grain, 4 fruit, 5 vegetable, 2 dairy, 2 nuts/legumes/protein, 2 added fat, ½ sweets

||||||||||||||||||||||||||||||||||||||||||||||||||||||||||||||||||||||||||||||||||||||||||||

2,000 CALORIES: DAY 5
Target: 7 grain, 4 fruit, 4 vegetable, 2½ dairy, 2 nuts/legumes/protein, 2 added fat, ½ sweets

Breakfast *(425 calories)*
1 cup low-fat fruited yogurt, *1 dairy (200 calories)*
1 ounce low-fat granola (about ¼ cup), *1 grain (110 calories)*
2 tablespoons chopped walnuts, *¼ nuts/legumes/protein (80 calories)*
½ cup mixed fresh berries, *1 fruit (35 calories)*

Morning Snack *(155 calories)*
1 cup sliced mango, *2 fruit (120 calories)*
¾ ounce low-fat cheddar cheese (1 small slice), *½ dairy (35 calories)*

Lunch *(520 calories)*
1⅓ cups Quinoa, Corn, and Black Bean Salad (see recipe), *½ vegetable, 2 grain, ½ nuts/legumes/protein (250 calories)*
3 ounces crumbled tempeh, *¼ nuts/legumes/protein (160 calories)*
½ cup sliced red pepper and ½ cup sliced carrots, *2 vegetable (30 calories)*
2 tablespoons low-fat ranch dressing, *½ added fat (80 calories)*

Afternoon Snack *(300 calories)*
1 medium pear, *1 fruit (100 calories)*
1½ ounces low-fat cheddar cheese, *1 dairy (70 calories)*
1 ounce whole-wheat snack crackers, *1 grain (130 calories)*

Dinner *(445 calories)*
3 ounces Poached Salmon (see recipe), *1 nuts/legumes/protein (145 calories)*
1 cup steamed corn kernels, *2 vegetable (135 calories)*
½ teaspoon trans-fat-free margarine, *½ added fat (15 calories)*
1 small (2-ounce) whole-wheat dinner roll, *2 grain (150 calories)*
OR **Dinner 2** *(445 calories)*
3 ounces sautéed herbed seitan,* *1 nuts/legumes/protein (130 calories)*
1 cup cooked green peas, *2 vegetable (120 calories)*
½ teaspoon trans-fat-free margarine, *½ added fat (15 calories)*
1 cup cooked whole-wheat couscous, *2 grain (180 calories)*

* Sauté seitan in 1 teaspoon olive oil over medium heat until seitan is firm. Sprinkle with fresh herbs (basil, rosemary, sage).

Evening Snack/Dessert *(140 calories)*
3 cups air-popped popcorn, *1 grain (100 calories)*
½ teaspoon trans-fat-free margarine, *½ added fat (15 calories)*
2 teaspoons cinnamon sugar, *½ sweets (25 calories)*

Nutrition analysis for the day: 1,985 calories, 7 grain, 4 fruit, 4½ vegetable, 2½ dairy, 2 nuts/legumes/protein, 1½ added fat, ½ sweets

||||||||||||||||||||||||||||||||||||||||||||||||||||||||||||||||||||||||||||||||||||||||||||||||||||||||

2,000 CALORIES: DAY 6
Target: 7 grain, 4 fruit, 4 vegetable, 2½ dairy, 2 nuts/legumes/protein, 2 added fat, ½ sweets

Breakfast *(275 calories)*
One 1-ounce slice cinnamon raisin bread, toasted, *1 grain (80 calories)*
1 teaspoon trans-fat-free margarine, *1 added fat (25 calories)*
½ cup sliced banana, *1 fruit (70 calories)*
½ cup unsweetened applesauce, *1 fruit (55 calories)*
½ cup nonfat milk, *½ dairy (45 calories)*

Morning Snack *(245 calories)*
¼ cup low-fat cottage cheese, *½ dairy (40 calories)*
½ cup cubed cantaloupe, *1 fruit (30 calories)*

2 tablespoons sliced almonds, *¼ nuts/legumes/protein (75 calories)*
1 small low-fat granola bar, *1 grain (100 calories)*

Lunch *(350 calories)*
Piled-High Veggie Pizza (⅙ of a 14-inch pizza) (see recipe), *2 grain, 2 vegetable, ½ dairy (250 calories)*
1 medium pear, *1 fruit (100 calories)*

Afternoon Snack *(370 calories)*
1 cup nonfat chocolate milk, *1 dairy (160 calories)*
1 tablespoon peanut butter, *½ nuts/legumes/protein (90 calories)*
2 graham cracker rectangles, *1 grain (120 calories)*

Dinner *(540 calories)*
1 cup cooked whole-wheat pasta, *2 grain (200 calories)*
1 cup low-sodium marinara sauce, *2 vegetable (80 calories)*
1 cup reconstituted TVP,* *1 nuts/legumes/protein (160 calories)*
1 cup Roasted Brussels Sprouts (see recipe), *2 vegetable (100 calories)*

*See Chapter 10 for more on TVP (texturized vegetable protein).

Evening Snack/Dessert *(205 calories)*
Half a ¾-inch slice Gingerbread (see recipe), *½ sweets (75 calories)*
2 tablespoons chopped peanuts, *¼ nuts/legumes/protein (110 calories)*
2 tablespoons low-fat whipped topping, *1 added fat (20 calories)*

Nutrition analysis for the day: 1,985 calories, 7 grain, 4 fruit, 6 vegetable, 2½ dairy, 2 nuts/legumes/protein, 2 added fat, ½ sweets

||||||||||||||||||||||||||||||||||||||||||||||||||||||||||||||||||||||||||||||||||||||||||||||||||||||

2,000 CALORIES: DAY 7
Target: 7 grain, 4 fruit, 4 vegetable, 2½ dairy, 2 nuts/legumes/protein, 2 added fat, ½ sweets

Breakfast *(535 calories)*
Apple, onion, and cheddar omelet (cooked with cooking spray):
   2 whole eggs, *⅔ nuts/legumes/protein (160 calories)*
   ½ cup diced apple, *1 fruit (30 calories)*
   ½ cup diced white onion (cooked until soft), *1 vegetable (50 calories)*
   1½ ounces shredded low-fat cheddar cheese (about ⅓ cup), *1 dairy (70 calories)*
½ large (about 4-inch) whole-wheat bagel, *2 grain (200 calories)*
1 teaspoon trans-fat-free margarine, *1 added fat (25 calories)*

Morning Snack *(170 calories)*
2 graham cracker rectangles, *1 grain (120 calories)*
½ cup unsweetened applesauce, *1 fruit (50 calories)*

Lunch *(435 calories)*
1 Veggie Melt Panini (see recipe), *2 grains, 2 vegetable, 1 dairy (335 calories)*
¼ cup dried cherries, *1 fruit (100 calories)*

Afternoon Snack *(105 calories)*
1½ cups air-popped popcorn, *½ grain (55 calories)*
1 kiwi, *1 fruit (50 calories)*

Dinner *(470 calories)*
5 ounces Poached Cod (see recipe), *1⅔ nuts/legumes/protein (150 calories)*
½ cup brown rice pilaf, *1 grain (100 calories)*
1½ cups mixed raw leafy greens with ½ cup sliced roasted red bell peppers,
    2 vegetable (60 calories)
2 tablespoons low-fat balsamic vinaigrette, *1 added fat (60 calories)*
½ small (2-ounce) whole-wheat dinner roll, *1 grain (75 calories)*
1 teaspoon trans-fat-free margarine, *1 added fat (25 calories)*
OR Dinner 2 *(470 calories)*
5 ounces sautéed seitan,* *1⅔ nuts/legumes/protein (190 calories)*
1 cup sautéed peppers and onion, *1 vegetable (20 calories)*
2 tablespoons low-fat balsamic vinaigrette, *1 added fat (60 calories)*
½ cup brown rice pilaf, *1 grain (100 calories)*
½ small (2-ounce) whole-wheat dinner roll, *1 grain (75 calories)*
1 teaspoon trans-fat-free margarine, *1 added fat (25 calories)*

*Sauté peppers and onion in 1 teaspoon olive oil until soft. Add seitan and sauté until firm.
Drizzle with vinaigrette.

Evening Snack/Dessert *(200 calories)*
½ cup low-fat frozen yogurt, *1 dairy (140 calories)*
½ Baked Banana (see recipe), *1 fruit, ½ sweets (60 calories)*

*Nutrition analysis for the day: 1,915 calories, 7½ grain, 5 fruit, 5 vegetable,
3 dairy, 2⅓ nuts/legumes/protein, 3 added fat, ½ sweets*

III

2,200 CALORIES: DAY 1

Target: 8 grain, 4 fruit, 5 vegetable, 3 dairy, 2½ nuts/legumes/protein, 2½ fat, 1 sweets

Breakfast *(340 calories)*
1 ounce uncooked oatmeal, cooked with water (cooks to about ¾ cup), *1 grain (100 calories)*
2 tablespoons chopped walnuts, *¼ nuts/legumes/protein (80 calories)*
½ cup sliced banana, *1 fruit (70 calories)*
1 cup nonfat milk, *1 dairy (90 calories)*

Morning Snack *(275 calories)*
1 cup low-fat fruited yogurt, *1 dairy (200 calories)*
2 tablespoons slivered almonds, *¼ nuts/legumes/protein (75 calories)*

Lunch *(540 calories)*
One 7-inch whole-wheat pita pocket, *2 grain (170 calories)*
4 ounces grilled seitan, *1⅓ nuts/legumes/protein (120 calories)*
1 teaspoon deli mustard *(5 calories)*
1 cup grilled zucchini and summer squash, *2 vegetable (30 calories)*
1 cup mixed raw leafy greens, *1 vegetable (15 calories)*
2 tablespoons reduced-fat balsamic vinaigrette, *1 added fat (50 calories)*
1 ounce unsalted mini pretzels (about ½ cup), *1 grain (110 calories)*
½ cup fresh blueberries, *1 fruit (40 calories)*

Afternoon Snack *(270 calories)*
2 ounces unsalted mini pretzels (about 1 cup), *2 grain (220 calories)*
1 medium apple, *1 fruit (50 calories)*

Dinner *(510 calories)*
1 cup Fruity Tofu Stir-Fry (see recipe), *1 fruit, 1 vegetable, ½ nuts/legumes/protein (235 calories)*
1 cup cooked whole-wheat couscous, *2 grains (180 calories)*
2 teaspoons trans-fat-free margarine, *2 added fat (50 calories)*
1 cup steamed cut green beans, *2 vegetable (45 calories)*

Evening Snack/Dessert *(240 calories)*
½ cup low-fat frozen yogurt, *1 dairy (140 calories)*
1½ ounces chocolate syrup (about 2 tablespoons), *1½ sweets (100 calories)*

Nutrition analysis for the day: 2,175 calories, 8 grain, 4 fruit, 6 vegetable, 3 dairy, 2⅓ nuts/legumes/protein, 3 added fat, 1½ sweets

2,200 CALORIES: DAY 2
Target: 8 grain, 4 fruit, 5 vegetable, 3 dairy, 2½ nuts/legumes/protein, 2½ fat,
*   1 sweets*

Breakfast *(305 calories)*
1 whole egg plus 4 egg whites, scrambled (cooked with cooking spray), *1 nuts/*
*   legumes/protein (150 calories)*
¾ ounce shredded low-fat cheddar cheese (about 3 tablespoons), *½ dairy (40 calories)*
One 1-ounce slice whole-wheat bread, toasted, *1 grain (80 calories)*
½ cup mixed fresh berries, *1 fruit (35 calories)*

Morning Snack *(275 calories)*
½ large (about 4-inch) whole-wheat bagel, *2 grain (200 calories)*
1 teaspoon trans-fat-free margarine, *1 added fat (25 calories)*
1 medium apple, *1 fruit (50 calories)*

Lunch *(550 calories)*
1 Tofu Caesar Wrap (see recipe), *2 vegetable, ⅓ nuts/legumes/protein, 2 grain, ½ dairy,*
*   1 added fat (500 calories)*
½ cup grapes, *1 fruit (50 calories)*

Afternoon Snack *(335 calories)*
1½ ounces (about 1½ slices) low-fat swiss cheese, *1 dairy (75 calories)*
2 ounces whole-wheat snack crackers, *2 grain (260 calories)*

Dinner *(575 calories)*
Black bean burrito:
        One 10-inch whole-wheat tortilla, *2 grain (180 calories)*
        ½ cup canned black beans, drained and rinsed, *1 nuts/legumes/protein*
        (115 calories)
        ½ ripe avocado, *1 vegetable (120 calories)*
        1½ ounces shredded low-fat cheddar cheese (about ⅓ cup), *1 dairy*
        (75 calories)
        ½ cup tomato salsa, *1 vegetable (30 calories)*
        1 tablespoon reduced-fat sour cream, *½ added fat (20 calories)*
½ cup chopped fresh tomato, *1 vegetable (15 calories)*
1 cup shredded lettuce, *1 vegetable (20 calories)*

Evening Snack/Dessert *(165 calories)*
1 slice angel food cake (¹⁄₁₂ of a 10-inch cake), *1 sweets (140 calories)*
½ cup fresh strawberries, *1 fruit (25 calories)*

Nutrition analysis for the day: 2,205 calories, 9 grain, 4 fruit, 6 vegetable, 3 dairy, 2⅓ nuts/legumes/protein, 2½ added fat, 1 sweets

||||||||||||||||||||||||||||||||||||||||||||||||||||||||||||||||||||||||||||||||||||||||||||||||||||||||||||||||

2,200 CALORIES: DAY 3

Target: 8 grain, 4 fruit, 5 vegetable, 3 dairy, 2½ nuts/legumes/protein, 2½ fat, 1 sweets

Breakfast *(325 calories)*
Peanut butter raspberry banana smoothie:
      1 medium (7-inch) banana, *2 fruit (105 calories)*
      ½ cup frozen raspberries, *1 fruit (30 calories)*
      1 tablespoon peanut butter, *½ nuts/legumes/protein (100 calories)*
      1 cup nonfat milk, *1 dairy (90 calories)*

Morning Snack *(295 calories)*
1 large (about 4 inches) cinnamon raisin bagel, *2 grain (200 calories)*
2 tablespoons reduced-fat cream cheese, *1 added fat (70 calories)*
½ cup cubed cantaloupe, *1 fruit (25 calories)*

Lunch *(585 calories)*
1 Veggie Melt Panini (see recipe), *2 grain, 2 vegetable, 1 dairy (335 calories)*
¼ cup hummus, *½ nuts/legumes/protein (140 calories)*
1 ounce unsalted pretzels, *1 grain (110 calories)*

Afternoon Snack *(310 calories)*
1 cup low-fat fruited yogurt, *1 dairy (200 calories)*
1 ounce low-fat granola (about ¼ cup), *1 grain (110 calories)*

Dinner *(510 calories)*
3 ounces grilled seitan, *1 nuts/legumes/protein (90 calories)*
¼ cup low-sodium teriyaki sauce (for marinade) *(50 calories)*
1 cup steamed broccoli, *2 vegetable (60 calories)*
1 small (2-ounce) whole-wheat dinner roll, *2 grain (150 calories)*
1 teaspoon trans-fat-free margarine, *1 added fat (25 calories)*
1 cup baby arugula, *1 vegetable (5 calories)*
¾ ounce shredded parmesan cheese (about ¼ cup), *½ dairy (85 calories)*
Dressing: 1 teaspoon olive oil, 2 teaspoons white wine vinegar, 1½ teaspoons lemon
    juice, *1 added fat (45 calories)*

Evening Snack/Dessert *(150 calories)*
One ¾-inch slice Gingerbread (see recipe), *1 sweets (150 calories)*

Nutrition analysis for the day: 2,175 calories, 8 grain, 4 fruit, 5 vegetable, 3½ dairy, 2 nuts/legumes/protein, 3 added fat, 1 sweets

---

2,200 CALORIES: DAY 4
Target: 8 grain, 4 fruit, 5 vegetable, 3 dairy, 2½ nuts/legumes/protein, 2½ fat, 1 sweets

Breakfast *(320 calories)*
2 ounces bran flakes (about 1½ cup), *2 grain (180 calories)*
½ cup fresh raspberries, *1 fruit (30 calories)*
1 cup low-fat milk, *1 dairy (110 calories)*

Morning Snack *(270 calories)*
2 graham cracker rectangles, *1 grain (120 calories)*
1 tablespoon peanut butter, *½ nuts/legumes/protein (100 calories)*
½ cup sliced pears, *1 fruit (50 calories)*

Lunch *(595 calories)*
Spinach salad pocket:
    One 7-inch whole-wheat pita pocket, *2 grain (170 calories)*
    2 cup raw spinach, *2 vegetable (20 calories)*
    ½ cup chopped fresh tomato, *1 vegetable (15 calories)*
    ½ cup sliced cucumber, *1 vegetable (10 calories)*
    3 ounces firm tofu (about ¼ block), *⅓ nuts/legumes/protein (70 calories)*
    1½ ounces shredded parmesan cheese (about ⅓ cup), *1 dairy (170 calories)*
    Dressing: 2 teaspoons olive oil, 4 teaspoons white wine vinegar, 1 tablespoon
        lemon juice, *2 added fat (90 calories)*
1 cup sliced fresh strawberries, *2 fruit (50 calories)*

Afternoon Snack *(290 calories)*
1 cup low-fat vanilla yogurt, *1 dairy (180 calories)*
1 ounce low-fat granola (about ¼ cup), *1 grain (110 calories)*

Dinner *(590 calories)*
1⅓ cup reconstituted TVP,* *1⅓ nuts/legumes/protein (215 calories)*
1½ cup cooked brown rice pilaf, *3 grain (300 calories)*
½ cup chopped fresh tomato, *1 vegetable (15 calories)*
2 tablespoons chopped fresh basil *(0 calories)*
2 tablespoons "lite" balsamic vinaigrette, *1 added fat (60 calories)*

*See Chapter 10 for more on TVP (texturized vegetable protein).

Evening Snack/Dessert *(110 calories)*
2 fig bars, *1 sweets (110 calories)*

Nutrition analysis for the day: 2,175 calories, 9 grain, 4 fruit, 5 vegetable, 3 dairy,
2 nuts/legumes/protein, 3 added fat, 1 sweets

||||||||||||||||||||||||||||||||||||||||||||||||||||||||||||||||||||||||||||||||||||||||||||||||||||||||

2,200 CALORIES: DAY 5

Target: 8 grain, 4 fruit, 5 vegetable, 3 dairy, 2½ nuts/legumes/protein, 2½ fat,
1 sweets

Breakfast *(395 calories)*
2 ounces shredded wheat squares (about 1¼ cups), *2 grain (200 calories)*
1 medium (7-inch) banana, *2 fruit (105 calories)*
1 cup nonfat milk, *1 dairy (90 calories)*

Morning Snack *(150 calories)*
½ cup sliced fresh peaches, *1 fruit (30 calories)*
1½ ounces reduced-fat cheddar cheese (2 thin slices), *1 dairy (120 calories)*

Lunch *(665 calories)*
1⅓ cups Quinoa, Corn, and Black Bean Salad (see recipe), *2 grain, ½ vegetable, ½ nuts/*
    legumes/protein (250 calories)
4½ ounces firm tofu (about ¼ block), *½ nuts/legumes/protein (115 calories)*
1 ounce honey whole-wheat pretzels, *1 grain (110 calories)*
½ cup sliced red bell pepper, *1 vegetable (20 calories)*
1 cup shredded carrots, *2 vegetable (50 calories)*
3 tablespoons reduced-fat ranch dressing, *1½ added fat (120 calories)*

Afternoon Snack *(230 calories)*
1 ounce unsalted pretzels, *1 grain (110 calories)*
½ cup low-fat cottage cheese, *1 dairy (80 calories)*
½ cup fresh pineapple, *1 fruit (40 calories)*

Dinner *(530 calories)*
4½ ounces Poached Salmon (see recipe), *1½ nuts/legumes/protein (220 calories)*
1 cup steamed corn kernels, *2 vegetable (135 calories)*
1 teaspoon trans-fat-free margarine, *1 added fat (25 calories)*
1 small (2-ounce) whole-wheat dinner roll, *2 grain (150 calories)*
OR Dinner 2 *(525 calories)*
4½ ounces sautéed herbed seitan,* *1½ nuts/legumes/protein (215 calories)*
1 cup steamed corn kernels, *2 vegetable (135 calories)*

1 teaspoon trans-fat-free margarine, *1 added fat (25 calories)*
1 small (2-ounce) whole-wheat dinner roll, *2 grain (150 calories)*

*Sauté seitan in 2 teaspoons olive oil over medium heat until seitan is firm. Sprinkle with fresh herbs (basil, rosemary, sage).

Evening Snack/Dessert *(160 calories)*
4 dark chocolate kisses, *1 sweets (80 calories)*
¼ cup dried apricots, *1 fruit (80 calories)*

Nutrition analysis for the day: 2,130 calories, 8 grain, 5 fruit, 5½ vegetable, 3 dairy, 2½ nuts/legumes/protein, 2½ added fat, 1 sweets

||||||||||||||||||||||||||||||||||||||||||||||||||||||||||||||||||||||||||||||||||||||||||||||||||||||

2,200 CALORIES: DAY 6
Target: 8 grain, 4 fruit, 5 vegetable, 3 dairy, 2½ nuts/legumes/protein, 2½ fat, 1 sweets

Breakfast *(390 calories)*
1 whole-wheat English muffin, *2 grain (130 calories)*
1 tablespoon peanut butter, *½ nuts/legumes/protein (100 calories)*
1 cup nonfat milk, *1 dairy (90 calories)*
½ cup sliced banana, *1 fruit (70 calories)*

Morning Snack *(215 calories)*
¼ ripe avocado, mashed with a fork, *½ vegetable (60 calories)*
½ cup chopped fresh tomato, *1 vegetable (15 calories)*
One 1-ounce snack bag baked tortilla chips, *1 grain (140 calories)*

Lunch *(550 calories)*
Piled-High Veggie Pizza (⅙ of a 14-inch pizza) (see recipe), *2 grain, 2 vegetable, ½ dairy (250 calories)*
1 cup low-fat fruited yogurt, *1 dairy (200 calories)*
2 small chocolate chip cookies, *1 sweets (100 calories)*

Afternoon Snack *(290 calories)*
1 ounce unsalted mini pretzels (about ½ cup), *1 grain (110 calories)*
3 tablespoons hummus, *½ nuts/legumes/protein (130 calories)*
1 medium apple, *1 fruit (50 calories)*

Dinner *(585 calories)*
5 ounces Poached Cod (see recipe), *1⅔ nuts/legumes/protein (150 calories)*
1 cup brown rice pilaf, *2 grain (200 calories)*

¼ cup raisins, *1 fruit (110 calories)*
2 cups mixed raw leafy greens, *2 vegetable (25 calories)*
2 tablespoons balsamic vinaigrette, *2 added fat (100 calories)*
OR Dinner *2 (585 calories)*
5 ounces pan-seared seitan,* *1⅔ nuts/legumes/protein (190 calories)*
1 cup brown rice pilaf, *2 grain (200 calories)*
2 cups mixed raw leafy greens, *2 vegetable (25 calories)*
2 tablespoons balsamic vinaigrette, *2 added fat (100 calories)*
One 4-ounce snack cup peaches in juice, *1 fruit (70 calories)*

*Sear seitan in 1 teaspoon of olive oil over medium heat until crisp and warm throughout.

Evening Snack/Dessert *(175 calories)*
½ cup low-fat frozen yogurt, *1 dairy (140 calories)*
½ cup fresh strawberries, *1 fruit (25 calories)*
1 tablespoon low-fat whipped topping, *½ added fat (10 calories)*

Nutrition analysis for the day: 2,205 calories, 8 grain, 4 fruit, 5½ vegetable, 3½ dairy, 2⅔ nuts/legumes/protein, 2½ added fat, 1 sweets

‖‖

2,200 CALORIES: DAY 7
Target: 8 grain, 4 fruit, 5 vegetable, 3 dairy, 2½ nuts/legumes/protein, 2½ fat, 1 sweets

Breakfast *(455 calories)*
2 ounces shredded wheat squares (about 1 cup), *2 grain (200 calories)*
½ cup fresh blueberries, *1 fruit (40 calories)*
One 1-ounce slice cinnamon raisin bread, toasted, *1 grain (80 calories)*
1 teaspoon trans-fat-free margarine, *1 added fat (25 calories)*
1 cup low-fat milk, *1 dairy (110 calories)*

Morning Snack *(160 calories)*
1 cup apple slices, *2 fruit (60 calories)*
1 tablespoon peanut butter, *½ nuts/legumes/protein (100 calories)*

Lunch *(455 calories)*
½ cup canned pinto beans, drained and rinsed, *1 nuts/legumes/protein (105 calories)*
½ cup tomato salsa, *1 vegetable (30 calories)*
1 cup cooked brown rice, *2 grain (200 calories)*
1½ ounces shredded reduced-fat cheddar cheese (about ⅓ cup), *1 dairy (120 calories)*

Afternoon Snack *(205 calories)*

3 tablespoons whole roasted almonds, *½ nuts/legumes/protein (150 calories)*

½ cup sliced mango, *1 fruit (55 calories)*

Dinner *(760 calories)*

1 cup cooked whole-wheat pasta, *2 grain (200 calories)*

1 cup low-sodium marinara sauce, *2 vegetable (60 calories)*

½ cup reconstituted TVP,* *½ nuts/legumes/protein (80 calories)*

1½ ounces shredded parmesan cheese (about ⅓ cup), *1 dairy (160 calories)*

1 small (2-ounce) whole-wheat dinner roll, *2 grain (150 calories)*

1 teaspoon trans-fat-free margarine, *1 added fat (25 calories)*

2 cups chopped romaine lettuce, *2 vegetable (40 calories)*

1 tablespoon reduced-fat caesar dressing, *½ added fat (45 calories)*

* See Chapter 10 for more on TVP (texturized vegetable protein).

Evening Snack/Dessert *(100 calories)*

2 chocolate sandwich cookies, *1 sweets (100 calories)*

Nutrition analysis for the day: 2,135 calories, 9 grain, 4 fruit, 5 vegetable, 3 dairy, 2½ nuts/legumes/protein, 2½ added fat, 1 sweets

2,400 CALORIES: DAY 1

Target: 9 grain, 5 fruit, 5 vegetable, 3 dairy, 2½ nuts/legumes/protein, 3 added fat, 1 sweets

Breakfast *(530 calories)*

2 ounces uncooked oatmeal, cooked with water (cooks to about 1½ cups), *2 grain (200 calories)*

2 tablespoons chopped walnuts, *¼ nuts/legumes/protein (80 calories)*

¼ cup raisins, *1 fruit (110 calories)*

1 cup nonfat milk, *1 dairy (90 calories)*

1 medium apple, *1 fruit (50 calories)*

Morning Snack *(235 calories)*

1 cup nonfat vanilla yogurt, *1 dairy (160 calories)*

2 tablespoons slivered almonds, *¼ nuts/legumes/protein (75 calories)*

Lunch *(570 calories)*

One 7-inch whole-wheat pita pocket, *2 grain (170 calories)*

4 ounces grilled seitan, *1⅓ nuts/legumes/protein (120 calories)*

1 teaspoon deli mustard *(5 calories)*

1 cup grilled zucchini and summer squash, *2 vegetable (30 calories)*
1 cup mixed raw leafy greens, *1 vegetable (15 calories)*
2 tablespoons low-fat creamy Italian dressing, *1 added fat (80 calories)*
One 1-ounce snack bag honey wheat pretzels, *1 grain (110 calories)*
½ cup fresh blueberries, *1 fruit (40 calories)*

Afternoon Snack *(160 calories)*
1 ounce unsalted mini pretzels, *1 grain (110 calories)*
1 medium apple, *1 fruit (50 calories)*

Dinner *(660 calories)*
1 cup Fruity Tofu Stir-Fry (see recipe), *1 fruit, 1 vegetable, ½ nuts/legumes/protein
    (235 calories)*
1 cup cooked whole-wheat couscous, *2 grain (180 calories)*
1 cup steamed cut green beans, *2 vegetable (45 calories)*
2 teaspoons trans-fat-free margarine, *2 added fat (50 calories)*
1 small (2-ounce) whole-wheat dinner roll, *2 grain (150 calories)*

Evening Snack/Dessert *(240 calories)*
½ cup low-fat frozen yogurt, *1 dairy (140 calories)*
1½ ounces chocolate syrup (about 2 tablespoons), *1½ sweets (100 calories)*

*Nutrition analysis for the day: 2,395 calories, 10 grain, 5 fruit, 6 vegetable, 3 dairy,
2⅓ nuts/legumes/protein, 3 added fat, 1½ sweets*

|||||||||||||||||||||||||||||||||||||||||||||||||||||||||||||||||||||||||||||||||||||||||||||||||||||||||||||||||||||

2,400 CALORIES: DAY 2
*Target: 9 grain, 5 fruit, 5 vegetable, 3 dairy, 2½ nuts/legumes/protein, 3 added fat,
    1 sweets*

Breakfast *(410 calories)*
1 whole egg plus 4 egg whites, scrambled (cooked with cooking spray), *1 nuts/
    legumes/protein (150 calories)*
¾ ounce shredded low-fat cheddar cheese (about 3 tablespoons), *½ dairy (40 calories)*
Two 1-ounce slices whole-wheat bread, *2 grain (160 calories)*
1 teaspoon trans-fat-free margarine, *1 added fat (25 calories)*
½ cup mixed fresh berries, *1 fruit (35 calories)*

Morning Snack *(325 calories)*
½ large (about 4-inch) whole-wheat bagel, *2 grain (200 calories)*
1 teaspoon trans-fat-free margarine, *1 added fat (25 calories)*
1 cup cubed cantaloupe, *2 fruit (100 calories)*

Lunch *(550 calories)*
1 Tofu Caesar Wrap (see recipe), *2 vegetable, ⅓ nuts/legumes/protein, 2 grain, ½ dairy,*
   1 added fat (500 calories)
½ cup grapes, *1 fruit (50 calories)*

Afternoon Snack *(330 calories)*
1 cup low-fat fruited yogurt, *1 dairy (200 calories)*
1 ounce whole-wheat snack crackers, *1 grain (130 calories)*

Dinner *(580 calories)*
Black bean burrito:
>   One 10-inch whole-wheat tortilla, *2 grain (180 calories)*
>   ½ cup canned black beans, drained and rinsed, *1 nuts/legumes/protein*
>   *(115 calories)*
>   ½ ripe avocado, *1 vegetable (120 calories)*
>   1½ ounces shredded low-fat cheddar cheese (about ⅓ cup), *1 dairy*
>   *(75 calories)*
>   ¼ cup tomato salsa, *½ vegetable (15 calories)*
>   2 tablespoons reduced-fat sour cream, *1 added fat (40 calories)*
½ cup chopped fresh tomato, *1 vegetable (15 calories)*
1 cup shredded lettuce, *1 vegetable (20 calories)*

Evening Snack/Dessert *(165 calories)*
1 slice angel food cake (1⁄12 of a 10-inch cake), *1 sweets (140 calories)*
½ cup fresh strawberries, *1 fruit (25 calories)*

Nutrition analysis for the day: 2,360 calories, 9 grain, 5 fruit, 5½ vegetable, 3 dairy,
2⅓ nuts/legumes/protein, 4 added fat, 1 sweets

||||||||||||||||||||||||||||||||||||||||||||||||||||||||||||||||||||||||||||||||||||||||||||||||||||||||||

2,400 CALORIES: DAY 3
Target: 9 grain, 5 fruit, 5 vegetable, 3 dairy, 2½ nuts/legumes/protein, 3 added fat,
   1 sweets

Breakfast *(445 calories)*
Peanut butter raspberry banana smoothie:
>   1 medium (7-inch) banana, *2 fruit (105 calories)*
>   1 tablespoon peanut butter, *½ nuts/legumes/protein (100 calories)*
>   1 cup frozen raspberries, *1 fruit (60 calories)*
>   1 cup low-fat vanilla yogurt, *1 dairy (180 calories)*

Morning Snack *(320 calories)*
1 large (about 4 inches) cinnamon raisin bread, toasted, *2 grain (200 calories)*
2 tablespoons reduced-fat cream cheese, *1 added fat (70 calories)*
1 cup cubed cantaloupe, *2 fruit (50 calories)*

Lunch *(585 calories)*
1 Veggie Melt Panini (see recipe), *2 grain, 2 vegetable, 1 dairy (335 calories)*
¼ cup hummus, *½ nuts/legumes/protein (140 calories)*
1 ounce unsalted pretzels, *1 grain (110 calories)*

Afternoon Snack *(310 calories)*
1 cup low-fat fruited yogurt, *1 dairy (200 calories)*
1 ounce low-fat granola (about ¼ cup), *1 grain (110 calories)*

Dinner *(575 calories)*
6 ounces grilled firm tofu (about ½ block), *⅔ nuts/legumes/protein (155 calories)*
¼ cup low-sodium teriyaki sauce (for marinade) *(50 calories)*
1 cup steamed broccoli, *2 vegetable (60 calories)*
1 small (2-ounce) whole-wheat dinner roll, *2 grain (150 calories)*
1 teaspoon trans-fat-free margarine, *1 added fat (25 calories)*
1 cup baby arugula, *1 vegetable (5 calories)*
¾ ounce shredded parmesan cheese (about ¼ cup), *½ dairy (85 calories)*
Dressing: 1 teaspoon olive oil, 2 teaspoons white wine vinegar, 1½ teaspoons lemon
   juice, *1 added fat (45 calories)*

Evening Snack/Dessert *(150 calories)*
One ¾-inch slice Gingerbread (see recipe), *1 sweets (150 calories)*

*Nutrition analysis for the day: 2,385 calories, 8 grain, 5 fruit, 5 vegetable, 3½ dairy,
1⅔ nuts/legumes/protein, 3 added fat, 1 sweets*

2,400 CALORIES: DAY 4
*Target: 9 grain, 5 fruit, 5 vegetable, 3 dairy, 2½ nuts/legumes/protein, 3 added fat,
   1 sweets*

Breakfast *(505 calories)*
2 ounces bran flakes (about 1½ cups), *2 grain (180 calories)*
¼ cup golden raisins, *1 fruit (110 calories)*
1 medium (7-inch) banana, sliced, *2 fruit (105 calories)*
1 cup low-fat milk, *1 dairy (110 calories)*

Morning Snack *(270 calories)*
2 graham cracker rectangles, *1 grain (120 calories)*
1 tablespoon peanut butter, *½ nuts/legumes/protein (100 calories)*
½ cup sliced pears, *1 fruit (50 calories)*

Lunch *(640 calories)*
Spinach salad pocket:

> One 7-inch whole-wheat pita pocket, *2 grain (170 calories)*
> 2 cup raw spinach, *2 vegetable (20 calories)*
> ½ cup chopped fresh tomato, *1 vegetable (15 calories)*
> ½ cup sliced cucumber, *1 vegetable (10 calories)*
> 3 ounces stir-fried firm tofu (about ⅓ block), *⅓ nuts/legumes/protein (115 calories)*
> 1½ ounces shredded parmesan cheese (about ⅓ cup), *1 dairy (170 calories)*
> Dressing: 2 teaspoons olive oil, 4 teaspoons white wine vinegar, 1 tablespoon lemon juice, *2 added fat (90 calories)*

1 cup sliced fresh strawberries, *2 fruit (50 calories)*

Afternoon Snack *(270 calories)*
1 cup nonfat vanilla yogurt, *1 dairy (160 calories)*
1 ounce low-fat granola (about ¼ cup), *1 grain (110 calories)*

Dinner *(590 calories)*
1⅓ cup reconstituted TVP,* *1⅓ nuts/legumes/protein (215 calories)*
1½ cup cooked brown rice pilaf, *3 grain (300 calories)*
½ cup chopped fresh tomato, *1 vegetable (15 calories)*
2 tablespoons chopped fresh basil *(0 calories)*
2 tablespoons "lite" balsamic vinaigrette, *1 added fat (60 calories)*

* See Chapter 10 for more on TVP (texturized vegetable protein).

Evening Snack/Dessert *(110 calories)*
2 fig bars, *1 sweets (110 calories)*

Nutrition analysis for the day: 2,385 calories, 9 grain, 6 fruit, 5 vegetable, 3 dairy, 2 nuts/legumes/protein, 3 added fat, 1 sweets

|||||||||||||||||||||||||||||||||||||||||||||||||||||||||||||||||||||||||||||||||||||||||||||||||||||||||||||||||||||||||||

2,400 CALORIES: DAY 5
Target: 9 grain, 5 fruit, 5 vegetable, 3 dairy, 2½ nuts/legumes/protein, 3 added fat, 1 sweets

Breakfast *(490 calories)*
1 Low-Fat Blueberry Muffin (see recipe), *2 grain (200 calories)*
1 teaspoon trans-fat-free margarine, *1 added fat (25 calories)*
1 cup nonfat vanilla yogurt, *1 dairy (160 calories)*
1 cup grapes, *2 fruit (105 calories)*

Morning Snack *(345 calories)*
1 cup sliced fresh peaches, *2 fruit (65 calories)*
1½ ounces smoked gouda cheese, *1 dairy (150 calories)*
1 ounce whole-wheat snack crackers, *1 grain (130 calories)*

Lunch *(610 calories)*
1⅓ cups Quinoa, Corn, and Black Bean Salad (see recipe), *2 grain, ½ vegetable, ½ nuts/ legumes/protein (250 calories)*
4½ ounces stir-fried firm tofu (about ¼ block), *½ nuts/legumes/protein (140 calories)*
1 ounce honey whole-wheat pretzels, *1 grain (110 calories)*
½ cup sliced red bell pepper, *1 vegetable (20 calories)*
½ cup sliced carrots, *1 vegetable (25 calories)*
2 tablespoons reduced-fat ranch dressing, *1 added fat (65 calories)*

Afternoon Snack *(230 calories)*
1 ounce unsalted mini pretzels (about ½ cup), *1 grain (110 calories)*
½ cup low-fat cottage cheese, *1 dairy (80 calories)*
½ cup fresh pineapple, *1 fruit (40 calories)*

Dinner *(530 calories)*
4½ ounces Poached Salmon (see recipe), *1½ nuts/legumes/protein (220 calories)*
1 cup steamed corn kernels, *2 vegetable (135 calories)*
1 teaspoon trans-fat-free margarine, *1 added fat (25 calories)*
1 small (2-ounce) whole-wheat dinner roll, *2 grain (150 calories)*
OR Dinner 2 *(525 calories)*
4½ ounces sautéed herbed seitan,* *1½ nuts/legumes/protein (215 calories)*
1 cup steamed corn kernels, *2 vegetable (135 calories)*
1 teaspoon trans-fat-free margarine, *1 added fat (25 calories)*
1 small (2-ounce) whole-wheat dinner roll, *2 grain (150 calories)*

* Sauté seitan in 2 teaspoons olive oil over medium heat until seitan is firm. Sprinkle with fresh herbs (basil, rosemary, sage).

Evening Snack/Dessert *(185 calories)*
2-inch square Low-Fat Brownie (see recipe), *1 sweets (155 calories)*
½ cup fresh raspberries, *1 fruit (30 calories)*

Nutrition analysis for the day: 2,390 calories, 9 grain, 6 fruit, 4½ vegetable, 3 dairy, 2½ nuts/legumes/protein, 3 added fat, 1 sweets

||||||||||||||||||||||||||||||||||||||||||||||||||||||||||||||||||||||||||||||||||||||||||||

2,400 CALORIES: DAY 6
Target: 9 grain, 5 fruit, 5 vegetable, 3 dairy, 2½ nuts/legumes/protein, 3 added fat, 1 sweets

Breakfast *(495 calories)*
½ large (about 4-inch) whole-wheat bagel, *2 grain (200 calories)*
1 tablespoon peanut butter, *½ nuts/legumes/protein (100 calories)*
1 cup nonfat milk, *1 dairy (90 calories)*
1 medium (7-inch) banana, *2 fruit (105 calories)*

Morning Snack *(275 calories)*
½ ripe avocado, mashed with a fork, *1 vegetable (120 calories)*
½ cup chopped fresh tomato, *1 vegetable (15 calories)*
One 1-ounce snack bag baked tortilla chips, *1 grain (140 calories)*

Lunch *(560 calories)*
Piled-High Veggie Pizza (⅙ of a 14-inch pizza) (see recipe), *2 grain, 2 vegetable, ½ dairy (250 calories)*
1 cup sliced pears, *2 fruit (100 calories)*
One 1-ounce snack bag honey wheat pretzels, *1 grain (110 calories)*
2 small chocolate chip cookies, *1 sweets (100 calories)*

Afternoon Snack *(240 calories)*
1 ounce unsalted mini pretzels (about ½ cup), *1 grain (110 calories)*
3 tablespoons hummus, *½ nuts/legumes/protein (130 calories)*

Dinner *(605 calories)*
5 ounces Poached Cod (see recipe), *1⅔ nuts/legumes/protein (150 calories)*
1 cup brown rice pilaf, *2 grain (200 calories)*
1 medium (5-inch) baked sweet potato, *2 vegetable (180 calories)*
1 tablespoon trans-fat-free margarine, *3 added fat (75 calories)*
OR **Dinner 2** *(610 calories)*
5 ounces pan-seared seitan,* *1⅔ nuts/legumes/protein (190 calories)*
1 small (2-ounce) whole-wheat dinner roll, *2 grain (150 calories)*

1 tsp. olive oil (for dipping), *1 added fat (40 calories)*
1 medium (5-inch) baked sweet potato, *2 vegetable (180 calories)*
2 teaspoons trans-fat-free margarine, *2 added fat (50 calories)*

*Sear seitan in 1 teaspoon of olive oil over medium heat until crisp and warm throughout.

Evening Snack/Dessert *(165 calories)*
½ cup low-fat frozen yogurt, *1 dairy (140 calories)*
½ cup fresh strawberries, *1 fruit (25 calories)*

Nutrition analysis for the day: 2,340 calories, 9 grain, 5 fruit, 6 vegetable, 2½ dairy, 2⅔ nuts/legumes/protein, 3 added fat, 1 sweets

||||||||||||||||||||||||||||||||||||||||||||||||||||||||||||||||||||||||||||||||||||||||||||||||||||||

2,400 CALORIES: DAY 7
Target: 9 grain, 5 fruit, 5 vegetable, 3 dairy, 2½ nuts/legumes/protein, 3 added fat, 1 sweets

Breakfast *(605 calories)*
2 ounces shredded wheat squares (about 1 cup), *2 grain (200 calories)*
¼ cup raisins, *1 fruit (110 calories)*
One 1-ounce slice cinnamon raisin bread, toasted, *1 grain (80 calories)*
1 teaspoon trans-fat-free margarine, *1 added fat (25 calories)*
¾ cup 100% orange juice, *1 fruit (80 calories)*
1 cup low-fat milk, *1 dairy (110 calories)*

Morning Snack *(160 calories)*
1 cup apple slices, *2 fruit (60 calories)*
1 tablespoon peanut butter, *½ nuts/legumes/protein (100 calories)*

Lunch *(575 calories)*
1 cup cooked brown rice, *2 grain (200 calories)*
½ cup canned pinto beans, drained and rinsed, *1 nuts/legumes/protein (105 calories)*
½ cup tomato salsa, *1 vegetable (30 calories)*
½ ripe avocado, *1 vegetable (120 calories)*
1½ ounces shredded reduced-fat cheddar cheese (about ⅓ cup), *1 dairy (120 calories)*

Afternoon Snack *(230 calories)*
3 tablespoons whole roasted almonds, *½ nuts/legumes/protein (150 calories)*
¼ cup dried apricots, *1 fruit (80 calories)*

Dinner *(760 calories)*

1 cup cooked whole-wheat pasta, *2 grain (200 calories)*
1 cup low-sodium marinara sauce, *2 vegetable (80 calories)*
½ cup reconstituted TVP,* *½ nuts/legumes/protein (80 calories)*
1½ ounces shredded parmesan cheese (about ⅓ cup), *1 dairy (160 calories)*
1 small (2-ounce) whole-wheat dinner roll, *2 grain (150 calories)*
1 teaspoon trans-fat-free margarine, *1 added fat (25 calories)*
1 cup chopped romaine lettuce, *1 vegetable (20 calories)*
1 tablespoon reduced-fat caesar dressing, *1 added fat (45 calories)*

*See Chapter 10 for more on TVP (texturized vegetable protein).

Evening Snack/Dessert *(100 calories)*
2 chocolate sandwich cookies, *1 sweets (100 calories)*

Nutrition analysis for the day: 2,430 calories, 9 grain, 5 fruit, 5 vegetable, 3 dairy, 2½ nuts/legumes/protein, 3 added fat, 1 sweets

|||||||||||||||||||||||||||||||||||||||||||||||||||||||||||||||||||||||||||||||||||||||||||||||||||||||||||||

2,600 CALORIES: DAY 1
Target: 10 grain, 5 fruit, 5 vegetable, 3 dairy, 3½ nuts/legumes/protein, 3 added fat, 1½ sweets

Breakfast *(580 calories)*
2 ounces uncooked oatmeal, cooked with water (cooks to about 1½ cups), *2 grain (200 calories)*
2 tablespoons chopped walnuts, *¼ nuts/legumes/protein (80 calories)*
¼ cup raisins, *1 fruit (110 calories)*
1 cup nonfat milk, *1 dairy (90 calories)*
1 medium pear, *1 fruit (100 calories)*

Morning Snack *(275 calories)*
1 cup low-fat fruited yogurt, *1 dairy (200 calories)*
2 tablespoons slivered almonds, *¼ nuts/legumes/protein (75 calories)*

Lunch *(615 calories)*
One 7-inch whole-wheat pita pocket, *2 grain (170 calories)*
4½ ounces grilled seitan, *1½ nuts/legumes/protein (135 calories)*
1 teaspoon deli mustard *(5 calories)*
1 cup grilled zucchini and summer squash, *2 vegetable (30 calories)*
1 cup mixed raw leafy greens, *1 vegetable (15 calories)*
2 tablespoons low-fat creamy Italian dressing, *1 added fat (80 calories)*

1 ounce unsalted mini pretzels (about ½ cup), *1 grain (110 calories)*
One 4-ounce snack cup peaches in juice, *1 fruit (70 calories)*

Afternoon Snack *(235 calories)*
½ cup cooked brown rice, *1 grain (100 calories)*
½ cup canned black beans rinsed and drained, *1 nuts/legumes/protein (120 calories)*
¼ cup tomato salsa, *½ vegetable (15 calories)*

Dinner *(660 calories)*
1 cup Fruity Tofu Stir-Fry (see recipe), *1 fruit, 1 vegetable, ½ nuts/legumes/protein*
   (235 calories)
1 cup cooked whole-wheat couscous, *2 grain (180 calories)*
1 cup steamed green beans, *2 vegetable (45 calories)*
2 teaspoons trans-fat-free margarine, *2 added fat (50 calories)*
1 small (2-ounce) whole-wheat dinner roll, *2 grain (150 calories)*

Evening Snack/Dessert *(240 calories)*
½ cup low-fat frozen yogurt, *1 dairy (140 calories)*
1½ ounces chocolate syrup (about 2 tablespoons), *1½ sweets (100 calories)*

Nutrition analysis for the day: 2,605 calories, 10 grain, 4 fruit, 6½ vegetable,
3 dairy, 3½ nuts/legumes/protein, 3 added fat, 1½ sweets

||||||||||||||||||||||||||||||||||||||||||||||||||||||||||||||||||||||||||||||||||||||||||||||||||||||

2,600 CALORIES: DAY 2
Target: 10 grain, 5 fruit, 5 vegetable, 3 dairy, 3½ nuts/legumes/protein, 3 added
   fat, 1½ sweets

Breakfast *(535 calories)*
Cheese omelet (cooked with cooking spray):
      3 whole eggs, *1 nuts/legumes/protein (240 calories)*
      ¾ ounce shredded low-fat cheddar cheese (about 3 tablespoons), *½ dairy*
         (40 calories)
Two 1-ounce slices whole-wheat bread, *2 grain (160 calories)*
1 teaspoon trans-fat-free margarine, *1 added fat (25 calories)*
1 cup mixed fresh berries, *1 fruit (70 calories)*

Morning Snack *(350 calories)*
½ large (about 4-inch) whole-wheat bagel, *2 grain (200 calories)*
1 tablespoon peanut butter, *½ nuts/legumes/protein (100 calories)*
1 cup cantaloupe, *2 fruit (50 calories)*

Lunch *(610 calories)*
1 Tofu Caesar Wrap (see recipe), *2 vegetable, ⅓ nuts/legumes/protein, 2 grain, ½ dairy, 1 added fat (500 calories)*
1 ounce honey whole-wheat pretzels, *1 grain (110 calories)*

Afternoon Snack *(330 calories)*
1 cup low-fat fruited yogurt, *1 dairy (200 calories)*
1 ounce whole-wheat snack crackers, *1 grain (130 calories)*

Dinner *(640 calories)*
Black bean burrito:
    One 10-inch whole-wheat tortilla, *2 grain (180 calories)*
    ¾ cup canned black beans, drained and rinsed, *⅔ nuts/legumes/protein (175 calories)*
    ½ ripe avocado, *1 vegetable (120 calories)*
    1½ ounces shredded low-fat cheddar cheese (about ⅓ cup), *1 dairy (75 calories)*
    ¼ cup tomato salsa, *½ vegetable (15 calories)*
    2 tablespoons reduced-fat sour cream, *1 added fat (40 calories)*
½ cup chopped fresh tomato, *1 vegetable (15 calories)*
1 cup shredded lettuce, *1 vegetable (20 calories)*

Evening Snack/Dessert *(190 calories)*
1 slice angel food cake (½₂ of a 10-inch cake), *1 sweets (140 calories)*
½ cup fresh strawberries, *1 fruit (25 calories)*
1½ teaspoons sugar, *½ sweets (25 calories)*

Nutrition analysis for the day: 2,655 calories, 10 grain, 5 fruit, 5½ vegetable, 3 dairy, 3⅓ nuts/legumes/protein, 3 added fat, 1½ sweets

||||||||||||||||||||||||||||||||||||||||||||||||||||||||||||||||||||||||||||||||||||||||||||||||||

2,600 CALORIES: DAY 3
Target: 10 grain, 5 fruit, 5 vegetable, 3 dairy, 3½ nuts/legumes/protein, 3 added fat, 1½ sweets

Breakfast *(330 calories)*
1 whole-wheat English muffin, *2 grain (130 calories)*
2 tablespoons reduced-fat cream cheese, *1 added fat (70 calories)*
1 cup cubed cantaloupe, *2 fruit (50 calories)*
¾ cup 100% orange juice, *1 fruit (80 calories)*

Morning Snack *(345 calories)*
Peanut butter, flaxseed, and banana smoothie:
      1 medium (7-inch) banana, *2 fruit (105 calories)*
      1 tablespoon peanut butter, *½ nuts/legumes/protein (100 calories)*
      1 tablespoon flaxseeds, *½ nuts/legumes/protein (50 calories)*
      1 cup nonfat milk, *1 dairy (90 calories)*

Lunch *(695 calories)*
1 Veggie Melt Panini (see recipe), *2 grain, 2 vegetable, 1 dairy (335 calories)*
2 ounces unsalted pretzel sticks, *2 grain (220 calories)*
¼ cup hummus, *½ nuts/legumes/protein (140 calories)*

Afternoon Snack *(420 calories)*
1 cup low-fat fruited yogurt, *1 dairy (200 calories)*
2 ounces low-fat granola (about ½ cup), *2 grain (220 calories)*

Dinner *(670 calories)*
6 ounces grilled seitan, *2 nuts/legumes/protein (180 calories)*
¼ cup low-sodium teriyaki sauce (for marinade) *(50 calories)*
1 cup cooked green peas, *2 vegetable (130 calories)*
1 small (2-ounce) whole-wheat dinner roll, *2 grain (150 calories)*
1 teaspoon trans-fat-free margarine, *1 added fat (25 calories)*
1 cup baby arugula, *1 vegetable (5 calories)*
¾ ounce shredded parmesan cheese (about ¼ cup), *½ dairy (85 calories)*
Dressing: 1 teaspoon olive oil, 2 teaspoons white wine vinegar, 1½ teaspoons lemon
    juice, *1 added fat (45 calories)*

Evening Snack/Dessert *(150 calories)*
One ¾-inch slice Gingerbread (see recipe), *1 sweets (150 calories)*

*Nutrition analysis for the day: 2,610 calories, 10 grain, 5 fruit, 5 vegetable,
3½ dairy, 3½ nuts/legumes/protein, 3 added fat, 1 sweets*

2,600 CALORIES: DAY 4
*Target: 10 grain, 5 fruit, 5 vegetable, 3 dairy, 3½ nuts/legumes/protein, 3 added
fat, 1½ sweets*

Breakfast *(610 calories)*
2 ounces bran flakes (about 1½ cup), *2 grain (180 calories)*
One 1-ounce slice whole-wheat bread, toasted, *1 grain (80 calories)*
1½ teaspoons fruit preserves, *½ sweets (25 calories)*

¼ cup golden raisins, *1 fruit (110 calories)*
1 medium (7-inch) banana, sliced, *2 fruit (105 calories)*
1 cup low-fat milk, *1 dairy (110 calories)*

Morning Snack *(370 calories)*
2 graham cracker rectangles, *1 grain (120 calories)*
2 tablespoons peanut butter, *1 nuts/legumes/protein (200 calories)*
½ cup sliced pears, *1 fruit (50 calories)*

Lunch *(615 calories)*
Spinach salad pocket:
    One 7-inch whole-wheat pita pocket, *2 grain (170 calories)*
    2 cups raw spinach, *2 vegetable (20 calories)*
    ½ cup chopped fresh tomato, *1 vegetable (15 calories)*
    ½ cup sliced cucumber, *1 vegetable (10 calories)*
    3 ounces stir-fried firm tofu (about ⅕ block), *⅓ nuts/legumes/protein*
        (115 calories)
    1½ ounces shredded parmesan cheese (about ⅓ cup), *1 dairy (170 calories)*
    Dressing: 2 teaspoons olive oil, 4 teaspoons white wine vinegar, 1 tablespoon
        lemon juice, *2 added fat (90 calories)*
½ cup sliced fresh strawberries, *1 fruit (25 calories)*

Afternoon Snack *(270 calories)*
1 cup nonfat vanilla yogurt, *1 dairy (160 calories)*
1 ounce low-fat granola (about ¼ cup), *1 grain (110 calories)*

Dinner *(655 calories)*
1⅔ cup reconstituted TVP,* *1⅔ nuts/legumes/protein (265 calories)*
1½ cup cooked brown rice pilaf, *3 grain (300 calories)*
1 cup chopped fresh tomato, *2 vegetable (30 calories)*
2 tablespoons chopped fresh basil *(0 calories)*
2 tablespoons "lite" balsamic vinaigrette, *1 added fat (60 calories)*

*See Chapter 10 for more on TVP (texturized vegetable protein).

Evening Snack/Dessert *(110 calories)*
2 fig bars, *1 sweets (110 calories)*

Nutrition analysis for the day: 2,630 calories, 10 grain, 5 fruit, 6 vegetable, 3 dairy, 3 nuts/legumes/protein, 3 added fat, 1½ sweets

||||||||||||||||||||||||||||||||||||||||||||||||||||||||||||||||||||||||||||||||||||||||||||||||||||||||||||||||||||||||||||||||||||||||

2,600 CALORIES: DAY 5

Target: 10 grain, 5 fruit, 5 vegetable, 3 dairy, 3½ nuts/legumes/protein, 3 added fat, 1½ sweets

Breakfast *(530 calories)*
1 Low-Fat Blueberry Muffin (see recipe), *2 grain (200 calories)*
1 teaspoon trans-fat-free margarine, *1 added fat (25 calories)*
1 cup low-fat fruited yogurt, *1 dairy (200 calories)*
1 cup grapes, *2 fruit (105 calories)*

Morning Snack *(380 calories)*
1 cup sliced mango, *2 fruit (110 calories)*
2 reduced-fat string cheese sticks, *1⅓ dairy (140 calories)*
1 ounce whole-wheat snack crackers, *1 grain (130 calories)*

Lunch *(575 calories)*
1⅓ cups Quinoa, Corn, and Black Bean Salad (see recipe), *2 grain, ½ vegetable, ½ nuts/ legumes/protein (250 calories)*
3 ounces stir-fried seitan, *1 nuts/legumes/protein (110 calories)*
¼ ripe avocado, mashed with a fork, *½ vegetable (60 calories)*
1 ounce honey whole-wheat pretzels, *1 grain (110 calories)*
½ cup sliced red bell pepper, *1 vegetable (20 calories)*
½ cup sliced carrots, *1 vegetable (25 calories)*

Afternoon Snack *(215 calories)*
1 ounce unsalted mini pretzels, *1 grain (110 calories)*
1½ teaspoons fruit preserves, *½ sweets (25 calories)*
½ cup low-fat cottage cheese, *1 dairy (80 calories)*

Dinner *(670 calories)*
6 ounces Poached Salmon (see recipe), *2 nuts/legumes/protein (290 calories)*
1 cup (10–12 small spears) Roasted Asparagus (see recipe), *2 vegetable (80 calories)*
½ cup cooked brown rice, *1 grain (100 calories)*
2 teaspoons trans-fat-free margarine, *2 added fat (50 calories)*
1 small (2-ounce) whole-wheat dinner roll, *2 grain (150 calories)*
OR Dinner 2 *(665 calories)*
6 ounces sautéed herbed seitan,* *2 nuts/legumes/protein (260 calories)*
1 cup (10–12 small spears) Roasted Asparagus (see recipe), *2 vegetable (80 calories)*
1 cup cooked brown rice pilaf, *2 grain (200 calories)*

2 teaspoons trans-fat-free margarine, *2 added fat (50 calories)*
½ small (2-ounce) whole-wheat dinner roll, *1 grain (75 calories)*

*Sauté seitan in 2 teaspoons olive oil over medium heat until seitan is firm. Sprinkle with fresh herbs (basil, rosemary, sage).

Evening Snack/Dessert *(185 calories)*
2-inch square Low-Fat Brownie (see recipe), *1 sweets (155 calories)*
½ cup fresh raspberries, *1 fruit (30 calories)*

Nutrition analysis for the day: 2,560 calories, 10 grain, 5 fruit, 5 vegetable, 3⅓ dairy, 3½ nuts/legumes/protein, 3 added fat, 1½ sweets

||||||||||||||||||||||||||||||||||||||||||||||||||||||||||||||||||||||||||||||||||||||||||||||||||||||||||||

2,600 CALORIES: DAY 6
Target: 10 grain, 5 fruit, 5 vegetable, 3 dairy, 3½ nuts/legumes/protein, 3 added fat, 1½ sweets

Breakfast *(620 calories)*
½ large (about 4-inch) whole-wheat bagel, *2 grain (200 calories)*
2 tablespoons peanut butter, *1 nuts/legumes/protein (200 calories)*
1½ teaspoons fruit preserves, *½ sweets (25 calories)*
1 cup nonfat milk, *1 dairy (90 calories)*
1 medium (7-inch) banana, *2 fruit (105 calories)*

Morning Snack *(275 calories)*
½ ripe avocado, mashed with a fork, *1 vegetable (120 calories)*
½ cup chopped fresh tomato, *1 vegetable (15 calories)*
One 1-ounce snack bag baked tortilla chips, *1 grain (140 calories)*

Lunch *(560 calories)*
Piled-High Veggie Pizza (⅙ of a 14-inch pizza) (see recipe), *2 grain, 2 vegetable, ½ dairy (250 calories)*
1 medium pear, *1 fruit (100 calories)*
One 1-ounce snack bag honey wheat pretzels, *1 grain (110 calories)*
2 small chocolate chip cookies, *1 sweets (100 calories)*

Afternoon Snack *(280 calories)*
1 ounce unsalted mini pretzels (about ½ cup), *1 grain (110 calories)*
¾ ounce low-fat cheddar cheese (1 small slice), *½ dairy (40 calories)*
3 tablespoons hummus, *½ nuts/legumes/protein (130 calories)*

Dinner *(635 calories)*
6 ounces Poached Cod (see recipe), *2 nuts/legumes/protein (180 calories)*
1 cup brown rice pilaf, *2 grain (200 calories)*
1 medium (5-inch) baked sweet potato, *2 vegetable (180 calories)*
1 tablespoon trans-fat-free margarine, *3 added fat (75 calories)*
OR Dinner 2 *(640 calories)*
6 ounces pan-seared seitan,* *2 nuts/legumes/protein (220 calories)*
1 small (2-ounce) whole-wheat dinner roll, *2 grain (150 calories)*
1 tsp. olive oil (for dipping), *1 added fat (40 calories)*
1 medium (5-inch) baked sweet potato, *2 vegetable (180 calories)*
2 teaspoons trans-fat-free margarine, *2 added fat (50 calories)*

*Sear seitan in 1 teaspoon of olive oil over medium heat until crisp and warm throughout.

Evening Snack/Dessert *(165 calories)*
½ cup low-fat frozen yogurt, *1 dairy (140 calories)*
½ cup fresh strawberries, *1 fruit (25 calories)*

Nutrition analysis for the day: 2,535 calories, 9 grain, 4 fruit, 6 vegetable, 3 dairy, 3½ nuts/legumes/protein, 3 added fat, 1½ sweets

||||||||||||||||||||||||||||||||||||||||||||||||||||||||||||||||||||||||||||||||||||||||||||||||||||||||||

2,600 CALORIES: DAY 7
Target: 10 grain, 5 fruit, 5 vegetable, 3 dairy, 3½ nuts/legumes/protein, 3 added fat, 1½ sweets

Breakfast *(655 calories)*
2 ounces shredded wheat squares (about 1 cup), *2 grain (200 calories)*
1 tablespoon flaxseeds, *½ nuts/legumes/protein (50 calories)*
¼ cup raisins, *1 fruit (110 calories)*
One 1-ounce slice cinnamon raisin bread, toasted, *1 grain (80 calories)*
1 teaspoon trans-fat-free margarine, *1 added fat (25 calories)*
¾ cup 100% orange juice, *1 fruit (80 calories)*
1 cup low-fat milk, *1 dairy (110 calories)*

Morning Snack *(160 calories)*
1 cup apple slices, *2 fruit (60 calories)*
1 tablespoon peanut butter, *½ nuts/legumes/protein (100 calories)*

Lunch *(525 calories)*
1 cup cooked brown rice, *2 grain (200 calories)*
½ cup pinto beans, drained and rinsed, *1 nuts/legumes/protein (105 calories)*

½ cup tomato salsa, *1 vegetable (30 calories)*
½ ripe avocado, *1 vegetable (120 calories)*
1½ ounces shredded low-fat cheddar cheese (about ⅓ cup), *1 dairy (70 calories)*

Afternoon Snack *(325 calories)*
Mango–black bean salsa:
    ½ cup chopped mango, *1 fruit (60 calories)*
    2 tablespoons finely chopped red onion, *¼ vegetable (10 calories)*
    ½ cup canned black beans, drained and rinsed, *1 nuts/legumes/protein
      (115 calories)*
    Squeeze of lime *(0 calories)*
One 1-ounce snack bag baked tortilla chips, *1 grain (140 calories)*

Dinner *(760 calories)*
1 cup cooked whole-wheat pasta, *2 grain (200 calories)*
1 cup low-sodium marinara sauce, *2 vegetable (80 calories)*
½ cup reconstituted TVP*, *½ nuts/legumes/protein (80 calories)*
1½ ounces shredded parmesan cheese (about ⅓ cup), *1 dairy (160 calories)*
1 small (2-ounce) whole-wheat dinner roll, *2 grain (150 calories)*
1 teaspoon trans-fat-free margarine, *1 added fat (25 calories)*
1 cup chopped romaine lettuce, *1 vegetable (20 calories)*
1 tablespoon reduced-fat caesar dressing, *1 added fat (45 calories)*

* See Chapter 10 for more on TVP (texturized vegetable protein).

Evening Snack/Dessert *(150 calories)*
3 chocolate sandwich cookies, *1½ sweets (150 calories)*

***Nutrition analysis for the day: 2,575 calories, 10 grain, 5 fruit, 5¼ vegetable,
3 dairy, 3½ nuts/legumes/protein, 3 added fat, 1½ sweets***

Part 4

Recipes

Main Dishes

||||||||||||||||||||||||||||||||||||||||||||||||||||||||||||||||||||||||||||||||||||||||||||||||||||||||||||||||||||||||||

Veggie Melt Panini

1 teaspoon deli mustard
Two 1-ounce slices whole-wheat bread
1½ ounces sliced low-fat cheese (cheddar and swiss work well)
7 asparagus spears, grilled
7 strips red and yellow bell pepper, grilled
Nonstick cooking spray

1. Spread the mustard on one side of each slice of bread. Place the cheese evenly over the mustard on one slice of bread. Arrange the asparagus and peppers on top of the cheese. Top with the second slice of bread, mustard side down.
2. Heat a panini press until ready or heat a cast-iron skillet over medium heat until hot. Spray the press plates or skillet very lightly with cooking spray.
3. If using a press, place the sandwich on the bottom plate and close the top. If using a skillet, place the sandwich in it and place a second skillet on top. (You might want to wrap the outside of the second skillet with foil first.)
4. Grill the sandwich until the cheese is melted. Serve hot.

DASH servings (per sandwich)
2 grain
2 vegetable
1 dairy
Calories: 335

II

Piled-High Veggie Pizza

Nonstick cooking spray
2 teaspoons cornmeal (optional)
1 tablespoon olive oil
1 cup broccoli florets
2 cups sliced mushrooms
1 red bell pepper, stemmed, seeded, and cut into strips
1 small white onion, peeled and chopped
One 12-ounce package pizza dough (found in the freezer or
    refrigerated sections of most supermarkets; thaw if frozen)
1 cup low-sodium tomato sauce
½ cup shredded low-fat mozzarella

1. Preheat the oven to 450°F. Lightly spray a baking sheet with cooking spray, or if using a pizza stone, sprinkle the dry stone with the cornmeal.
2. Heat the oil in a skillet over medium heat until hot but not smoking. Add the broccoli, mushrooms, bell pepper, and onion and cook, stirring occasionally, just until tender. Remove from the heat.
3. Roll out the pizza dough to a round 14 inches in diameter and ¼-inch thick. Place on the prepared baking sheet or stone.
4. Spread the tomato sauce over the dough. Top the sauce evenly with the cooked veggies. Sprinkle the cheese over the veggies.
5. Bake for 15 to 20 minutes, until the crust is baked through and golden crisp on the edges, and the cheese is melted and bubbling.

DASH servings (per ⅙ pizza)
2 grain
2 vegetable
½ dairy
Calories: 250

Fruity Chicken Stir-Fry

1½ tablespoons sesame oil
1¼ pounds boneless, skinless chicken breasts, cut in thin strips
½ cup peeled and sliced onions
1 cup peeled and grated carrots
1 teaspoon dried basil
1 cup snow peas or sugar snap peas
1 tablespoon water
¼ cup pine nuts or 2 tablespoons cashew nuts
¼ cup chopped dried apricots
2 tablespoons seedless raisins
1 large unpeeled Golden Delicious apple, quartered, cored, and cut
    into lengthwise slices
¾ cup prepared duck sauce

1. Heat 1 tablespoon of the sesame oil in a skillet or wok over medium-high heat until hot but not smoking. Add the chicken and stir-fry until lightly browned and cooked through (about 4 minutes).
2. Transfer the chicken to a plate and set aside, covering it lightly with foil to keep warm.
3. Pour the remaining 1½ teaspoons oil into the skillet and add onion, carrots, and basil. Stir-fry until the carrots are tender.
4. Add the snow peas and water and stir-fry for 2 minutes more.
5. Stir in the pine nuts, apricots, and raisins. Remove from the heat and stir in the apples.
6. Add the chicken back to the pan along with the duck sauce and stir to combine. Serve immediately.

Makes 5 cups

(continued on next page)

DASH servings (per 1 cup stir-fry, without rice)
1 vegetable
1 fruit
½ meat
Calories: 330

Fruity Tofu Stir-Fry

Substitute 1 pound firm tofu, drained, for the chicken.

DASH servings (per 1 cup stir-fry, without rice)
1 vegetable
1 fruit
½ nuts/seeds/legumes
Calories: 235

||||||||||||||||||||||||||||||||||||||||||||||||||||||||||||||||||||||||||||||||||||||||||||

Chicken Caesar Wrap

2 cups shredded romaine lettuce
1½ ounces grilled skinless chicken breast, shredded
2 tablespoons Lite Caesar Dressing (recipe follows)
Half a 12-inch whole-wheat pita pocket (sliced into 2 rounds through
    the edge), or one 12-inch whole-wheat wrap
¼ cup shredded parmesan cheese

1. Combine the lettuce and chicken in a medium bowl. Drizzle over the dressing and toss well to mix.
2. Lay the pita half on a work surface, cut side (inside) up. Spoon the lettuce-chicken mixture onto the pita. Sprinkle evenly with the parmesan. Roll up. Cut in half on an angle, if desired. Serve immediately.

DASH servings (per wrap with dressing)
2 grain
2 vegetable
½ meat
½ dairy
Calories: 395

Lite Caesar Dressing

¼ cup "lite" mayonnaise
1 teaspoon olive oil
¼ teaspoon lemon juice
½ teaspoon vinegar
¼ teaspoon Dijon mustard
Dash of Worcestershire sauce
2 tablespoons nonfat milk
1 clove garlic, peeled and minced
⅛ teaspoon ground black pepper
2 tablespoons grated parmesan cheese

Stir together all ingredients in a small bowl. Cover and store in the refrigerator.

Tofu Caesar Wrap

Substitute 3 ounces stir-fried firm tofu or grilled seitan for the chicken.

DASH servings (per wrap with dressing)
2 grain
2 vegetable
½ nuts/seeds/legumes
½ dairy
Calories with stir-fried tofu: 500

||||||||||||||||||||||||||||||||||||||||||||||||||||||||||||||||||||||||||||||||||||||||||||||||||||||||||||||||||||

Shrimp Scampi

1 tablespoon plus 1 teaspoon olive oil
1 pound peeled and deveined shrimp
½ medium onion, peeled and chopped
2 cloves garlic, peeled and minced
1 cup low-sodium fish or vegetable stock
½ cup dry white wine
1 tablespoon lemon juice
¼ cup chopped fresh parsley

1. Heat 1 tablespoon of the olive oil in a large skillet over medium heat until hot but not smoking. Add the shrimp and cook, stirring constantly, just until they turn pink (about 3 minutes). Transfer the shrimp to a plate and set aside.
2. Add the remaining teaspoon of oil to the pan and heat. Add the onion and cook, stirring occasionally, until just tender (about 5 minutes).
3. Stir in the garlic and cook for 1 minute more.
4. Add the stock, wine, and lemon juice, raise the heat, and bring to a boil. Reduce the heat so the mixture simmers and cook, stirring occasionally, until the liquid is reduced to about 1 cup.
5. Add the shrimp back and simmer for about 3 minutes or until the shrimp are heated through.
6. Sprinkle with the parsley and serve immediately.

Makes four 4-ounce portions

DASH servings (per 4 ounces shrimp, with sauce)
1⅓ meat
Calories: 185

Poached Salmon

Nonstick cooking spray
½ white onion, peeled and sliced
1 tablespoon chopped fresh dill
½ cup dry white wine
1 cup low-sodium fish or vegetable stock
1 pound skinless wild salmon fillet

1. Spray a medium skillet with cooking spray and heat over medium heat. Add the onion and cook, stirring occasionally, until softened but not browned (about 5 minutes).
2. Stir in the dill and cook 30 seconds more.
3. Add the wine and stock and raise the heat to bring to a boil.
4. Reduce to a simmer and add the fish, skin-side down.
5. Cover the skillet and simmer for 5 to 10 minutes, depending on thickness, until the fish is cooked through and barely flakes with a fork.
6. Use a slotted spoon to portion the fish onto plates, but don't worry if some of the cooking liquid comes with it.

DASH servings (per 4½ ounces cooked fish)
1½ meat
Calories: 215

Poached Cod

Substitute 1 pound skinless cod fillet for the salmon.

DASH servings (per 4½ ounces cooked fish)
1½ meat
Calories (cod): 135

|||||||||||||||||||||||||||||||||||||||||||||||||||||||||||||||||||||||||||||||||||||||||||||||||||||||||||||||||||||||||

Beef and Vegetable Stir-Fry

2 tablespoons sesame oil
2 cups broccoli florets
2 red bell peppers, stemmed, seeded, and cut into strips
2 yellow bell peppers, stemmed, seeded, and cut into strips
1 cup snow peas
1 pound top sirloin, cut into thin strips
½ cup 100% orange juice
¼ cup low-sodium soy sauce
¼ teaspoon ground ginger

1. Heat 1 tablespoon of the oil in a skillet or wok over medium heat until very hot but not smoking.
2. Add the broccoli, bell peppers, and snow peas. Stir-fry until the broccoli is tender. Transfer the veggies to a bowl and set aside.
3. Pour the remaining 1 tablespoon oil into the pan and heat again until very hot but not smoking. Add the beef and stir-fry to the desired doneness. Remove the meat from the pan and add it to the vegetables.
4. Pour the orange juice, soy sauce, and ginger and stir constantly over medium-high heat until liquid reduces to about one-third cup.
5. Add back the vegetables and meat, toss to coat, and continue cooking until they're heated through, about 3 minutes. Serve immediately.

DASH servings (per 1 cup stir-fry with sauce)
2 vegetable
½ meat
Calories: 200

Tofu and Vegetable Stir-Fry

Substitute one 14- to 16-ounce block firm tofu, drained well and cubed, for the beef.

DASH servings (per 1 cup stir-fry with sauce)
2 vegetable
½ nuts/seeds/legumes
Calories: 180

Turkey Soft Tacos

1 teaspoon vegetable oil
½ cup peeled and diced onion
3 ounces ground turkey breast meat
2 teaspoons ground cumin
½ teaspoon chili powder
½ teaspoon cayenne pepper
1 teaspoon paprika
½ teaspoon onion powder
½ cup canned diced tomatoes
½ cup low-sodium canned black beans, drained and rinsed
Two 4-inch whole-wheat or corn tortillas
½ cup diced fresh tomatoes
½ cup shredded lettuce
1 tablespoon low-fat sour cream

1. Heat the vegetable oil in a skillet over medium heat. Add the onion and cook, stirring occasionally, until soft but not browned (about 5 minutes).
2. Crumble in the ground turkey. Stir the cumin, chili powder, cayenne, paprika, and onion powder, and canned tomatoes. Cook for about 5 minutes, stirring occasionally.

(continued on next page)

3. When the turkey is cooked through and no longer pink, stir in the beans and heat until warmed through. The mixture may become dry during cooking; add a little water as needed just to keep it moist.
4. Meanwhile, wrap the tortillas in a paper towel and heat in the microwave.
5. Divide the filling between the tortillas and top with the fresh tomatoes, lettuce, and sour cream.

DASH servings (per 2 tacos)
2 grain
2 vegetable
1 meat
Calories: 500

Tempeh Soft Tacos

Substitute 4 ounces crumbled tempeh for the turkey.

DASH servings (per 2 tacos)
2 grain
2 vegetable
1 nuts/seeds/legumes
Calories: 595

||||||||||||||||||||||||||||||||||||||||||||||||||||||||||||||||||||||||||||||||||||||||||||||

Pasta Primavera

2 teaspoons vegetable oil
1 onion, peeled and chopped
1 clove garlic, peeled and minced
2 cups nonfat milk
1 cup low-sodium or homemade chicken broth
3 tablespoons all-purpose flour or Wondra*

---

*Wondra is a brand of flour that is partially cooked and granulated to dissolve easily in liquids without lumping.

½ teaspoon salt
¼ teaspoon ground black pepper
½ cup grated parmesan cheese
16 ounces uncooked whole-grain fettuccine pasta
2 cups broccoli florets
1 cup sliced zucchini
1 cup peeled and chopped carrots
1 cup chopped fresh tomatoes

1. Set a large pot of water over high heat to come to a boil.
2. In a medium saucepan, heat the oil over medium heat. Add the onion and garlic and cook, stirring occasionally, until golden brown.
3. In the meantime, in a small saucepan stir together the milk, chicken broth, flour, salt, and pepper over low heat until smooth and thick. Stir into the onion mixture.
4. Continue to cook the sauce over medium-low heat, stirring frequently, until the sauce is thick. Stir in parmesan cheese. Turn down the heat to very low to keep warm.
5. Cook pasta in the boiling water according to package directions. Add the broccoli, zucchini, and carrots to the pasta for the last several minutes of cooking. Continue cooking until the pasta is al dente.
6. Drain the pasta and vegetables and transfer to a large bowl. Add the tomatoes. Pour over the sauce and toss until everything is coated. Serve immediately.

DASH servings (per 1½ cups)
2 grain
2 vegetable
½ dairy
Calories: 410

Tempeh Burger

8 ounces tempeh
2 tablespoons olive oil
¾ cup chopped peeled onion
2 cloves garlic, peeled and chopped
½ cup chopped mushrooms
1 tablespoon rice vinegar
½ teaspoon ground ginger
¼ cup whole-wheat flour
2 tablespoons low-sodium tamari or soy sauce
Nonstick cooking spray
4 whole-wheat sandwich buns

1. Fill a medium saucepan with about an inch of water and place a steamer basket in it. Bring to a boil. Place the tempeh in the basket, cover the pot, and steam the tempeh for 15 minutes. Drain and set aside to cool.
2. Heat 1 tablespoon of the oil in a skillet over medium-high heat until hot but not smoking. Add the onion and garlic and cook, stirring often, until soft but not browned (about 3 minutes).
3. Add the mushrooms and cook for 3 minutes.
4. Add the vinegar and ginger and cook for another 2 minutes. Remove from the heat and set aside to cool slightly.
5. Using your fingers, crumble the steamed tempeh into a bowl. Add the cooked vegetables, flour, tamari, and the remaining 1 tablespoon olive oil. Stir well to combine. Portion into four burgers and place on a plate.
6. Chill the burgers for at least 1 hour; this helps them hold together better.
7. When you are ready to cook the burgers, heat a skillet over medium heat. Spray it lightly with cooking spray. Cook the burgers until well browned and warmed through, 3 to 4 minutes per side.

8. If you like, while the burgers are cooking, toast the buns. Serve each burger on a bun.

DASH servings (per burger, including bun)
2 grains
1 nuts/seeds/legumes
Calories: 330

Soups, Salads, Dressing, and Dips

||||||||||||||||||||||||||||||||||||||||||||||||||||||||||||||||||||||||||||||||||||||||||||||||||||||||||||||||||||||

Butternut Squash and Apple Soup

1 small butternut squash (about 1 pound)
3 tart green apples, such as Granny Smith or Crispin
1 medium onion
¼ teaspoon dried rosemary
¼ teaspoon dried marjoram
Three 10.5-ounce cans low-sodium chicken broth
2 cans water
2 slices whole-wheat bread, crumbled
Salt and ground black pepper
1 tablespoon chopped fresh parsley

1. Cut the butternut squash in half. With a sharp paring knife or vegetable peeler, remove the peel. Scoop out and discard the seeds. Cut the squash into cubes with a chef's knife. Peel, core, and coarsely chop the apples. Peel the onion and chop coarsely.
2. Combine the squash, apples, onion, rosemary, marjoram, chicken broth, water, bread, and salt and pepper to taste in a large, heavy saucepan. Bring to a boil, then reduce the heat and simmer uncovered for 45 minutes.
3. Working in small batches, never filling the blender more than a quarter full each time, puree the soup in a blender until smooth. Transfer each batch to a clean saucepan.
4. Bring the pureed soup to a boil, then reduce the heat and simmer briefly.
5. Serve hot with a sprinkle of parsley.
6. This recipe makes 6 to 8 servings, and can be multiplied for greater quantities. Refrigerate any leftover soup to reheat gently within the next couple of days.

DASH servings (per 1 cup)
1 vegetable
1 fruit
Calories: 180

|||||||||||||||||||||||||||||||||||||||||||||||||||||||||||||||||||||||||||||||||||||||||||||||||||||||||||

Tortellini and Bean Soup

1 teaspoon olive oil

2 cups coarsely chopped peeled white onions

1 small red bell pepper, stemmed, seeded, and coarsely chopped

3 cloves garlic, peeled and minced

1 teaspoon Italian seasoning

2 cups loosely packed, coarsely chopped raw spinach

One 15- to 16-ounce can no-salt-added navy beans

One 14.5-ounce can low-sodium vegetable broth

⅔ cup water

One 14.5-ounce can no-salt-added whole tomatoes, with their juice

One 14-ounce can water-packed artichoke hearts, drained

One 9-ounce package cheese tortellini

1. Heat the oil in a soup pot over medium-high heat. Add the onion, bell pepper, garlic, and Italian seasoning. Cook, stirring occasionally, until the vegetables are tender but not browned (about 5 minutes).
2. Add the spinach, beans, broth, water, tomatoes and their juice, and artichokes.
3. Raise the heat to high and bring to a boil, then reduce the heat and simmer for 2 minutes.
4. Add the tortellini and simmer until thoroughly cooked, according to package directions.
5. Serve immediately.

(continued on next page)

DASH servings (per 1½ cups; about 6 servings per recipe)
2 vegetables
½ dairy
½ grain
Calories: 330

||||||||||||||||||||||||||||||||||||||||||||||||||||||||||||||||||||||||||||||||||||||||||||||||||||||||||||||||||||||||||||

Quinoa, Corn, and Black Bean Salad

Dressing
1½ teaspoons sugar
½ cup chopped fresh cilantro
½ teaspoon dried oregano
¼ teaspoon chili powder (optional, for extra spice)
2 tablespoons lime or lemon juice
1 tablespoon white vinegar
¾ cup low-sodium vegetable juice

1 cup canned black beans, drained and rinsed
2 cups cooked quinoa
1 cup corn kernels (cooked fresh or thawed frozen)
½ cup diced peeled red onion
¼ cup thinly sliced scallions (green onions)
½ cup chopped red bell pepper

1. Whisk together the dressing ingredients in a medium bowl. Add the beans, quinoa, corn, onion, scallions, and bell pepper. Mix well.
2. Serve immediately, or cover and refrigerate for 30 minutes before serving.

DASH servings (per ⅔ cup)
1 grain
¼ vegetable
¼ nuts/seeds/legumes
Calories: 125

||||||||||||||||||||||||||||||||||||||||||||||||||||||||||||||||||||||||||||||||||||||||||||||||||||||||||||||||||||

Simple Spinach Salad

Dressing
2 teaspoons vegetable oil
4 teaspoons distilled white vinegar
1½ teaspoons sugar
1 teaspoon ketchup
Dash of Worcestershire sauce

3 cups loosely packed fresh spinach leaves (remove heavy stems
   before measuring)
½ cup grape tomatoes
1 ounce shredded low-fat cheddar cheese (about ¼ cup)

1. Combine the dressing ingredients in tightly covered jar or salad
   dressing shaker and shake until well mixed. Set aside.
2. Rinse the spinach thoroughly and spin dry. Place in a large bowl.
3. Rinse the tomatoes and pat dry with paper towels. Add to the
   spinach.
4. Shake the dressing to recombine it and pour over the spinach and
   tomatoes. Toss well. Add the cheese and toss again. Serve immediately.

DASH servings (per 2 cup portion)
2 vegetable
¼ dairy
1 added fat
Calories: 115

Cobb Salad

6 cups baby arugula, rinsed and spun dry
1 cup grape tomatoes, cut in half
Whites of 3 hard-boiled eggs, very coarsely chopped
½ cup cubed peeled avocado
¼ cup low-fat balsamic vinaigrette dressing
2 tablespoons crumbled blue cheese
3 tablespoons bacon bits

1. Combine the arugula, tomatoes, egg whites, and avocado in a large bowl. Toss to combine. Add the vinaigrette and toss again to coat everything.
2. Divide the salad between two serving bowls. Sprinkle each with 1 tablespoon cheese and 1½ tablespoons bacon bits. Serve immediately.

DASH servings (per ½ recipe)
4 vegetable
½ dairy
½ meat
1 added fat
Calories: 225

Lemon Caper Vinaigrette

½ cup extra virgin olive oil
¼ cup flaxseed oil
¼ cup white balsamic vinegar
4 teaspoons lemon juice

¼ cup capers, rinsed and drained
Freshly ground pepper

1. Combine the olive and flaxseed oils, vinegar, lemon juice, and capers in a blender. Blend until pureed. Add pepper to taste and blend again.
2. Alternatively, combine all ingredients in a tightly capped jar and shake.
3. Toss 1 tablespoon with each serving of the salad of your choice. Store any remaining dressing in a covered jar in the fridge and shake well before each use.

DASH servings (per 1 tablespoon; about 16 servings per recipe)
1 added fat
Calories: 60

||||||||||||||||||||||||||||||||||||||||||||||||||||||||||||||||||||||||||||||||||||||||||||||||||||||||||||||||

"Dill"icious Dill Dip

One 16-ounce carton low-fat cottage cheese
1 tablespoon chopped fresh dill
1 tablespoon chopped fresh parsley
½ teaspoon garlic powder

Whip cottage cheese in a blender until smooth. Transfer to a small bowl and stir in the remaining ingredients. Cover and refrigerate at least 1 hour or preferably overnight. Serve with fresh vegetables.

DASH servings (per 2 tablespoons; 16 portions per recipe)
¼ dairy
Calories: 20

‖‖

Black Bean Dip

One 14- to 16-ounce can black beans, drained and rinsed
One 16-ounce can corn kernels (white, yellow, or Mexican corn),
   drained
One 14.5-ounce can diced tomatoes
½ cup prepared salsa
1 tablespoon chopped cilantro
½ cup diced avocado (optional)

1. Toss together the beans, corn, tomatoes with their juice, and salsa
   in a medium bowl. Cover and refrigerate at least 1 hour or preferably overnight.
2. Just before serving, stir in the cilantro, and avocado if using.

DASH servings (per ⅔ cup; 8 servings per recipe)
1 vegetable
1 nuts/seeds/legumes
Calories: 105

Vegetables

||||||||||||||||||||||||||||||||||||||||||||||||||||||||||||||||||||||||||||||||||||||||||||||||||||||||||||||||||||||||||||||||||||

Roasted Brussels Sprouts

Nonstick cooking spray
1 pound brussels sprouts
½ yellow onion, peeled and finely chopped
1 tablespoon olive oil
½ teaspoon ground black pepper

1. Preheat the oven to 425°F. Lightly spray a baking sheet with cooking spray. Place a steamer basket in a large pot, add about 1 inch of water, cover, and bring to a boil.
2. Wash and trim the brussels sprouts for cooking.
3. Place the brussels sprouts in the steamer basket and steam for about 4 minutes, until barely tender.
4. Remove the brussels sprouts from the pot and drain well. Transfer to a large bowl and toss with the onion, olive oil, and pepper to coat.
5. Spread the vegetables in a single layer on the prepared baking sheet and bake for 15 to 20 minutes, tossing periodically until crisp-tender and very lightly browned. Do not overcook.

DASH servings (per 1 cup)
2 vegetable
Calories: 100

Roasted Asparagus

Substitute 1 pound asparagus for the brussels sprouts. Break off the woody ends and trim the spears. It is not necessary to steam asparagus before roasting.

(continued on next page)

DASH servings (per 1 cup—10–12 small spears)
2 vegetable
Calories: 80

Variations

Also try carrots (peel and halve crosswise) and winter squash (peel, seed, and cut into large cubes).

DASH servings (per 1 cup)
2 vegetable
Calories: 80–120 calories

||||||||||||||||||||||||||||||||||||||||||||||||||||||||||||||||||||||||||||||||||||||||||||||||||||||||||||||||||||||

Roasted Cauliflower

4 cups cauliflower florets
4 teaspoons olive oil
¼ cup Italian seasoned bread crumbs

1. Preheat the oven to 400°F.
2. Place the cauliflower on a large baking sheet. Drizzle with the olive oil and sprinkle with the bread crumbs. Toss to coat. Spread out in a single layer.
3. Bake until crisp-tender and lightly browned (about 20 minutes), stirring occasionally. Serve hot.

DASH servings (per 1 cup; 4 cups per recipe)
2 vegetable
Calories: 100

Desserts, Snacks, and Smoothies

||||||||||||||||||||||||||||||||||||||||||||||||||||||||||||||||||||||||||||||||||||||||||||||||||||||||||||

Low-Fat Brownies

6 ounces semisweet chocolate
½ cup hot water
4 egg whites
1 teaspoon vanilla extract
⅔ cup granulated sugar
1½ cups all-purpose flour
1 teaspoon baking powder
½ cup chopped walnuts (optional)

1. Preheat oven to 350°F.
2. In large heatproof bowl set over simmering water, melt the choco-late with the hot water, stirring until smooth. Remove from heat and let cool slightly. Whisk in egg whites and mix in the vanilla. In a separate bowl, mix together the sugar, flour, and baking powder; stir into chocolate batter until just combined. Stir in walnuts. Spray an 8-inch square cake pan with cooking spray. Pour into cake pan.
3. Bake in preheated oven for 20 to 30 minutes, or until edges pull away from pan. Let cool on rack, then serve.

DASH servings (per 2×2-inch brownie; makes 16 brownies)
1 sweets
Calories: 155

||||||||||||||||||||||||||||||||||||||||||||||||||||||||||||||||||||||||||||||||||||||||||||||||||||||

Strawberry Shortcake

2 pounds fresh strawberries, sliced
¾ cup sugar
1 10-inch angel food cake, sliced into 10 slices
Low-fat whipped topping (optional)

1. In a large mixing bowl, combine sugar and strawberries and set aside.
2. Once strawberries have "bled" to make a sweet juice, spoon about ½ cup strawberries (with juice) over each slice of cake.

Makes 10 portions.

DASH servings (per one slice cake with strawberries)
1 sweet
1 fruit
Calories: 265

||||||||||||||||||||||||||||||||||||||||||||||||||||||||||||||||||||||||||||||||||||||||||||||||||||||

Low-Fat Blueberry Muffins

Nonstick cooking spray (optional)
4 tablespoons trans-fat-free soy margarine, softened
½ cup unsweetened applesauce
1 cup granulated sugar
1 teaspoon pure vanilla extract
½ cup 1% low-fat milk
¾ cup all-purpose flour (stir with a fork before measuring)
¾ cup whole-wheat flour (stir with a fork before measuring)
1 tablespoon baking powder

½ cup wheat germ
2 cups fresh blueberries

1. Preheat the oven to 350°F. Line 12 muffin pan cups with paper liners or spray with cooking spray.
2. Beat together the margarine, applesauce, sugar, vanilla, and milk in a large bowl.
3. Combine the all-purpose and whole-wheat flours, baking powder, and wheat germ in a separate large bowl. Stir with a fork to combine and lighten them.
4. Slowly stir dry ingredients into wet mixture just until all the dry ingredients are moistened. Do not overmix.
5. Gently fold in the blueberries.
6. Spoon the batter into the prepared muffin cups, filling each three-quarters full.
7. Bake 35 minutes or until the tops are firm. Cool slightly on rack.

DASH servings (per muffin; makes 12 muffins)
2 grain
Calories: 200

||||||||||||||||||||||||||||||||||||||||||||||||||||||||||||||||||||||||||||||||||||||||||||||||||||||||||||

Gingerbread

Nonstick cooking spray
⅓ cup granulated sugar
4 tablespoons trans-fat-free soy margarine, softened
⅓ cup molasses
1 large egg
¾ cup all-purpose flour (measured using spoon-and-sweep method)

(continued on next page)

¾ cup whole-wheat flour (measured using spoon-and-sweep
    method)
1 teaspoon ground ginger
½ teaspoon baking soda
¼ teaspoon ground nutmeg
⅛ teaspoon ground cloves
¾ cup 1% low-fat milk
2 teaspoons powdered sugar

1. Preheat the oven to 350°F. Spray an 8-inch loaf pan with cooking
   spray.
2. Beat the granulated sugar and margarine with an electric mixer at
   medium speed in a large bowl until well-blended (about 5 minutes). Add molasses and egg; beat well.
3. In a separate bowl, stir together the all-purpose and whole-wheat
   flours, ginger, baking soda, nutmeg, and cloves to combine and aer-
   ate them.
4. Add the flour mixture to sugar mixture alternately with the milk,
   beginning and ending with flour mixture. Stir until just combined;
   do not overmix.
5. Pour the batter into the prepared loaf pan. Bake for 30 minutes or
   until a wooden pick inserted in the center comes out clean.
6. Cool in the pan on a wire rack. Sift powdered sugar over top of cake
   and serve warm.
7. Remove any leftover gingerbread from the pan, slice, wrap well in
   plastic wrap, and store at room temperature in a sealed heavy-duty
   plastic bag for up to 3 days. Freeze for longer storage and thaw at
   room temperature before serving.

DASH servings (per ¾-inch slice; makes about 10 slices)
1 sweets
Calories: 150

Baked Banana

Nonstick cooking spray
1 medium (7-inch) banana
1½ teaspoons brown sugar

1. Preheat the oven to 400°F. Spray a baking dish with cooking spray.
2. Peel the banana and slice in half lengthwise. Place in the baking dish cut side up. Sprinkle with the brown sugar. Bake for 10 to 15 minutes, until the sugar is melted and bubbling. Serve warm.

DASH servings (per whole banana)
2 fruit
1 sweets
Calories: 120

Mango Smoothie

2 cups diced mango (frozen is easiest)
½ cup low-fat vanilla yogurt
1 cup low-fat buttermilk
4 teaspoons lime juice
2 tablespoons honey

Combine all ingredients in a blender and blend until smooth. Serve immediately.

DASH servings (per 1 cup; 4 cups per recipe)
1 fruit
1 dairy
½ sweets
Calories: 140

Appendix A

Calculating Your Daily Calorie Target

You can use this formula to calculate how many calories you need each day to maintain your current weight. Then we'll subtract 500 calories from that to get your daily calorie goal for weight loss.

The formula is called the Mifflin-St. Jeor equation.

STEP 1. CALCULATE BASAL CALORIE NEEDS.

"Basal" means the number of calories you would need if you were sedentary all the time.

For Men

$$\text{Basal calories} = (4.545 \times \text{weight in pounds}) + (15.875 \times \text{height in inches}) - (5 \times \text{age in years}) + 5$$

For Women

$$\text{Basal calories} = (4.545 \times \text{weight in pounds}) +$$
$$(15.875 \times \text{height in inches}) - (5 \times \text{age in years}) - 161$$

Write your basal calories here: _____

STEP 2. ADJUST BASAL CALORIES FOR YOUR ACTIVITY LEVEL.

This gives you your activity-adjusted calorie needs to maintain your current weight.

Multiply your basal calories from Step 1 times your activity factor:

- Sedentary (little or no exercise, desk job) = basal calories × 1.2
- Lightly active (light exercise 1 to 3 days/week) = basal calories × 1.375
- Moderately active (moderate exercise 3 to 5 days/week) = basal calories × 1.55
- Very active (hard exercise 6 to 7 days/week) = basal calories × 1.725
- Extremely active (hard daily exercise or very physical job) = basal calories × 1.9

Write activity-adjusted calories here: _____

STEP 3. CALCULATE YOUR CALORIE GOAL FOR WEIGHT LOSS.

Subtract 500 calories for your activity-adjusted calories from Step 2. This is your weight-loss calorie goal. Write that number here:

_____

STEP 4. GO TO TABLE 4.3 TO FIND YOUR DAILY DASH SERVINGS FOR YOUR CALORIE TARGET.

If your calorie goal in Step 3 is less than 1,200 calories, use the daily servings for 1,200 calories in the table.

If your calorie goal in Step 3 is greater than 2,600 calories, use the daily servings for 2,600 calories in the table.

Appendix B

The DASH for Health® Program

The DASH for Health® program is our online nutrition and exercise education program. We teach people the DASH Diet and give them tips on how to follow it. Exercise advice in this online program is based upon standard, well-accepted exercise practices. The type of information that we provide in our online program is very similar to the information in this book. We publish new articles on the DASH for Health website twice each week. Each time we publish a new article, we send a reminder e-mail to everyone who is enrolled in the program, giving them a brief summary of what the recently published article is about. The website also provides the ability for enrollees to monitor their weight, their blood pressure, and their food intake.

Since we began this program in 2002, over 18,000 people have enrolled. In many instances, employers have asked us to offer the program to all of their employees. However, individuals can also sign up for the program for a three- or six-month enrollment fee.

Many of the suggestions and helpful hints in this book were

learned from these 18,000 enrollees. People in the program send us e-mails with helpful suggestions or, in some cases, ask us questions. Questions that are raised often are covered in Part 2, Section V of this book, Frequently Asked Questions.

In our research, we investigated whether, at the end of 12 months in the DASH for Health program, people have lost weight, lowered their blood pressure, or changed their eating habits. We found that people who were interested in losing weight had lost on average 4.1 pounds. People with a blood pressure concern who were interested in lowering their blood pressure reduced their systolic pressure by 6.8 points (about the same blood pressure lowering as is typically achieved by blood pressure medication). And based upon their self-entered food surveys on the website, enrollees at the end of 12 months were eating significantly more fruits and vegetables, and reduced their consumption of carbonated beverages.

We also looked at the effect of enrollment in the DASH for Health program on the amount of money people spend on health care. We compared nearly 2,000 people who signed up for the DASH for Health program versus 15,000 people who did not. We examined health care spending in people who had one or more of three medical conditions which the DASH Diet should benefit: high blood pressure, high cholesterol, and diabetes. Compared to people with these conditions who did not sign up for the DASH program, DASH enrollees spent $827 less per year on health care. The amount of health care savings was dependent upon how often a person visited the DASH website.

To our knowledge, the DASH for Health program is the only on-line program which has been proven to provide health benefits (such as weight loss, blood pressure lowering, and improved eating habits) as well as proven reductions in health care spending.

Appendix C

Scientific Papers About the DASH Diet

You may be interested in reading the scientific articles that the DASH group and others have written about the DASH Diet. Following is a list of many such articles. More are being published all the time, so we apologize that this list is not complete and current. If you are interested in a more current list and you have access to Medline searching, search on the terms "DASH Diet." This should provide references to almost all the published literature.

ARTICLES BY MEMBERS OF THE DASH TEAM

Appel LJ, Miller ER III, Jee SH, Stolzenberg-Solomon R, Lin PH, Erlinger T, Nadeau MR, Selhub J. Effect of dietary patterns on serum homocysteine: results of a randomized, controlled feeding study. *Circulation* 102(8):852–57 (2000).

Appel LJ, Moore TJ, Obarzanek E, Vollmer WM, Svetkey LP, Sacks FM, Bray GA, Vogt TM, Cutler JA, Windhauser MM, Lin PH, Karanja N. A clinical trial of the effects of dietary patterns on blood pressure. DASH Collaborative Research Group. *New England Journal of Medicine* 336(16):1117–24 (1997).

Appel LJ, Vollmer WM, Obarzanek E, Aicher KM, Conlin PR, Kennedy BM, Charleston JB, Reams PM, for the DASH Collaborative Research Group. Recruitment and baseline characteristics of participants in the Dietary Approaches to Stop Hypertension trial. *Journal of the American Dietetic Association* 99:S69–75 (1999).

Appel LJ. Nonpharmacologic therapies that reduce blood pressure: a fresh perspective. *Clinical Cardiology* 22(Suppl III):III-1–III-5 (1999). Review.

Chen L, Appel LJ, Loria C, Lin PH, Champagne CM, Elmer PJ, Ard JD, Mitchell D, Batch BC, Svetkey LP, Caballero B. Reduction in consumption of sugar-sweetened beverages is associated with weight loss: the PREMIER trial. *American Journal of Clinical Nutrition* 89(5):1299–306 (2009). Epub April 1, 2009.

Conlin PR, Chow D, Miller ER III, Svetkey LP, Lin PH, Harsha DW, Moore TJ, Sacks FM, Appel LJ. The effect of dietary patterns on blood pressure control in hypertensive patients: results from the Dietary Approaches to Stop Hypertension (DASH) trial. *American Journal of Hypertension* 13(9):949–55 (2009).

Conlin PR, Erlinger TP, Bohannon A, Miller ER III, Appel LJ, Svetkey LP, Moore TJ. The DASH diet enhances the blood pressure response to losartan in hypertensive patients. *American Journal of Hypertension* 16(5, pt 1):337–42 (2003).

DASH Collaborative Research Group. The effect of dietary patterns on blood pressure: results from the Dietary Approaches to Stop Hypertension (DASH) clinical trial. *Current Concepts in Hypertension* 2:4–5 (1998).

Elmer PJ, Obarzanek E, Vollmer WM, Simons-Morton D, Stevens VJ, Young DR, Lin PH, Champagne C, Harsha DW, Svetkey LP, Ard J, Brantley PJ, Proschan MA, Erlinger TP, Appel LJ; PREMIER Collaborative Research Group. Effects of comprehensive lifestyle modification on diet, weight, physical fitness, and blood pressure control: 18-month results of a randomized trial. *Annals of Internal Medicine* 144(7):485–95 (2006).

Harsha DW, Pao-Hwa L, Obarzanek E, Karanja NM, Moore TJ, Caballero B. Dietary Approaches to Stop Hypertension: A summary of results. *Journal of the American Dietetic Association* 99:S35–39 (1999).

Hollis JF, Gullion CM, Stevens VJ, Brantley PJ, Appel LJ, Ard JD, Champagne CM, Dalcin A, Erlinger TP, Funk K, Laferriere D, Lin PH, Loria CM, Samuel-Hodge C, Vollmer WM, Svetkey LP; Weight Loss Maintenance Trial Research Group. Weight loss during the intensive intervention phase of the weight-loss maintenance trial. *American Journal of Preventive Medicine* 35(2):118–26 (2008).

Jacobs DR Jr, Gross MD, Steffen L, Steffes MW, Yu X, Svetkey LP, Appel LJ, Vollmer WM, Bray GA, Moore T, Conlin PR, Sacks F. The effects of dietary patterns on urinary albumin excretion: results of the Dietary Approaches to Stop Hypertension (DASH) Trial. *American Journal of Kidney Disease* 53(4):638–46 (2009). Epub January 23, 2009.

Karanja NM, McCullough ML, Kumanyika SK, Pedula KL, Windhauser MM, Obarzanek E, Lin PH, Champagne CM, Swain J, for the DASH Collaborative Research Group. Pre-enrollment diets of Dietary Approaches to Stop Hypertension trial participants. *Journal of the American Dietetic Association* 99:S28–34 (1999).

Karanja NM, Obarzanek E, Lin PH, McCullough ML, Phillips KM, Swain JF, Champagne CM, Hoben KP, for the DASH Collaborative Research Group. Descriptive characteristics of the dietary patterns used in the Dietary Approaches to Stop Hypertension trial. *Journal of the American Dietetic Association* 99:S19–27 (1999).

Lien LF, Brown AJ, Ard JD, Loria C, Erlinger TP, Feldstein AC, Lin PH, Champagne CM, King AC, McGuire HL, Stevens VJ, Brantley PJ, Harsha DW, McBurnie MA, Appel LJ, Svetkey LP. Effects of PREMIER lifestyle modifications on participants with and without the metabolic syndrome. *Hypertension* 50(4):609–16 (2007). Epub August 13, 2007.

Lin PH, Windhauser MM, Plaisted CS, Hoben KP, McCullough ML, Obarzanek E, for the DASH Collaborative Research Group. The linear index model for establishing nutrient goals in the Dietary Approaches to Stop Hypertension trial. *Journal of the American Dietetic Association* 99:S40–44 (1999).

McCullough ML, Karanja NM, Lin PH, Obarzanek E, Phillips KM, Laws RL, Vollmer WM, O'Connor EA, Champagne CM, Windhauser MM, for the DASH Collaborative Research Group. Comparison of 4 nutrient databases with chemical composition data from the Dietary Approaches to Stop Hypertension trial. *Journal of the American Dietetic Association* 99:S45–53 (1999).

Miller ER III, Appel LJ, Risby TH. Effect of dietary patterns on measures of lipid peroxidation: results from a randomized clinical trial. *Circulation* 98(22):2390–95 (1998).

Moore TJ for the DASH Steering Committee (letter to editor). *Science* 282:1049–50 (1998).

Moore TJ, Alsabeeh N, Apovian CM, Murphy MC, Coffman GA, Cullum-Dugan D, Jenkins M, Cabral H. Weight, blood pressure, and dietary benefits after 12 months of a web-based nutrition education program (DASH for Health): longitudinal observational study. *Journal of Medical Internet Research* 10(4):e52 (2008).

Moore TJ, Conlin PR, Ard J, Svetkey LP. DASH (Dietary Approaches to Stop Hypertension) diet is effective treatment for stage 1 isolated systolic hypertension. *Hypertension* 38(2):155–8 (2001).

Moore TJ, Vollmer WM, Apell LJ, Sacks FM, Svetkey LP, Vogt TM, Conlin PR, Simons-Morton DG, Carter-Edwards L, Harsha DW. Effect of dietary patterns on ambulatory blood pressure: results from the Dietary Approaches to Stop Hypertension (DASH) trial. *Hypertension* 34(3):472–77 (1999).

Obarzanek E, Moore TJ. Foreword: Using feeding studies to test the efficacy of dietary interventions: Lessons from the Dietary Approaches to Stop Hypertension Trial. *Journal of the American Dietetic Association* 99:S9–10 (1999).

Obarzanek E, Proschan MA, Vollmer WM, Moore TJ, Sacks FM, Appel LJ, Svetkey LP, Most-Windhauser MM, Cutler JA. Individual blood pressure responses to changes in salt intake: results from the DASH-Sodium trial. *Hypertension* 42(4):459–67 (2003).

Phillips KM, Stewart KK, Karanja NM, Windhauser MM, Champagne CM, Swain JF, Lin PH, Evans MA, for the DASH Collaborative Research Group. Validation of diet composition for the Dietary Approaches to Stop Hypertension trial. *Journal of the American Dietetic Association* 99:S60–68 (1999).

Plaisted CS, Lin PH, Ard JD, McClure ML, Svetkey LP. The effects of dietary patterns on quality of life: a substudy of the Dietary Approaches to Stop Hypertension trial. *Journal of the American Dietetic Association* 99:S84–89 (1999).

Sacks FM, Appel LJ, Moore TJ, Obarzanek E, Vollmer WM, Svetkey LP, Bray GA, Vogt TM, Cutler JA, Windhauser MM, Lin PH, Karanja N. A dietary approach to prevent hypertension: a review of the Dietary Approaches to Stop Hypertension (DASH) Study. *Clinical Cardiology* 22(Suppl III):III6–III10 (1999).

Sacks FM, Obarzanek E, Windhauser MM, Svetkey LP, Vollmer WM, McCullough M, Karanja N, Lin PH, Steele P, Proschan MA, et al. Rationale and design of the Dietary Approaches to Stop Hypertension trial (DASH). A multicenter controlled-feeding study of dietary patterns to lower blood pressure. *Annals of Epidemiology* 5(2):108–18 (1995).

Sacks N, Cabral H, Kazis LE, Jarrett KM, Vetter D, Richmond R, Moore TJ. A web-based nutrition program reduces health care costs in employees with cardiac risk factors: before and after cost analysis. *Journal of Medical Internet Research* 11(4):e43 (2009).

Svetkey LP, Harris EL, Martin E, Vollmer WM, Meltesen GT, Ricchiuti V, Williams G, Appel LJ, Bray GA, Moore TJ, Winn MP, Conlin PR. Modulation of the BP response to diet by genes in the renin-angiotensin system and the adrenergic nervous system. *American Journal of Hypertension* 24(2):209–17 (2011). Epub November 18, 2010.

Svetkey LP, Moore TJ, Simons-Morton DG, Appel LJ, Bray GA, Sacks FM, Ard JD, Mortensen RM, Mitchell SR, Conlin PR, Kesari M; DASH collaborative research group. Angiotensinogen genotype and blood pressure response in the Dietary Approaches to Stop Hypertension (DASH) study. *Journal of Hypertension* 19(11):1949–56 (2001).

Svetkey LP, Sacks FM, Obarzanek E, Vollmer WM, Appel LJ, Lin PH, Karanja NM, Harsha DW, Bray GA, Aickin M, Proschan MA, Windhauser MM, Swain JF, McCarron PB, Rhodes DG, Laws RL, for the DASH-Sodium Collaborative Research Group. The DASH diet, sodium intake and blood pressure trial (dash-sodium): rationale and design. *Journal of the American Dietetic Association* 1999; 99:S96–104.

Svetkey LP, Simons-Morton D, Vollmer WM, Appel LJ, Conlin PR, Ryan DH, Ard J, Kennedy BM. Effects of dietary patterns on blood pressure: subgroup analysis of the Dietary Approaches to Stop Hypertension (DASH) randomized clinical trial. *Archives of Internal Medicine* 159(3):285–93 (1999).

Svetkey LP, Stevens VJ, Brantley PJ, Appel LJ, Hollis JF, Loria CM, Vollmer WM, Guillion CM, Funk K, Smith P, Samuel-Hodge C, Myers V, Lien LF, Laferriere D, Kennedy B, Jerome GJ, Heinith F, Harsha DW, Evans P, Erlinger TP, Dalcin AT, Coughlin J, Charleston J, Champagne CM, Bauck A, Ard JD, Aicher K; Weight Loss Maintenance Collaborative Research Group. Comparison of strategies for sustaining weight loss: the weight loss maintenance randomized controlled trial. *Journal of the American Medical Association* 299(10):1139–48 (2008).

Swain JF, Windhauser MM, Hoben KP, Evans MA, McGee BB, Steele PD, for the DASH Collaborative Research Group. Menu design and selection for multicenter controlled feeding studies: process used in the Dietary Approaches to Stop Hypertension trial. *Journal of the American Dietetic Association* 99:S54–59 (1999).

Vogt TM, Appel LJ, Obarzanek E, Moore TJ, Vollmer WM, Svetkey LP, Sacks FM, Bray GA, Cutler JA, Windhauser MM, Lin PH, Karanja NM, for the DASH Collaborative Research Group. Dietary Approaches to Stop Hypertension: rationale, design and methods. *Journal of the American Dietetic Association* 99:S12–18 (1999).

Vollmer WM, Sacks FM, Ard J, Appel LJ, Bray GA, Simons-Morton DG, Conlin PR, Svetkey LP, Erlinger TP, Moore TJ, Karanja N; DASH-Sodium Trial Collaborative Research Group. Effects of diet and sodium intake on blood pressure: subgroup analysis of the DASH-sodium trial. *Annals of Internal Medicine* 135(12):1019–28 (2001).

Windhauser MM, Ernst DB, Karanja NM, Crawford SW, Redican SE, Swain JF, Karimbakas JM, Champagne CM, Hoben KP, Evans MA, for the DASH Collaborative Research Group. Translating the Dietary Approaches to Stop Hypertension diet from research to practice: dietary and behavior change techniques. *Journal of the American Dietetic Association* 99:S90–95 (1999).

Windhauser MM, Evans MA, McCullough ML, Swain JF, Lin PH, Hoben KP, Plaisted CS, Karanja NM, Vollmer WM, for the DASH Collaborative Research Group. Dietary adherence in the Dietary Approaches to Stop Hypertension trial. *Journal of the American Dietetic Association* 99: S76–83 (1999).

BY OTHER INVESTIGATORS

de Koning L, Chiuve SE, Fung TT, Willett WC, Rimm EB, Hu FB. Diet-quality scores and the risk of type 2 diabetes in men. *Diabetes Care* 34(5)1150–6 (2011).

Egan BM. Reproducibility of BP responses to changes in dietary salt: compelling evidence for universal sodium restriction? *Hypertension* 42(4):457–8 (2003).

Forman JP, Stampfer MJ, Curhan GC. Diet and lifestyle risk factors associated with incident hypertension in women. *Journal of the American Medical Association* 302(4):401–11 (2009).

Fraser GE. Nut consumption, lipids, and risk of a coronary event. *Clinical Cardiology* 22(7 Suppl):III-11–III-15 (1999). Review.

Fung TT, Hu FB, Wu K, Chiuve SE, Fuchs CS, Giovannucci E. The Mediterranean and Dietary Approaches to Stop Hypertension (DASH) diets and colorectal cancer. *American Journal of Clinical Nutrition* 92(6):1429–35 (2010).

Fung TT, Chiuve SE, McCullough ML, Rexrode KM, Logroscino G, Hu FB. Adherence to a DASH-style diet and risk of coronary heart disease and stroke in women. *Archives of Internal Medicine* 168(7):713–20 (2008).

Hermansen K. Diet, blood pressure and hypertension. *British Journal of Nutrition* 83 Suppl 1:S113–9 (2000). Review.

Kolasa KM. Dietary Approaches to Stop Hypertension (DASH) in clinical practice: a primary care experience. *Clinical Cardiology* 22 (Suppl III):III16–III22 (1999). Review.

Levitan EB, Wolk A, Mittleman MA. Consistency with the DASH diet and incidence of heart failure. *Archives of Internal Medicine* 169(9):851–57 (2009).

Miller GD, DiRienzo DD, Reusser ME, McCarron DA. Benefits of dairy product consumption on blood pressure in humans: a summary of the biomedical literature. *Journal of the American College of Nutrition* 19(2 Suppl):147S–164S. Review.

Smith PJ, Blumenthal JA, Babyak MA, Craighead L, Welsh-Bohmer KA, Browndyke JN, Strauman TA, Sherwood A. Effects of the dietary approaches to stop hypertension diet, exercise, and caloric restriction on neurocognition in overweight adults with high blood pressure. *Hypertension* 55(6):1331–8 (2010).

Stevens VJ, Funk KL, Brantley PJ, Erlinger TP, Myers VH, Champagne CM, Bauck A, Samuel-Hodge CD, Hollis JF. Design and implementation of an interactive website to support long-term maintenance of weight loss. *Journal of Medical Internet Research* 10(1):e1 (2008).

Taylor EN, Fung TT, Curhan GC. DASH-style diet associates with reduced risk for kidney stones. *Journal of the American Society of Nephrology* 20(10):2253–59 (2009).

The DASH diet. It may benefit your blood pressure, and more. *Mayo Clinic Health Letter* 16(4):7.

Tucker K. Dietary patterns and blood pressure in African Americans. *Nutrition Reviews* 57 (11):356–58 (1999). Review.

US Department of Agriculture and US Department of Health and Human Services. *Dietary Guidelines for Americans, 2010.* 7th ed. Washington, DC: US Government Printing Office, 2010.

Zemel MB. Dietary pattern and hypertension: the DASH study. Dietary Approaches to Stop Hypertension. *Nutrition Reviews* 55(8):303–5 (1997). Review.

Index

aerobics, 128, 129–30
affirmation visualization exercise, 146–47, 148
age, calorie intake targets and, 34–35
Agriculture Department, U.S. (USDA), 5, 6
alcoholic beverages, 88–89, 160, 209
American Heart Association, 5, 6, 27
American Journal of Preventive Medicine, portion study in, 24
Annals of Internal Medicine, DASH Diet study in, 7
arthritis. *See* osteoarthritis
artificial sweeteners, 87, 88
Asparagus, Roasted (recipe), 355–56

Baked Banana (recipe), 361
bakeries/baked goods
    avoiding, 10
    carbohydrates in, 188
    fat in, 74–75
    low-fat, 56
    salt/sodium in, 98
    shopping at, 163

Banana, Baked (recipe), 361
Beef and Vegetable Stir Fry (recipe), 342
behavior change strategies. *See* skillpower
Bel Air car story, 11–13
bikes, 128, 131, 132, 134
Black Bean Dip (recipe), 354
blindness, 20
blood pressure
    DASH Diet and, 5, 6, 8
    doing it for life and, 179
    lifestyle exercise and, 131
    obesity and, 19
    salt and, 95
    vegetable juice and, 87
    vegetarians and, 109
    weight-loss pills and, 183
blood sugar
    carbohydrates and, 187, 188
    obesity and, 19
body mass index (BMI), 16–18, 208
    table for calculating, 17, 18
body temperature, 193

boiling
  eggs, 67
  vegetables, 45
bone strength, DASH Diet and, 5
bread
  in brown bag lunches, 198, 199
  as carbohydrate, 187
  dining out and, 169, 171
  fiber and, 203
  as Hi-Lo-Slo food, 55–56
  low-fat, 56
  Nutrition Facts Panel for, 52
  serving size for, 51–52
  skipping meals and, 203
  as snacks, 85
  stocking up on, 165
  vegetarians and, 117
  See also grains; sandwiches
breakfast, skipping, 203
breast cancer, 19
brown bag lunches, FAQ's about,
      198–200
Brownies, Low-Fat (recipe), 357
brushing teeth, 160
Brussels Sprouts, Roasted (recipe),
      355
Burger, Tempeh (recipe), 346–47
butter, 62, 63, 67, 69, 75–76, 78, 117,
      168, 169, 170, 171
Butternut Squash and Apple Soup
      (recipe), 348–49

caffeine, 161, 209
calcium, 60, 110, 116, 189
calorie intake target
  charts for, 34, 35, 37, 41
  dairy products and, 60
  DASH Diet credentials and, 27
  determining your (tables), 33–36
  determining your (formula),
      363–65
  doing it for life and, 176
  fat and oil and, 37, 75
  fruit and, 46, 184
  grain and, 50
  meal plans and, 105–6, 214
  meat, fish, and poultry and, 65
  My DASH Diet program for weight
      loss and, 41

number of servings and, 36–37
nuts, seeds, and legumes and,
      71
serving size and, 37–39
snacks and, 83
sweets and, 79
vegetables and, 43, 184
See also specific food group
calories
  in alcoholic beverages, 88–89
  carbohydrates and, 188
  causes of obesity and, 20–23, 26
  in cereals, 54
  cost of food and, 22, 205–8
  cravings and, 159, 160
  cutting of, 13–14
  differences between DASH Diet
      and other weight-loss programs
      and, 9
  dining out and, 171
  in drinks, 86–91
  emotional eating and, 156
  exercise and, 160, 193, 209–10
  fat and oil and, 57, 58, 59, 75, 76,
      78
  fiber and, 187
  in fruit, 46, 48, 184
  in fruit juice, 88
  grains and, 55, 57–58
  increase in daily intake of, 21
  low-fat foods and, 189–90
  meal plans and, 105, 119, 213,
      214
  meat and, 65, 68, 69, 112, 206
  in milk, 62, 88, 90
  in nuts, seeds and legumes, 71
  physical activity and, 119, 120, 128,
      129
  pizza and, 190
  in sandwiches, 203–5
  science of weight loss and, 12–14
  in snacks, 83, 84–85, 86
  in soups, 93
  sugar and, 189
  sweets and, 80
  vegans and, 113
  vegetables and, 43
  vegetarians and, 110, 112, 114, 115,
      116, 117, 272

walking and, 122, 125, 126
weekend eating and, 201
in yogurt, 189
See also calorie intake target; Hi-Lo-
Slo foods; *specific food or food
group*
cancer, 8, 19, 27, 88, 120, 179
carbohydrates, 57–58, 74, 187–88
cardiovascular exercise, 128, 129
casseroles, 73, 110
Cauliflower, Roasted (recipe),
356
Centers for Disease Control and
Prevention, U.S. (CDC), 16
cereals
calories in, 54
cold, 51, 52–54, 207
cost of, 206, 207
fat in, 77
fiber in, 203
as Hi-Lo-Slo food, 55, 56
low-fat, 56
nutrition/food labels on, 52–53
seeds in, 73
selection and preparation of, 53–54,
63, 64
serving size for, 51, 52–54, 56
skipping meals and, 203
as snacks, 85
stocking up on, 165
sugar in, 54, 59, 206
See also grains
cheese
in brown bag lunches, 199
calories in, 116
dining out and, 169, 170
"down-shifting" and, 63
fat and oil in, 94
hard, 60–61
as Hi-Lo-Slo food, 61, 63
lactose intolerance and, 189
low-fat/nonfat, 61, 64, 98, 107, 116,
166, 199, 204
meal plans and, 107
in mixed dishes, 92–93
in pizza, 191
and preparing ingredients ahead of
time, 107
salt/sodium in, 98

in sandwiches, 204, 205
selection and preparation of, 64
serving size of, 61
as snacks, 85
stocking up on, 166
vegetarians and, 114–15, 116
See also cottage cheese; dairy
products
chewing
food, 150–51
gum, 158, 160
Chicken Caesar Wrap (recipe),
338–39
chili: as mixed dish, 93
chips, 45, 199
See also potato chips
chocolate, 10, 80, 199
cholesterol
carbohydrates and, 187
DASH Diet and, 5, 6, 8, 111
eggs and, 67
fat and oil and, 76, 77
fiber and, 187
obesity and, 19
vegetarians and, 111, 114
weight loss pills and, 183
CICO (calories in, calories out), 20–23,
119
clothing, exercise, 124, 210
Cobb Salad (recipe), 352
cocoa, 64
Cod, Poached (recipe), 341
coffee, 62, 63, 64, 87, 90, 206–7
colon cancer, 6, 19
comfort foods, 156
condiments, 98
conscious eating
benefits of, 150, 152
cravings and, 160
feeling fuller and, 151
Hi-Lo-Slo foods and, 149–52
as key to weight loss, 149
marriage and, 150
convenience foods: salt/sodium in,
98
cornbread, 117
costs
of dining out, 105
FAQ's about food, 205–8

costs (*cont.*)
  obesity and, 22
  of snacks, 83, 85
  vegetarian DASH Diet and, 110
cottage cheese, 60, 61, 166
counseling, nutrition, 158
crackers
  in brown bag lunches, 199
  food label for, 97
  Hi-Lo-Slow index and, 55
  low-fat, 41, 56, 165
  salt/sodium in, 98
  serving size for, 51
  as snack foods, 45, 54, 77, 85
  stocking up on, 165
  trans fats in, 77
  whole-grain, 54, 57
cravings
  emotional eating and, 158
  how to avoid, 159–61
  visualization exercise and, 147
crunchy foods, 117
  See also specific food

"daily values," 97
dairy products
  in brown bag lunches, 199, 200
  calorie intake target and, 37, 60
  cost of, 22, 207
  as drinks, 87–88
  FAQ's about, 188–89
  as Hi-Lo-Slo food, 61
  importance of, 60
  lactose intolerance and, 188–89
  low-fat/nonfat, 60, 80, 83, 200
  in mixed dishes, 93
  number of servings each day of, 37,
    60, 200
  selection and preparation of,
    63–65
  serving sizes of, 38
  shopping for, 163
  as snacks, 83
  as sweets, 80
  vegan version of DASH Diet and,
    70
  vegetarians and, 110
  weight loss and, 188–89
  See also cheese; milk; yogurt

dancing, 134
DASH Diet
  benefits of, 5–7, 175–76
  credentials of, 27–28
  differences between other
    weight loss programs and,
    8–10
  endorsements of, 4–5, 6, 27
  feedback about, 137
  food tracking study for, 100–101
  health benefits of, 5–6, 8, 27
  and how it works, 6–7
  initial design/participants of, 5, 109,
    189
  key questions about, 3–10
  long-term emphasis of, 10, 175–80
  and losing weight, 7–8
  "magic bullet" of, 6–7
  as new "habit," 180
  ovo-lacto vegetarian version of,
    110
  principles of, 176–77
  scientific evidence supporting, 5, 6,
    8, 27
  specialness of, 4–6
  vegan version of, 70, 113
  vegetarian revisions to, 70, 110–13,
    271–72
  website for, 114
  See also DASH for Health
DASH for Health (online program),
  7–8, 9, 28, 103, 176, 181, 184,
  367–8
depression: obesity and, 19, 20
desserts
  dining out and, 170
  frozen, 166
  fruit on, 186
  low-fat, 190
  recipes for, 357–58
  stoking up on, 166
  See also bakeries/baked goods;
    sweets
diabetes, 6, 8, 19–20, 27, 179,
  183
"diet saboteurs," 194–95
diet soda, 88
diet studies, FAQ's about contradictory,
  181–82

dieting
   controlling your environment and,
      177–78
   for life, 10, 26, 27, 175–80
   as a positive experience, 177
   practicing the principles of,
      176–77
   progress in, 179–80
   sticking to the basics and, 178–79
   on weekends, 200–202
   See also specific topic
"Dill"icious Dill Dip (recipe), 353
dining out
   business lunches and, 155
   calories and, 171
   causes of obesity and, 22
   choice words when, 167–68, 171
   conscious eating when, 150
   consumer demands and, 168–69,
      171
   costs of, 105, 207
   "doggy-bags" from, 199
   fat and oil and, 78, 167, 169, 170,
      172
   learning about, 167–73
   meal plans and, 105
   mixed dishes and, 92, 93–94
   portions when, 167
   restaurant dish descriptions and,
      167–68, 171
   restaurant quiz and, 170–72
   salt and, 167
   sugar and, 167
   tools for learning about, 144
   on vacations, 210
   vegetarians and, 170
   weight loss and, 167–73
   what to ask for when, 169–70
   See also fast-food restaurants;
      restaurants
dinner plates: size of, 24
dips
   dairy products and, 64
   oil and fat and, 78
   recipes for, 353–54
   snacks and, 83, 85
   vegetarian DASH Diet and,
      110
dogs: walking, 132

doing it for life
   being positive and, 177
   benefits of DASH Diet and, 10,
      175–80
   controlling your environment and,
      177
   goals and, 179–80
   inspiration for, 32
   perfection and, 179–80
   principles of DASH Diet and,
      176–77
dressings, salad
   dining out and, 169, 172
   fat and oil in, 75, 76, 77, 78,
      172
   and preparing ingredients ahead of
      time, 107
   recipes for, 352–53
   at salad bars, 184
   salt/sodium in, 98
   serving size of, 75
   stocking up on, 165
   vegetarians and, 117
drinks
   to avoid, 90–91
   in brown bag lunches, 199
   caffeinated, 161, 209
   calories in, 86–91
   conditionally recommended, 88
   conscious eating and, 151
   cravings and, 160
   diet, 208
   diet soda, 88
   in moderation, 88–90
   recommended, 87–88
   with sandwiches, 205
   sugar-sweetened, 79, 86–87,
      90–91
   warm, 151, 160
   weight loss and, 86–91
   See also alcoholic beverages; coffee;
      diet soda; juice; milk; soda; tea;
      water

eating habits
   changing, 137
   differences between DASH Diet and
      other weight-loss programs and,
      8–9

eating habits (*cont.*)
  long-term, 32, 175–80
  skillpower and, 137
  weight loss and, 26–27
eating plans/program. *See* meal plans
eggs
  calorie intake target and, 37
  calories and, 112
  cholesterol and, 67
  fat in, 67
  as meat substitute, 67
  milk and, 67
  number of servings each day of, 37,
    65, 67
  preparation pointers for, 67,
    68–69
  protein in, 70
  serving sizes of, 38, 66, 112
  as snacks, 85
  stocking up on, 166
  vegetables and, 67
  vegetarians and, 110, 111, 112
emotional eating
  conquering, 156–58
  conscious eating and, 151
  degrees of, 158
  distractions for helping overcome,
    157–58
  identifying triggers for, 157
  reasons for, 156–57
energy
  carbohydrates as source of, 187,
    188
  exercise and, 192
environment
  controlling the, 177
  doing it for life and, 177
evolution: causes of obesity and, 25
exercise
  amount of, 128
  calories and, 160, 193, 209–10
  cardiovascular, 128, 129
  clothing for, 124, 210
  for core muscles, 127–28
  cravings and, 160
  DASH Diet and, 7
  doing it for life and, 176, 177,
    179–80
  emotional eating and, 158

energy and, 192
FAQ's about, 121, 129, 191–94
Food and Exercise Log, 102
growing your own vegetables as,
    206
guideline for, 135
in gyms, 127, 128, 129, 192
health and, 120–21
at home, 127–28, 132, 134–35
hunger and, 193–94
importance of, 119–21
for legs, 127
lifestyle, 131–35
in morning, 192
100-calorie workout and, 133–35
perfect, 135
regular, 135
science of weight loss and, 14
shoes for, 124, 133
sleep and, 209
strength training and, 128–30
time for, 191–93
vegetarians and, 113
visualization, 146–47
on weekends, 201, 202
where to do, 127
in workplace, 132, 192
See also fitness program; physical
    activity; walking
exercise balls, 128

FAQs (Frequently Asked Questions)
  about brown bag lunches,
    198–200
  about carbohydrates, 51, 187–88
  about contradicting diet studies, 8,
    181–82
  about cost of food, 205–8
  about dairy products, 64, 188–89
  about dealing with temptation, 155,
    194–95
  about exercise, 121, 129, 191–94
  about fruit, 45, 49, 183–87
  about grocery shopping, 189–90
  about hunger, 193–94
  about lactose intolerance, 64
  about low-fat foods, 76
  about pedometers, 144, 194
  about pizza, 190–91

about sandwiches, 203–5
about seafood, 196–98
about skipping meals, 203
about sleep-weight connection,
    208–9
about tempting foods, 194–95
about vegetables, 45, 183–86
about vitamin supplements, 196
about weekend eating, 200–202
about weight-loss goals, 209–10
about weight-loss pills, 26,
    182–83
farmers' markets, 207
fast-food restaurants, 22, 23, 25, 65,
    168–69
fat and oil
    added, 37, 38, 74–79
    in brown bag lunches, 199
    calorie intake target and, 37, 75
    calories and, 57, 58, 59, 75, 76, 78
    in cheese, 94
    choice index for, 76
    cholesterol and, 76, 77
    cravings and, 159
    dining out and, 78, 167, 169, 170,
        172
    in eggs, 67
    emotional eating and, 156
    in fish, 196
    heart disease and, 77, 78
    as Hi-Lo-Slo foods, 76
    meal plans and, 105
    in meat, 66, 68, 74, 94, 204, 206
    in mixed dishes, 93, 94
    monounsaturated, 77, 78
    number of servings each day of, 37,
        75
    in pastries, 74–75
    pizza and, 190
    polyunsaturated, 77, 78
    saturated, 59, 65, 66, 68, 77, 78, 115,
        116, 196, 206
    selection and preparation of, 78
    serving sizes of, 38, 75
    stocking up on, 165
    trans-, 59, 77–78
    vegans and, 113
    vegetarians and, 113, 115, 116, 117
    See also low-fat foods

fiber
    benefit of eating, 10
    calories and, 187
    carbohydrates and, 187–88
    cholesterol and, 187
    cravings and, 161
    fruit as source of, 47, 88, 187,
        203
    grains as source of, 50, 55, 203
    in Hi-Lo-Slo foods, 10
    legumes as source of, 69, 74
    in nuts, 69
    in seeds, 69
    skipping meals and, 203
    vegetables as source of, 13, 187
    vegetarians and, 111, 117
First Three Steps concept
    calorie target intake and, 33–36
    doing it for life and, 178
    number of servings from each food
        group and, 36–37
    size of servings in each food group
        and, 37–39
fish
    calorie intake target and, 37, 65
    calories and, 68, 112
    chemicals in, 196–98
    cost of, 22
    dining out and, 169
    fat and oil in, 196
    as Hi-Lo-Slo food, 66
    number of servings each day of, 37,
        65
    protein in, 68, 196
    selection and preparation of,
        68–69
    serving sizes of, 38, 66
    stocking up on, 166
    vegetarians and, 110
    See also meat
fitness program
    beginning a, 129
    motivation and, 128
    partners for, 128
    personal trainers and, 128
    ramping up your, 127–30
    reps and sets in, 130
    strength training and, 127,
        128–30

fitness program (*cont.*)
    stretching in, 130
    weight loss and, 127–30
    See also exercise
food
    cost of, 22, 83, 85, 110, 205–8
    measuring, 37–39
    preparation of, 22
    wasting, 105
    See also specific food or food group
food allergies, 4
Food and Drug Administration, U.S.
    (FDA), 27, 196, 197–98
Food and Exercise Log
    doing it for life and, 179
    emotional eating and, 157
    Food and Exercise Log, 102
    importance of, 100–103
    sample log for, 101, 102
    support and, 154
    tips for keeping, 103
    as tool for weight loss, 100–103,
        143–44
    walking and, 125
    when you eat and, 143
    why you eat and, 143
    why you eat certain foods and,
        143–44
food groups, DASH
    number of servings from, 33,
        36–37
    and serving size, 38
    specialness of DASH Diet and, 4
    tools for learning about, 144
    See also specific food group
food labels
    cereals and, 52–53
    "daily values" on, 97
    fat and oil and, 78
    grains and, 50, 57, 58, 59
    salt/sodium content on, 97–98
food tracking
    doing it for life and, 179
    emotional eating and, 157
    Food and Exercise Log, 102
    importance of, 100–103
    sample log for, 101, 102
    support and, 154
    tips for keeping, 103

    as tool for weight loss, 100–103,
        143–44
    walking and, 125
    when you eat and, 143
    why you eat and, 143
    why you eat certain foods and,
        143–44
free samples, 163
freezers, stocking up, 166
french fries, 44, 114–15, 170
fried food
    dining out and, 168, 170
    meat as, 69, 77
    oil and fat and, 77, 78
friends/partners
    fitness program and, 128
    support from, 153–55
    walking with, 125
frozen food, 98, 105, 185, 186
    See also specific food or food group
fruit
    in brown bag lunches, 198, 200
    buying and storing, 186–87
    calorie intake target and, 37, 184
    calories in, 46, 48, 184
    canned, 47, 48
    carbohydrates in, 187
    cost of, 22, 207
    dried, 47, 48, 80, 83, 117, 165, 184,
        200
    as drinks, 91
    FAQ's about, 183–87
    fiber in, 47, 88, 187
    frozen, 47, 48
    goals and, 184
    grocery shopping for, 163, 185,
        207
    as Hi-Lo-Slo food, 46–50, 183, 184,
        207
    as juice, 47, 48, 49, 87, 88, 91, 184,
        200, 203
    multivitamins and, 196
    number of servings each day of, 37,
        46, 200
    portability of, 184
    post-exercise, 193
    in salads, 49, 85, 200
    selection and preparation of,
        48–49

serving sizes of, 38, 46, 47, 200
skipping meals and, 203
as snacks, 83, 84–85, 193
stocking up on, 165, 166
sugar-sweetened, 91
as sweets, 79, 80
as toppings, 186, 207
unripe, 186–87
vegetarians and, 113, 117
washing of, 186
Fruity Chicken Stir-Fry (recipe),
    337–38
fullness signals, 10, 150, 151–52, 172,
    187, 188, 190, 203

gelatin, 79, 83, 84
Gingerbread (recipe), 359–60
goals, diet
    doing it for life and, 179–80
    exercise for setting, 141–42
    fruit and vegetables and, 184
    meal plans and, 214
    Monday Mornings and, 202
    planning ahead and, 140
    realistic, 138–42
    rewards and, 140, 154
    setbacks and, 140–41
    SMART strategy and, 138–42
    support for reaching, 154
    on vacations, 209
grains
    calorie intake target and, 37
    calories and, 55, 57–58
    carbohydrates in, 57–58, 187,
        188
    eating at someone else's home and, 94
    fiber and, 50, 55, 203
    food labels and, 50, 57, 58, 59
    food varieties with, 50
    guide to recognizing, 56–60
    as Hi-Lo-Slo food, 55
    legumes and, 74
    low-fat, 54, 55, 56, 57, 58–59
    meat and, 68
    in mixed dishes, 92–93, 94
    multivitamins and, 196
    number of servings each day of, 37,
        50
    processed, 188

protein and, 57–58, 74
refined, 50, 55
in sandwiches, 204
selection and preparation of, 50,
    56
serving sizes for, 38, 51, 56
skipping meals and, 203
as snacks, 54, 83
terms that mean, 58
vegetarians and, 112, 113, 117
whole-, 50, 54, 55, 56–57, 67, 68, 83,
    94, 113, 117, 187, 196, 203
See also bread; cereals; pasta; rice
grocery shopping
    cost of food and, 207
    exercise/walking when, 132, 163
    FAQ's about, 189–90
    at farmers' markets, 207
    free samples when, 163
    for fruit and vegetables, 185
    hunger and, 162–63
    list for, 163, 164
    low-fat foods and, 189–90
    principles of, 162–63
    sticking to the perimeter of the store
        when, 163
    for weekend eating, 201, 202
    when to do, 163
gum, 158, 160
gyms: exercise in, 127, 128, 129, 192

health
    cost of food and, 205
    physical activity and, 120–21
    See also specific disease
heart disease/attacks
    DASH Diet and, 5, 8, 27
    doing it for life and, 179
    fat and oil and, 77, 78
    lifestyle exercise and, 131
    obesity and, 18, 19, 20
    physical activity and, 120
    salt and, 95
    seafood and, 196
herbal weight-loss preparations, 183
Hi-Lo-Slo foods (HIgh volume, LOw
        calorie, SLOw to eat)
    calorie intake targets and, 36
    conscious eating and, 149–52

Hi-Lo-Slo foods (HIgh volume, LOw calorie, SLOw to eat) (*cont.*)
  cost of food and, 207
  cravings and, 161
  dairy products as, 60–65
  dieting for life and, 175–80
  differences between DASH Diet and other weight-loss plans and, 9
  drinks and, 86–91
  fat and oil as, 74–79
  food groups and, 42–81
  fruit as, 46–50, 184
  grains as, 50–60
  grocery shopping for, 162–63
  introducing, 9–10
  meat, fish, poultry, and eggs as, 65–69
  mixed dishes and, 92–94
  nuts, seeds, and legumes as, 69–74
  pizza and, 190
  salads as, 94
  salt and, 95–99
  sandwiches and, 205
  selection of, 119, 176, 177
  serving size and, 37
  snacks as, 82–86
  soups as, 93, 94, 198
  stocking up on, 165–66
  structuring your own eating program and, 33
  sweets as, 78–81
  vegetables as, 42–46, 183, 184
  visualization techniques and, 145–48
  See also specific food group
high-density foods, examples of, 9, 10
home: exercise at, 127–28, 132, 134–35
household chores, 131, 132, 134, 158
hunger
  cravings and, 161
  exercise and, 193–94
  FAQ's about, 193–94
  grocery shopping and, 162–63
  at night, 161
hunger-fullness scale, 151–52
hydrogenation, 77, 78
hypertension, 19, 183
  and salt intake, 95

ice cream, 61, 189
ice packs: in brown bag lunches, 199
impulse buying, 105
impulse eating, 104–5
iron, 116

Journal of the American Dietetic Association: eating a healthy breakfast article in, 203
Journal of the American Medical Association: lifestyle exercise article in, 131
juice
  cubes of, 49
  fruit, 47, 48, 49, 87, 88, 91, 184, 200, 203
  vegetable, 87, 98, 184
  watering down, 88, 191
jumping rope, 134–35

kabobs, frozen fruit, 49
kidneys
  DASH Diet benefits and, 5
  obesity and, 20
kitchens
  exercising in, 193
  weight-loss friendly products for, 164–66

lactase supplements, 188–89
lactose intolerance, 188–89
lasagna, 92, 95, 110
leftovers: in brown bag lunches, 199
legumes
  calorie intake target and, 37, 71
  calories in, 71, 112
  carbohydrates in, 74
  cost of food and, 206
  examples of, 71
  fiber in, 69, 74
  grains and, 74
  health benefits of, 69, 71
  as Hi-Lo-Slo foods, 69, 71–74
  as low-fat, 74
  as meat alternatives, 73
  number of servings each day of, 37, 71
  protein in, 69, 70, 74
  in salad bars, 116–17

selection and preparation of,
72–74
serving sizes of, 38, 72, 112
vegetarians and, 71, 74, 110, 112, 113,
116–17
vitamins and minerals in, 74
Lemon Caper Vinaigrette (recipe),
352–53
life expectancy, 18, 120
lifestyle
exercise and, 131–35
Low-Fat Blueberry Muffins (recipe),
358–59
Low-Fat Brownies (recipe), 357
low-fat foods
calories and, 189–90
dairy products as, 60
grains as, 54, 55, 56, 57, 58–59
grocery shopping and, 189–90
legumes as, 74
meat and, 66, 68
Nutrition Facts Panel and, 59
snacks as, 54
sugar and, 189
vegetarians and, 113
See also fat and oil; specific food

macaroni and cheese, 92–93
magnesium, 74
main dishes: recipes for, 335–47
Mango Smoothie (recipe), 361
mayonnaise, 75, 76, 78, 117, 165, 169,
198, 204, 205
McDonald's, 25
meal plans
in action, 107–8
basic elements in structuring your
own, 33–41
benefits/purpose of, 41, 108, 213
calorie intake target and, 105–6, 214
calories and, 105, 119, 213, 214
creation of, 9, 27
DASH Diet credentials and, 27
definition of, 104
differences between DASH Diet and
other weight-loss plans and, 9
difficulty of following, 213–14
dining out and, 105
doing it for life and, 175–76

fat and oil and, 105
goals and, 214
grocery shopping and, 162
as guide, 106, 214
how to do, 105–8
impulse buying/eating and, 104–5
learning from, 106
meat eater, 215–69
number of servings and, 213
and preparing ingredients ahead of
time, 107
reasons to like, 105
shopping lists and, 107
snacks and, 105
sodium and, 105
substitutions in, 106, 214
support and, 153
swapping of, 214
as tools, 144, 213
variety in, 105, 144
for vegetarians, 106, 113, 271–331
for weekend eating, 201, 202
weight loss and, 104–8
and why it works, 104–5
meal plans—meat eater, 215–69
1,200 calories, 215–21
1,400 calories, 221–27
1,600 calories, 227–33
1,800 calories, 234–40
2,000 calories, 241–47
2,200 calories, 248–55
2,400 calories, 255–62
2,600 calories, 262–69
meal plans—vegetarian, 271–331
1,200 calories, 272–78
1,400 calories, 279–86
1,600 calories, 286–93
1,800 calories, 293–300
2,000 calories, 300–307
2,200 calories, 308–15
2,400 calories, 315–23
2,600 calories, 323–31
meals, quick-to-prepare, 105
measuring food, 37–39
meat
in brown bag lunches, 199
calorie intake target and, 37, 65
calories and, 65, 68, 69, 112, 206
cost of food and, 206

meat (*cont.*)
  deli, 66, 68, 166
  dining out and, 169
  eating at someone else's home and, 94
  eggs as substitute for, 67
  fat and oil in, 66, 68, 74, 94, 204, 206
  grain and, 68
  as Hi-Lo-Slo food, 66
  initial design of DASH Diet and, 109
  in mixed dishes, 93, 94
  number of servings each day of, 37, 65
  in pizza, 191
  processed, 68, 69, 98, 204
  protein in, 65, 68
  red, 10, 66, 206
  salt/sodium in, 68, 98
  in sandwiches, 204
  selection and preparation of, 68–69
  serving sizes of, 38, 66, 112
  shopping for, 163
  skinless, 66, 69
  stocking up on, 166
  vegetables with, 46, 68–69
  vegetarian DASH Diet and, 110, 112
meat alternatives, 110–13
  calories per serving for, 112
  cost of food and, 206
  going meatless and, 68, 70
  legumes as, 73
  number of servings of, 70
  serving sizes for, 38, 112
  vegetarian DASH Diet and, 110–11, 271, 272
media: reports of weight-loss studies in, 182
medical advice: about the DASH diet, 4
meditation, 158
men: calorie intake targets for, 33–36
mental health: obesity and, 20
mercury: in seafood, 196–97
metabolism, 19, 120, 129

microwaving, 45, 185–86
milk
  in brown bag lunches, 198, 199
  calories in, 62, 88, 90
  cost of food and, 207
  "down shifting" and, 63
  in drinks, 90
  as Hi-Lo-Slo food, 61, 63
  lactose intolerance and, 189
  nonfat/skim, 60, 62, 63, 64, 85, 87–88, 90, 166, 191, 198, 199, 205, 207
  nutrients in, 87, 88
  pizza and, 191
  with sandwiches, 205
  selection and preparation of, 63, 64
  serving size of, 61
  snacks and, 85
  soy, 115
  stocking up on, 166
  See also dairy products
mixed dishes
  definition of, 82
  dining out and, 92, 93–94
  estimating servings in, 92–94
  fat and oil in, 93, 94
  salt/sodium in, 98
  when eating at someone else's home, 94
Monday mornings: health goals and, 202
monounsaturated fats, 77, 78
mood: physical activity and, 120, 121
motivation
  fitness program and, 128
  food tracking and, 101
  physical activity and, 121
  tools for weight loss and, 143
Muffins, Low-Fat Blueberry (recipe), 358–59
multivitamins, 196
muscles
  core, 127
  exercise for building, 120, 127–28, 129
  lifestyle exercise and, 132
My DASH Diet Program for Weight Loss: form for, 41

naps, 209
National Cancer Institute, 18
National Health and Nutrition
    Examination Survey (NHANES),
    21, 208
National Heart, Lung, and Blood
    Institute (NHLBI), 24
National Institutes of Health (NIH), 5
National Weight Control Registry,
    203
New England Journal of Medicine, 5,
    18, 44
Nutrition Facts Panel
    for bread, 52
    grains and, 58
    low-fat products and, 59
    sodium and, 97
nuts
    calorie intake target and, 37, 71
    calories in, 71, 72
    examples of, 71
    fiber in, 69
    health benefits of, 69, 71
    as Hi-Lo-Slo foods, 73
    number of servings each day of, 37,
        71
    protein in, 69
    salt/sodium on, 98, 172
    selection and preparation of, 72–74
    serving sizes of, 38, 72
    as snacks, 83, 85
    stocking up on, 165
    as sweets, 80
    as toppings, 85, 207
    vegetarian DASH Diet and, 110,
        113

oatmeal, 51, 63, 73, 165, 206, 207
obesity
    American Journal of Preventive
        Medicine article about, 24
    causes of, 20–26
    classes of, 16, 18
    definition of, 16
    discrimination concerning, 206
    economics and, 22
    health problems and, 16, 18–20
    increase in, 15, 19–20, 21
    national concern about, 15

National Heart, Lung, and Blood
    Institute (NHLBI) and, 24
    physical activity and, 22–23
    reasons for worrying about, 18–20
    sleep and, 208
    soda and, 208
    toxic food and, 23–25
    vegetarians and, 113–14
    why we worry about, 18–20
olive oil, 75, 76, 77, 165
omega-3 fatty acids, 196, 197
osteoarthritis
    DASH Diet and, 27
    obesity and, 18–19
osteoporosis: DASH Diet and, 8
overweight: definition of, 16

Panini, Veggie Melt (recipe), 335
pantry
    removing items from, 159
    stocking Hi-Lo-Slo foods in,
        165–66
partners. See friends/partners
pasta
    carbohydrates in, 187, 188
    as Hi-Lo-Slo food, 55, 56
    low-fat, 56
    measuring of, 54–55, 56
    nuts in, 73
    recommendations for, 92–93
    sauces for, 59
    serving size for, 51, 54–55, 56
    stocking up on, 165
    vegetarians and, 114–15, 117
    whole grain, 54–56
    See also grains
Pasta Primavera (recipe), 344–45
pastries. See bakeries/baked goods
PCBs (polychlorinated biphenyls),
    seafood and, 197–98
peanuts, 80
pedometers, 133, 194, 210
perfection: dieting goals and, 179–80
personal trainers, 128, 202
physical activity
    calorie intake targets and, 34, 35, 36
    calories and, 119, 120, 128, 129
    causes of obesity and, 21, 22–23, 24,
        26

physical activity (*cont.*)
    decline in, 21, 22–23, 24, 26
    doing it for life and, 177
    health and, 120–21
    how much, 119–21
    muscle building and, 120
    strength and, 120
    time for, 192
    on vacation, 209–10
    See also exercise; fitness program;
        walking
Piled-High Veggie Pizza (recipe),
    336
pizza, 92–93, 98, 107, 114–15, 116,
    190–91, 336
Pizza, Piled-High Veggie (recipe),
    336
Poached Salmon (recipe), 341
polyunsaturated fats, 77, 78
popcorn, 83, 84, 85
portions
    definition of, 40
    dining out and, 167
    inflation in, 25
    of pizza, 190
    servings distinguished from, 40
    size of, 24–25, 40
    vegetarians and, 115–16
positive, being, 177
positive imagery exercise, 146
potassium, 74
potato chips, 44–45, 77, 161, 188,
    205
potatoes, 44–45, 94, 114–15, 187
poultry
    calorie intake target and, 37, 65
    calories and, 68
    as Hi-Lo-Slo food, 66
    number of servings each day of, 37,
        65
    protein in, 68
    salt/sodium in, 98
    selection and preparation of,
        68–69
    serving sizes of, 38, 66
    vegetarian DASH Diet and, 110
    See also meat
pretzels, 45, 54, 56, 80, 83, 84, 85, 98,
    166

processed food
    salt/sodium in, 96, 97
    shopping and, 163
protein
    cost of food and, 206
    dairy products and, 60
    in eggs, 70
    in fish, 196
    grains and, 57–58, 74
    legumes as source of, 69, 70, 74
    in meat, 65, 68
    in nuts and seeds, 69
    vegetarians and, 70, 110, 111, 112,
        114, 271–72
    in yogurt, 112

Quinoa, Corn, and Black Bean Salad
    (recipe), 350

recipes
    Baked Banana, 361
    Beef and Vegetable Stir-Fry, 342
    Black Bean Dip, 354
    Butternut Squash and Apple Soup,
        348–49
    Chicken Caesar Wrap, 338–39
    Cobb Salad, 352
    for desserts, 357–58
    "Dill"icious Dill Dip, 353
    for dips, 353–54
    for dressings, 352–53
    Fruity Chicken Stir-Fry, 337–38
    Gingerbread, 359–60
    Lemon Caper Vinaigrette, 352–53
    Low-Fat Blueberry Muffins,
        358–59
    Low-Fat Brownies, 357
    for main dishes, 335–47
    Mango Smoothie, 361
    Pasta Primavera, 344–45
    Piled-High Veggie Pizza, 336
    Poached Cod, 341
    Poached Salmon, 341
    Quinoa, Corn, and Black Bean Salad,
        350
    Roasted Brussels Sprouts, 355–56
    Roasted Cauliflower, 356
    for salads, 350–52
    Shrimp Scampi, 340

Simple Spinach Salad, 351
  for smoothies, 361
  for snacks, 358–60
  for soups, 348–54
  Strawberry Shortcake, 358
  Tempeh Burger, 346–47
  Tempeh Soft Tacos, 344
  Tortellini and Bean Soup, 349–50
  Turkey Soft Tacos, 343–44
  for vegetables, 355–56
  Veggie Melt Panini, 335
refrigerator
  fruits and vegetables in, 186
  removing items from, 159
  stocking Hi-Lo-Slo foods in, 166
relaxation exercises, 158
reps (repetitions), 130
restaurants
  consumer demands at, 168–69, 171
  costs of going to, 105, 207
  quiz about, 170–72
  on vacations, 210
  what to ask for at, 169–70
  See also dining out; fast-food
    restaurants
rewards, 140, 141, 154, 173, 201
rice
  carbohydrates in, 188
  cost of food and, 206
  dining out and, 170
  as Hi-Lo-Slo food, 55
  legumes and, 74
  low-fat, 56
  serving size for, 51
  stocking up on, 165
  See also grains
Roasted Brussels Sprouts (recipe),
    355–56
Roasted Cauliflower (recipe), 356
routines: weekend eating and, 201

salad bars, 116–17, 155, 172, 184
salads
  Cobb, 352
  dining out and, 169, 170
  fruit, 49, 85, 200
  as Hi-Lo-Slo foods, 94
  legumes in, 73
  as mixed dishes, 94

nuts in, 73
  pizza and, 190, 191
  Quinoa, Corn, and Black Bean,
    350
  recipes for, 350–52
  seeds in, 73
  Simple Spinach, 351
  vegetable, 46, 185, 190
  See also dressings, salad; salad bars
salmon, 197–98, 341
Salmon, Poached (recipe), 341
salt
  cooking with, 98–99
  dining out and, 167
  food labels and, 97–98
  getting enough, 96
  medical recommendations for, 96
  sodium distinguished from, 96–97
  in vegetable juice, 87
  weight loss and, 95–99
sandwiches
  in brown bag lunches, 198, 199
  calories in, 203–5
  FAQs about, 203–5
  See also bread
saturated fat, 65, 66, 68, 77, 78, 115, 116,
    196, 206
sauces
  calories and, 59
  choice words about, 168
  cost of food and, 206
  dining out and, 168, 169
  eating at someone else's home and,
    94
  low-fat, 190
  seeds in, 73
  vegetarians and, 117
scales, food, 39
seafood
  FAQ's about, 196–98
  heart disease/attacks and, 196
  mercury and, 196–97
  PCBs (polychlorinated biphenyls)
    and, 197–98
  See also fish
seeds
  calorie intake target and, 37, 71
  calories in, 71, 72
  examples of, 71

seeds (*cont.*)
  fiber in, 69
  health benefits of, 69, 71
  Hi-Lo-Slo foods and, 73
  number of servings each day of, 37,
    71
  protein in, 69
  selection and preparation of,
    72–74
  serving sizes of, 38, 72
  vegetarians and, 110, 113, 117
seitan, 70, 110, 111, 112
selection of foods. *See specific*
    food group
servings
  definition of, 40
  doing it for life and, 176
  measuring, 37–39
  My DASH Diet program for weight
    loss and, 41
  number of, 33, 36–37, 176,
    213
  portions distinguished from, 40
  size of, 4, 37–41, 176
  specialness of DASH Diet and, 4
  structuring your own eating program
    and, 33, 36–41
  tips for eyeballing, 39
  tools for learning about, 144
  what counts as, 33, 37–39
  See also specific food group
setbacks: goals and, 140–41
sets, 130
shoes, 124, 133, 210
shopping lists, 83, 107, 163, 164
Shrimp Scampi (recipe), 340
Simple Spinach Salad (recipe), 351
skewers, fruit, 49
skillpower
  building, 137
  definition of, 137
  doing it for life and, 176
  eating habits and, 137
  goals and, 138–42
  SMART strategy and, 138–42
  weight loss and, 137
skipping meals: FAQ's about, 203
sleep, 19, 161, 208–9
slow eating

  conscious eating as, 149–52
  dining out and, 172
  doing it for life and, 176
  See also Hi-Lo-Slo foods
SMART strategy, 138–42
Smoothie, Mango (recipe), 361
smoothies
  dairy products and, 64
  fruit, 49, 64
  recipes for, 361
  vegetarian DASH Diet and,
    110
snacks
  alternative, 83
  calorie intake target and, 83
  calories in, 83, 84–85, 86
  cost of, 83, 85
  cravings and, 161
  fruit as, 83, 84–85, 193
  grocery shopping and, 163
  as Hi-Lo-Slo foods, 83
  low-fat, 54
  meal plans and, 105, 106
  number of servings in common,
    84–85
  100-calorie, 83, 85–86
  post-exercise, 193–94
  recipes for, 358–60
  salt/sodium in, 98
  skipping meals and, 203
  smart, 82–86
  substituting, 106
  See also type of snack
soda, 79, 80, 86–87, 88, 89, 90–91, 191,
    199, 205, 207–8
sodium
  cravings and, 159
  food labels and, 97–98
  meal plans and, 105
  in meat, 68, 98
  in mixed dishes, 93
  salt distinguished from, 96–97,
    166
  in soups, 93
  stocking up the kitchen and, 165
soups
  calories in, 93
  canned, 98
  as Hi-Lo-Slo foods, 93, 94, 198

legumes in, 73
as mixed dishes, 93, 94
nuts and, 73
recipes for, 348–50
salt/sodium in, 98
suggestions for, 64, 93
vegetarian DASH Diet and,
    110
sports drinks, 91
spreads
    calories and, 59
    in sandwiches, 204
    selection and preparation of, 63
    on snacks, 85
    vegetarian DASH Diet and, 110
    See also specific spread
stairs, climbing, 133–34, 155, 193
Starbucks: specialty drinks from,
    90
stews
    as mixed dishes, 93
    vegetable, 69
    vegetarians and, 110
stir-fry
    chicken, 94
    as mixed dish, 93
    nuts in, 73
    oil and fat and, 78
    and preparing ingredients ahead of
        time, 107
    recipes for, 337–38, 342, 343
    vegetable, 69, 107
    vegetarians and, 110, 115
Strawberry Shortcake (recipe), 358
strength
    physical activity and, 120
    training for, 127, 128–30
stress: meal plans and, 105
stretching exercise, 130, 132, 158
strokes, 5, 18, 19, 20, 120
substitutions, in meal plans, 214
sugar
    calories and, 189
    carbohydrates and, 187, 188
    on cereals, 54, 59
    cost of foods and, 22, 206, 207
    dining out and, 167
    in drinks, 86–87, 91
    low-fat foods and, 189

stocking up the kitchen and, 165
    See also sweets
support
    from family and friends, 153–55
    pedometers and, 194
    for weight loss, 153–55
    at work, 155
swapping: of meal plans, 214
sweeteners, artificial, 87, 88
sweets
    in brown bag lunches, 199
    calorie intake target for, 37, 79
    calories and, 80
    grocery shopping and, 163
    as not Hi Lo Slo foods, 79
    number of servings each day of, 37,
        79, 80
    selection and preparation of,
        80–81
    serving sizes of, 38

Tacos, Tempeh Soft (recipe), 344
Tacos, Turkey Soft (recipe), 343–44
tea, 64, 87, 91, 160, 206–7
technology: causes of obesity and,
    23
teeth, brushing and flossing, 160
television
    cravings and, 159–60
    sleep and, 209
tempeh, 70, 110, 111, 112, 115, 344,
    346–47
Tempeh Burger (recipe), 346–47
Tempeh Soft Tacos (recipe), 344
tempting foods
    "diet saboteurs" and, 194–95
    FAQ's about avoiding, 194–95
    getting rid of, 161
thinking: DASH Diet benefits and, 6
tofu, 70, 110, 112, 115, 206, 343
Tofu and Vegetable Stir-fry (recipe),
    343
tools
    benefits of, 144
    doing it for life and, 176
    meal plans as, 144, 213
    for weight loss, 100–103, 143–44,
        176, 213
    See also Food and Exercise Log

toppings
  calories and, 59
  dairy products and, 64
  fruit as, 186
  See also specific food
Tortellini and Bean Soup (recipe),
    349–50
toxic foods
  *American Journal of Preventive
    Medicine* article about, 24
  causes of obesity and, 23–25, 26
  doing it for life and, 177–78
  and National Heart, Lung, and Blood
    Institute (NHLBI), 24
tracking, 100–103
  doing it for life and, 179
  emotional eating and, 157
  Food and Exercise Log, 102
  importance of, 100–103
  sample log for, 101, 102
  support and, 154
  tips for keeping, 103
  as tool for weight loss, 100–103,
    143–44
  walking and, 125
  when you eat and, 143
  why you eat certain foods and,
    143–44
trail mix, 80
trans fats, 59, 77–78
triglyceride levels, 19
Turkey Soft Tacos (recipe), 343–44
TVP (textured vegetable protein), 70,
    110, 111, 112, 115
Twain, Mark: quotation from, 175

unconscious eating, 159–60
University of Michigan: health and
    retirement study at, 205–6
University of Warwick (Britain): sleep-
    weight study at, 208
U.S. News & World Report magazine,
    5, 6

vacations: diet goals and, 209–10
vegans, 70, 113
vegetables
  in brown bag lunches, 198, 199
  calorie intake target and, 37, 43, 184

canned, 98
carbohydrates in, 187
color of, 172
conscious eating and, 151
cost of, 22, 206, 207
dining out and, 169, 170, 172
eating at someone else's home and,
    94
eggs and, 67
FAQ's about, 183–86
fiber in, 42, 187
fullness signals and, 151
goals and, 184
grocery shopping for, 163, 185, 207
growing your own, 206
as Hi-Lo-Slo foods, 42–46, 183, 184,
    207
importance of, 42
as juice, 87, 98, 184
to limit or avoid, 44
meal plans and, 107
meat and, 68–69
in mixed dishes, 93, 94
multivitamins and, 196
need for variety of, 43
number of servings each day of, 37,
    43
nuts and, 73
on pizza, 190, 191
portability of, 184
and preparing ingredients ahead of
    time, 107
raw, 46, 83, 151, 190
recipes for, 355–56
in salad bars, 116–17, 172
in salads, 46, 185, 190
salt/sodium in, 98
in sandwiches, 204
selection and preparation of, 45–46,
    185–86
serving sizes for, 38, 43
as snacks, 64, 83, 84–85
in stews, 69
stir-fry, 69
stocking up on, 166
vegetarians and, 112, 113, 115,
    116–17
washing of, 186
weight loss and, 42, 43

vegetarians
  adventurousness of, 115, 118
  blood pressure and, 109
  calories and, 114
  cheese and, 116
  dairy products and, 110
  DASH research and, 109
  dining out and, 170
  eggs and, 110
  exercise and, 113
  as expanding nutritional horizons,
    115, 118
  legumes and, 71, 74
  meal plans for, 106, 113, 271–331
  meat alternatives and, 110–11
  number of servings each day per food
    group for, 37
  obesity and, 113–14
  options for, 70
  ovo-lacto, 109–10
  pesco-, 271
  and pitfalls of vegetarianism, 114–18
  portion control and, 115–16
  protein and, 70, 271–72
  revisions to DASH Diet for, 70,
    110–13, 271–72
  salad bars and, 116–17
  weight loss and, 109–18
  weight of, 113–14
Veggie Melt Panini (recipe), 335
Vinaigrette, Lemon Caper (recipe),
  352–53
visualization techniques, 145–48
  exercises for, 146–47
vitamin A, 116
vitamin C, 116
vitamin supplements: FAQ's about,
  196

waist: circumference of, 19, 208
walking
  benefits of, 122
  calories and, 122, 125, 126
  cravings and, 160
  emotional eating and, 158
  Food and Exercise Log and, 125
  with friends, 125
  heavier people and, 125
  how far for, 123–24

  how long and how often to walk,
    123–24
  as lifestyle exercise, 131, 132
  program for, 123–24, 125
  speed for, 125, 126
  time for exercise and, 192, 193
  tips about, 124
  on vacations, 210
  weight loss and, 122–26
  and where to walk, 124, 125
water
  bottled, 207–8
  brown bag lunches and, 199
  cost of, 207–8
  emotional eating and, 158
  juice added to, 88, 191
  pizza and, 191
  as recommended drink, 87, 88, 91
  tonic, 89
weekends
  calories added on, 201
  exercise on, 201, 202
  FAQ's about eating on, 200–202
  grocery shopping for, 201, 202
  meal plans for, 201, 202
weight
  classes of obesity and, 16, 18
  discrimination concerning, 206
  sleep and, 208–9
  of vegetarians, 113–14
weight loss
  Bel Air car story and, 11–13
  calorie intake targets and, 33–36
  conscious eating as key to, 149–52
  contradictory studies about,
    181–82
  DASH Diet and, 15–28
  and DASH Diet differences from
    other weight-loss programs,
    8–10
  eating habits and, 26–27
  evidence of DASH Diet helping,
    7–8
  food tracking and, 100–103
  goals for, 138–42, 209–10
  and keeping it off, 10, 26
  kitchens as friendly to, 164–66
  lifestyle exercise and, 131–35
  long-term, 10, 26, 27, 175–80

weight loss (*cont.*)
  meal planning and, 104–8
  My DASH Diet program for, 41
  science of, 11–14
  short-term, 26
  skillpower and, 137
  successful programs for, 27
  support for, 153–55
  tools for, 100–103, 143–44
  vegetarians and, 109–18
  visualization techniques and, 145–48
  what you eat and, 33–41
  your weight and, 16–18
  See also specific topic
weight-loss pills, 26, 182–83
women: calorie intake targets for,
    33–36
workplace
  discrimination in, 20
  exercise in, 132, 192
  obesity and, 20
  salad bars in, 184
  support at, 155
Wrap, Chicken Caesar (recipe), 338–39

yard work, 131, 132, 134
yogurt
  in brown bag lunches, 198, 199
  calories in, 189
  in dips and dressings, 78
  "down shifting" and, 63
  frozen, 189
  Greek, 112
  as Hi-Lo-Slo food, 61
  lactose intolerance and, 189
  "live and active cultures" in, 189
  low-fat/nonfat, 60, 61, 63, 64, 78, 83,
      84, 85, 112, 161, 166, 186
  post-exercise, 193, 194
  protein in, 112
  as snack, 83, 84, 85, 161, 193,
      194
  stocking up on, 166
  as sweets, 80
  toppings on, 73, 186
  vegetarian DASH Diet and, 112
  See also dairy products

zinc, 74

About the Authors

Dr. Thomas J. Moore is professor of medicine at the Boston University School of Medicine and associate provost for the Boston University Medical Campus. His research team at Harvard Medical School worked with other teams at Johns Hopkins, Duke, Pennington Research Institute, and the University of Oregon to design the DASH Diet and prove its benefits. Dr. Moore is the founder of the online DASH for Health program.

Megan C. Murphy, MPH, earned her master's degree in public health at Boston University, where she focused her studies on how people make health and lifestyle choices. She has served as the program manager of the DASH for Health program since its inception in 2002, helping people make healthy choices every day.

Mark Jenkins is a freelance writer and the author of many successful books, including two Book-of-the-Month Club alternate selections. His writing has appeared in publications as diverse as *Rolling Stone* and *The Wall Street Journal*. Mark lives on the island of Martha's Vineyard, Massachusetts.